Recent Trends in Radiation Oncology
and Related Fields

# Recent Trends in Radiation Oncology and Related Fields

Proceedings of the Spring Symposium in Radiation Oncology:
Second Annual Conference, held on April 15-17, 1983, at the University
of Michigan Medical School, Ann Arbor, Michigan, U.S.A.

*Editors:*

## Beatriz E. Amendola, M.D.

Assistant Professor of Radiology, Acting Chairman, Department of Radiation
Therapy, University of Michigan Medical School, Ann Arbor, Michigan

and

## Marco A. Amendola, M.D.

Associate Professor of Radiology, Co-Director, Abdominal Radiology
Division, Department of Radiology, University of Michigan Medical School,
Ann Arbor, Michigan

Elsevier
New York • Amsterdam • Oxford

© 1983 by Elsevier Science Publishing Co., Inc.

Published by:

Elsevier Science Publishing Co., Inc.
52 Vanderbilt Avenue, New York, New York 10017

Sole distributors outside the USA and Canada:

Elsevier Science Publishers B.V.
P.O. Box 211, 1000 AE Amsterdam, The Netherlands

Library of Congress Cataloging in Publication Data

Spring Symposium in Radiation Oncology (2nd: 1983: University of Michigan
    Medical School)
    Recent trends in radiation oncology and related fields.

    Includes index.
    1. Cancer—Congresses. 2. Cancer—Radiotherapy—Congresses. I. Amendola,
    Beatriz E. II. Amendola, Marco A. III. Title.
RC261.A2S67   1983       616.99'40642     83-20570
ISBN 0-444-00846-2

Manufactured in the United States of America

DEDICATED

TO OUR PARENTS

AND

TO THE MEMORY OF
DR. ISADORE LAMPE

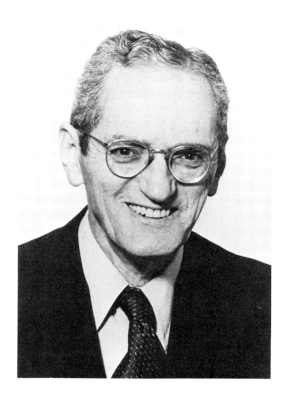

ISADORE LAMPE, M.D., Ph.D.   1906-1982.

# Contents

DEDICATION                                                              v

CONTRIBUTORS                                                           ix

PREFACE                                                               xv

ACKNOWLEDGMENTS                                                       xvii

SECTION I
   1.  Isadore Lampe                                                   1
      Juan A. Del Regato, M.D.

SECTION II   LYMPHOMA
   2.  Radical Radiation Therapy in the Treatment of
      Laparotomy Staged Hodgkin's Disease Patients                   21
      Seymour H. Levitt, M.D. and Chung K.K. Lee, M.D.
   3.  Chemotherapeutic Approach to Non-Hodgkin's Lymphomas           39
      Steven G. Roshon, M.D. and Kenneth S. Zuckerman, M.D.
   4.  Computed Tomography in Lymphoma                                53
      Marco A. Amendola, M.D. and Beatriz E. Amendola, M.D.

SECTION III   CENTRAL NERVOUS SYSTEM TUMORS
   5.  Progress and Problems of the Treatment of Brain Stem
      Glioma, Medulloblastoma and Craniopharyngioma in
      Childhood                                                      83
      J. Robert Cassady, M.D., Patricia Eifel, M.D. and
      James A. Belli, M.D.
   6.  Intermittent and Continuous Regional Chemotherapy for
      CNS Tumors                                                     95
      William F. Chandler, M.D., Harry S. Greenberg, M.D.
      and William D. Ensminger, M.D.
   7.  Management of CNS Tumors in Children:  Surgery             101
      Joan L. Venes, M.D.

SECTION IV.   GASTROINTESTINAL ONCOLOGY
   8.  Colorectal Cancer - Interactions of Surgery,
      Radiation, and Chemotherapy                                    111
      Leonard L. Gunderson, M.D., M.S., Michael J.
      O'Connell, M.D. and Robert W. Beart, M.D.
   9.  The Treatment of Liver Metastases                              127
      John E. Niederhuber, M.D.
  10. Pancreatic Cancer - A Multimodality Approach                   139
      Leonard L. Gunderson, M.D., M.S., J. Kirk Martin, M.D.
      and Lawrence K. Kvols, M.D.

SECTION V.   GENITOURINARY ONCOLOGY
    11. External Beam Irradiation in Adenocarcinoma of the
        Prostate    149
        Beatriz E. Amendola and Ihn H. Han, M.D., Ph.D.
    12. Prostate Cancer:  Staging and Its Effects on Therapy    159
        H. Barton Grossman, M.D.
    13. Computed Tomography of Prostatic Malignancy    169
        Marco A. Amendola, M.D., Beatriz E. Amendola, M.D.
        and H. Barton Grossman, M.D.
    14. Bladder Cancer:  Epidemiology and Recent
        Radiotherapeutic Directions    187
        M. Rotman, M.D., H. Aziz, M.D. and R. Yaes, M.D.
    15. Bladder Cancer:  Current Therapy and Future Prospects    197
        H. Barton Grossman, M.D.

SECTION VI.   GYNECOLOGIC ONCOLOGY
    16. Radiation Therapy of Stage IB Carcinoma of the
        Cervix:  Factors Influencing Prognosis    209
        M. Rotman, M.D., K. Choi, M.D. and J. Boyce, M.D.
    17. Radiation Therapy as Primary Treatment for Cancer of
        the Breast    221
        Luther W. Brady, M.D., John M. Bedwinek, M.D. and
        John R. Loughead, M.D.
    18. The Use of Computerized Tomography (CT) in Radiation
        Treatment Planning of Primary Breast Cancer    249
        Allen S. Lichter, M.D., Benedick A. Fraass, Ph.D.,
        Hal A. Fredrickson, and Jan van de Geijn, Ph.D.

SECTION VII   LUNG TUMORS
    19. Integration of Thoracic Radiation Therapy and
        Chemotherapy for Small Cell Carcinoma of the Lung.    261
        James D. Cox, M.D., Roger W. Byhardt, M.D., Ritsuko
        Komaki, M.D. Paul Y. Holoye, M.D.and John Norlund, M.D.

SECTION VIII   NEW DIAGNOSTIC TECHNIQUES
    20. Nuclear Magnetic Resonance:  Physical Principles and
        Instrumentation    273
        Alex M. Aisen, M.D.
    21. Nuclear Magnetic Resonance:  Clinical Applications    287
        Marco A. Amendola, M.D. and Alex M. Aisen, M.D.

SECTION IX
    22. Activities of the Radiation Therapy Oncology Group    301
        H. Gunter Seydel, M.D.
    23. Radiation Therapy Immobilization and Port Reproduction
        Techniques for Head and Neck Tumors.    307
        Cynthia A. Colwell, R.T.(T.)

INDEX    317

# Contributors

Alex M. Aisen, M.D.
Assistant Professor of Radiology
Department of Radiology
University of Michigan Medical School
Ann Arbor, Michigan

Beatriz E. Amendola, M.D.
Assistant Professor of Radiology
Acting Chairman, Department of Radiation Therapy
University of Michigan Medical School
Ann Arbor, Michigan

Marco A. Amendola, M.D.
Associate Professor, Department of Radiology
Co-Director, Division of Abdominal Radiology
University of Michigan Medical School
Ann Arbor, Michigan

H. Aziz, M.D.
Assistant Professor of Radiology
Department of Radiation Oncology
S.U.N.Y. Downstate Medical Center
Brooklyn, New York

Robert W. Beart, M.D.
Consultant in Surgery
Mayo Clinic
Associate Professor of Surgery
Mayo Medical School
Rochester, Minnesota

John M. Bedwineck, M.D.
Associate Professor
Division of Radiation Oncology
Mallinckrodt Institute of Radiology
Washington University School of Medicine
St. Louis, Missouri

James A. Belli, M.D.
Professor and Chairman
Department of Radiation Therapy
University of Texas at Galveston
Galveston, Texas

Roger Bighardt, M.D.
Associate Professor of Radiology
Radiation Oncology Division
Medical College of Wisconsin
Milwaukee, Wisconsin

J. Boyce, M.D.
Professor, Department of Obstetrics and Gynecology
S.U.N.Y. Downstate Medical Center
New York, New York

Luther W. Brady, M.D.
   Hylda Cohn/American Cancer Society Professor
   of Clinical Oncology
   Chairman Department of Radiation Therapy
   Hahnemann Medical College
   Philadelphia, Pennsylvania

James R. Cassady, M.D.
   Professor of Radiation Therapy and
   Peter Bent Brigham Women's and Children's Hospital Physician
   Joint Center for Radiation Therapy
   Harvard Medical School
   Boston, Massachusetts

William F. Chandler, M.D.
   Associate Professor Department of Surgery
   Section of Neurosurgery
   University of Michigan Medical School
   Ann Arbor, Michigan

K. Choi, M.D.
   Assistant Professor
   Department of Radiaion Oncology
   S.U.N.Y. Downstate Medical Center
   New York, New York

Cynthia A. Colwell, R.T.(T.)
   Chief Technologist
   Acting Administrative Associate
   Department of Radiation Therapy
   University of Michigan Medical School
   Ann Arbor, Michigan

James D. Cox, M.D.
   Professor of Radiology
   Chairman, Radiation Therapy Section
   Medical College of Wisconsin
   Milwaukee, Wisconsin

Patricia Eifel, M.D.
   Assistant Professor
   Joint Center for Radiation Therapy
   Harvard Medical School
   Boston, Massachusetts

William Ensminger, M.D., Ph.D.
   Professor of Medicine
   Department of Internal Medicine
   Division of Hematology-Oncology
   University of Michigan Medical School
   Ann Arbor, Michigan

Benedick A. Fraass, Ph.D.
    Radiation Oncology Branch
    Clinical Oncology Program
    Division of Cancer Treatment
    National Cancer Institute
    Bethesda, Maryland

Hal A. Fredrickson
    Computer Systems Laboratory
    Division of Computer Research and Technology
    National Institutes of Health
    Bethesda, Maryland

Harry Greenberg, M.D.
    Assistant Professor
    Department of Neurology
    University of Michigan Medical School
    Ann Arbor, Michigan

H. Barton Grossman, M.D.
    Assistant Professor
    Section of Urology/Oncology
    Department of Surgery
    University of Michigan Medical School
    Ann Arbor, Michigan

Leonard L. Gunderson, M.D.
    Consultant
    Department of Therapeutic Radiology
    Mayo Clinic
    Rochester, Minnesota

Ihn H. Han, M.D., Ph.D.
    Instructor of Radiology
    Department of Radiation Therapy
    University of Michigan Medical School
    Ann Arbor, Michigan

Paul Y. Holoye, M.D.
    Associate Professor of Medicine
    Department of Medicine
    Division of Hematology-Oncology
    Medical College of Wisconsin
    Milwaukee, Wisconsin

Ritsuko Komaki, M.D.
    Assistant Professor, Department of Radiology
    Radiation Oncology Division
    Medical College of Wisconsin
    Milwaukee, Wisconsin

Lawrence K. Kvols, M.D.
   Consultant in Medical Oncology
   Mayo Clinic
   Assistant Professor of Oncology
   Mayo Medical School
   Rochester, Minnesota

Chung K.K. Lee, M.D.
   Assistant Professor
   Department of Radiology
   University of Minnesota
   Minneapolis, Minnesota

Seymour H. Levitt, M.D.
   Professor and Head
   Department of Radiation Therapy
   University of Minnesota
   Minneapolis, Minnesota

John R. Loughead, M.D.
   Associate Professor
   Department of Obstetrics and Gynecology
   Hahnemann University
   Philadelphia, Pennsylvania

Allen S. Lichter, M.D.
   Head, Radiation Therapy Section
   Radiation Oncology Branch
   National Cancer Institute
   National Institutes of Health
   Bethesda, Maryland

J. Kirk Martin, M.D.
   Consultant in Surgical Oncology
   Mayo Clinic
   Assistant Professor Surgery
   Mayo Medical School
   Rochester Minnesota

John E. Niederhuber, M.D.
   Professor, Department of Surgery
   Head, Section of Surgical Oncology
   Professor, Department of Microbiology and Immunology
   Associate Dean for Research
   University of Michigan Medical School
   Ann Arbor, Michigan

John D. Norlund, M.D.
   Assistant Professor
   Department of Radiation Oncology
   Medical College of Wisconsin
   Milwaukee, Wisconsin

Michael J. O'Connell, M.D.
  Consultant in Medical Oncology
  Mayo Clinic
  Associate Professor in Oncology
  Mayo Medical School
  Rochester, Minnesota

Juan A. del Regato, M.D., FACR
  Professor, Department of Radiology
  University of Southern Florida College of Medicine
  Tampa Florida

Steven Roshon, M.D.
  Private Practice of Medicine
  1674 Sicamore Line
  Sandusky, Ohio

Marvin Rottman, M.D.
  Professor and Chairman
  Department of Radiation Oncology
  S.U.N.Y. Downstate Medical Center
  Brooklyn, New York

Gunter H. Seydel, M.D.
  Chairman, Department of Therapeutic Radiology
  Henry Ford Hospital
  Detroit, Michigan

Jan Van de Geijn, Ph.D.
  Radiation Oncology Branch
  Clinical Oncology Program
  Division of Cancr Treatment
  National Cancer Institute
  Bethesda, Maryland

Joan L. Venes, M.D.
  Assistant Professor Department of Surgery
  Section of Neurosurgery
  Chief of Pediatric Neurosurgery Section
  University of Michigan Medical School
  Ann Arbor, Michigan

R. Yaes, M.D.
  Assistant Instructor Department of Radiation Oncology
  S.U.N.Y. Downstate Medical Center
  Brooklyn, New York

Kenneth S. Zuckerman, M.D.
  Associate Professor Department of Internal Medicine
  Division of Hematology-Oncology
  University of Alabama Medical School
  Birmingham, Alabama

# Preface

This book is based on the proceedings of the Second Annual Symposium in Radiation Oncology held at the University of Michigan, Ann Arbor, in April, 1983. A highlight of this meeting was the third annual Isadore Lampe Lecture, masterfully delivered by Seymour Levitt, M.D. and included in this volume.

Needless to say, the caliber and quality of the participants in the program reflect their respect and admiration for Dr. Lampe, whose recent passing the entire community of radiation oncologists has mourned. We gratefully acknowledge Dr. Juan del Regato's contribution to this book in the form of a short biography of Dr. Lampe.

Radiation Oncology is a dynamic field; new approaches and techniques are continuously developing. Original investigation and analysis of results cast doubt on previous dogma and shed new light on the oncologic problem. Advances in the related fields of medical and surgical oncology, as well as diagnostic imaging, interact with radiation therapy and impact on its day to day practice. The editors thank all contributors for a lucid and timely review of recent advances in radiation oncology and related fields of medicine.

Beatriz E. Amendola, M.D.

Marco A. Amendola, M.D.

# Acknowledgments

The editors are grateful to:

Dimity Nelson for her invaluable contribution to the typing and editing of many manuscripts and to the final compilation of this book.

Dianne Pohrt for editorial assistance.

Recent Trends in Radiation Oncology
and Related Fields

ISADORE LAMPE


JUAN A. DEL REGATO, M.D.


Isadore Lampe was born in London, England on November 16th, 1906. He was the first child and only son of Anna Tamarkin (1886-1974) and Joseph Lampkovitz (1879-1964). His mother was born in Vitebsk, Russia; and was working in a London cigarette factory when she met Joseph Lampkovitz, a cabinet maker and former soldier from Plonsk, Poland. They were married on December 24th, 1905. They were both part of a remarkable massive migration of Eastern European Jews that took place around the turn of the century. Having endured the travail and spiritual deterioration of perennial poverty, torn between hopes of redemption and fears of western sacrilege, chanting Talmudic Hebrew but arguing hoarsely in Yiddish, people who considered themselves chosen decided to tear themselves from the lands that held the ashes of their revered ancestors.

When Isadore was only four and a half months old, he came to America wrapped in a tallith in his mother's arms, to join his father who had preceded them. For the immigrant, the vicissitudes of seasickness in the crossing of the Atlantic were pale in comparison to the anxiety of the nearest earthly likeness of the day of judgment: the burdening demands of the immigration officers. Beyond that they were to find friendly hospitality and opportunity. A fine artisan with a determination to succeed, Joseph Lampkovitz settled his family in the Woodland section of the city of Cleveland, on the southern shore of Lake Erie, where the immigrant baby became a beautiful child (Figure 1). There his sisters Helen (1910-), Lily (1913-1980), and Rose (1916-1974) were born. Kind, fervent and hardworking, Anna Lampkovitz kept her family well fed and stitched together by dividing her time between baking and cooking, sewing and knitting. Preserving their faith, they adopted the Conservative denomination of Orthodox Judaism developed in America. As their finances improved, they moved to the Kinsman and Mount Pleasant districts, and eventually to Cleveland Heights.

Young Isadore attended the Mount Pleasant Elementary School and simultaneously, the parochial Hebrew-Yiddish School. In 1920 he entered Central High School at Willson Avenue (2200 East 55the Street): the relatively

Reprinted with permission from the International Journal of Radiation Oncology Biology and Physics, J.A. del Regato, Isadore Lampe, Copyright (1983), Pergamon Press, Ltd.

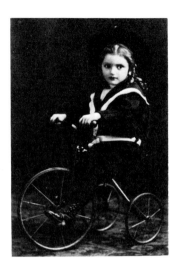

Fig. 1. With his long hair in curls and his sailor suit, young Isadore rode his tricycle (circa 1911). (Courtesy of Mrs. Isadore Lampe)

new building with well lit halls and central heating favored the students. The Central High School had acquired a wide reputation for its dedication to making good citizens of the immigrants; former graduates had achieved distinction in various fields. The school promoted debates as well as intercollegiate athletics. Isadore was a good student; his parents had instilled in him a respect for learning stemming from an old tradition by which the learned always sat by the eastern wall of the synagogue. He was a member of the track team, and although he privately favored the violin, he played the tuba in the school band. In 1923 he graduated with honors and especially excelled in chemistry (Figure 2).

Isadore Lampkovitz was admitted, within a restrictive quota, to Adelbert College. His scholarly dedication brought him membership in the oldest American fraternity, Phi Beta Kappa; he also played tennis and participated in swimming. He had long hoped to become a physician, and undoubtedly because of his scholarly performance, he was accepted at the end of his junior year to enter the School of Medicine of Western Reserve University. In 1927 he received his Bachelor of Arts degree from Adelbert College at the end of his first year of medicine.

There had been several medical schools in Cleveland at the turn of the century, but after the Flexner Report (1911), only the School of Medicine of Western Reserve University remained with a reinforced faculty and a demanding curriculum. Isadore's classmates nicknamed him "Lamp"; after reflection, he decided to heed their suggestion and petitioned the court to officially change his name to Lampe. His father thought it best to have all members of the family adopt the same name. In the second year of medical schools, Isadore was hospitalized at the Lakeside University Hospital of Cleveland with a serious bout of pneumonia and some underlying trouble; one would suspect tuberculosis. Whatever the pathology, the long hospitalization and the weakening effects of his illness interfered with Lampe's studies: he decided to repeat his second year. Thereafter, the handsome youngster lost his physical harmony; the serious setback affected the rest of his life. Lampe became a member of the Alpha Omega Alpha and Sigma Xi fraternities, and in 1931 he received his M.D. degree.

Isadore had confidently applied to serve his internship at the prestigious Mount Sinai Hospital of Cleveland; both he and his father were greatly disappointed when he was turned down. Instead, he was offered and accepted a position of intern at the Saint Vincent Hospital of Toledo, Ohio. This

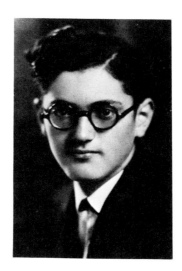

Fig. 2. A handsome graduate of high school (1923).
(Courtesy of Mrs. Isadore Lampe)

circumstance proved to be to Lampe's advantage, for in Toledo he was to meet a generous and inspiring man, John Thomas Murphy (1885-1944), who became his mentor and sponsor (Note A).

Dr. Murphy was Director of the Department of Radiology at Saint Vincent Hospital. A pioneer who had exposed himself excessively to radiation, he suffered from skin lesions which became worse with time. A handsome and eloquent man, he had a contagious enthusiasm for the growing specialty of radiology that impressed the young intern. Lampe decided to seek training in radiology. On Murphy's advice, he applied for a position as resident in the Department of Radiology at Harper Hospital in Detroit. This was one of the most prestigious departments in the midwest, headed by William A. Evans (1879-1940), a reputable radiodiagnostician, and by Traian Leucutia, a highly respected radiotherapist (Note C). Lampe was offered and accepted a position as resident in training: inexplicably, the offer was later withdrawn. However, again for Lampe's good fortune, the irksome reverse was to have fateful and advantageous consequences.

The Department of Radiology at the University of Michigan had lost its prestigious leader, Preston M. Hickey (Note B), and after a period of uncertainty, a successor had been chosen. Fred Jenner Hodges (1895-1977) was dedicated to developing a training program second to none. Former Hickey trainees and associates remained as assistant professors under Hodges' early chairmanship: Carleton Barnhart Peirce (1898-1979), Willis Seaman Peck (1900-1974), and Harold William Jacox (1904-).

Dr. Murphy had gone to Ann Arbor in December of 1931 to present to the University of Michigan, in the name of the American Roentgen Ray Society, a silver bas-relief as a memorial to Preston Hickey. Murphy used his influence with the new chairman on behalf of his protege; he brought Lampe and presented him personally to Hodges. An extra position of "assistant resident" was created to accommodate him. In all of the many years of their association, Hodges found no reason to regret it. By the account of his elders, Lampe was the most capable resident ever trained in the department. No one worked harder or longer. After two years, he was appointed instructor, and one year later, research instructor.

Lampe made a comparative study of cholecystographic appearances with proved pathology: it was published in co-authorship with Hodges.[1] With Pierce he reported observations on the treatment of giant-cell tumors of bone.[2] His interest in statistical methods led to his appointment as a part-time statistician in the Medical Records Division of the University Hospital. In this position, he set up the Medical Statistics Division of the University of Michigan. With the help of Hodges and John C. Bugher (1901-1970), he initiated a coding system that became a national model among tumor registries.[3]

In 1932 James Chadwick (1892-1974) identified and baptized as neutrons the highly penetrating chargeless particles dislodged from the atomic nucleus when bombarded by protons. Researchers sought to produce high energy electro-magnetic units that would enhance the effects. Ernest Thomas Sinton Walton (1903-) and John Cockcroft (1897-1967) produced in Cambridge, England a high energy accelerator hurling 50 million protons at high velocity; they achieved artificial transformation of lithium. At the same time, in Berkeley, California, Ernest Orlando Lawrence (1901-1958) and his graduate student, Milton Stanley Livingston (1905-), perfected their invention of the first cyclic accelerator: the cyclotron. It was capable of accelerating positive ions and repeated the artificial transformation of lithium.

The next logical step was to test the biologic effects of neutrons. Struggling against technical difficulties that had yet to be overcome, Ernest Lawrence, his graduate student, and collaborator Paul C. Aebersold (Note E) along with his brother, John Hindale Lawrence (1904-), succeeded in demonstrating relative biologic differences between x-rays and neutrons.[4] During the time when this work was done, Lampe spent six months in the Radiation Laboratory at Berkeley (Figure 3) and observed the procedures employed. "A very bright young man he was," recalled John H. Lawrence, M.D.

The Department of Physics of the University of Michigan developed a cyclotron capable of producing a low intensity beam of neutrons. Lampe arranged to be able to use it for biological research. Taking advantage of Aebersold's solution of the problem of collimation of neutrons[5] and aided by Raymond Elliot Zirkle (1902-), physicist, Lampe sought to investigate further the possible biologic differences between the effects of roentgen rays and neutrons. Their findings were reported by Lampe (1938) in his Ph.D. dissertation. They demonstrated that within the same species (Drosophila eggs of various ages) and within the same organism (shoot and tap root of wheat seedlings), there were obvious differences in the relative effectiveness of neutrons and roentgen rays in producing comparable biological effects. Under the circumstances of their work, the inevitable conclusion was that the selective effects of neutrons were inferior by a considerable margin - a conclusion that, in the opinion of Robert Parker (1925-), Lampe's distinguished student, was many years ahead of its time. The experiments also

6

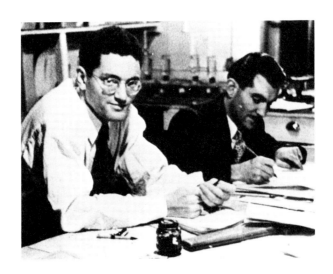

Fig. 3. Lampe in the company of Paul Aebersold at the Radiation Laboratories
of the University of California at Berkeley (1936).

suggested that neutrons may have their own characteristic selective effects
with probable significance in their use against malignant tumors.[6]

The strength of the Department of Radiology at the University of Michigan
rested on the skill of its radiodiagnosticians and the reputation of their
didactics. During Preston Hickey's tenure, the Division of Radiotherapy had
been headed briefly by a radiotherapist, Ernest A Pohle (Note D). After
Pohle's departure, the division became the charge of a succession of temporary
heads: William MacCawley Gilmore, Sr. (1903-), who returned to the practice
of general radiology in Canada; John McGregor Barnes (1899-1956), who left to
practice general radiology in Buffalo, New York; Harold William Jacox; William
Seaman Peck, a converted physical therapist, who left to practice general
radiology in Toledo. Of all these, only Jacox developed a genuine interest in
radiation therapy, held the position the longest (1932 to 1936), and chose to
remain in the specialty for the rest of his professional life (Note F). In
later years, Lampe wrote to "Jake" that the development of his department
stemmed from Jacox's early efforts.

In 1939, upon Peck's departure, Lampe was asked to assume charge of the
Division of Radiotherapy, a position which he held for 35 years. His interest
in radiotherapy had been aroused by Murphy in Toledo, and it was known that
Lampe frequently visited him on weekends, thus receiving continued stimulus.

His experimental work with neutrons had given him insight into radiobiology, yet he never received formal training in the various modalities of clinical radiation therapy: he was an autodidacta. This circumstance made him meticulous and fastidiously cautious. Also, he was a methodical reader of the world literature and developed an astute judgment of authors and of the value of their contributions.

In 1942 Lampe set out to test the possible advantages of neutrons in circumstances closely resembling clinical practice. Using 180 KV roentgen rays, Regaud and Ferroux[7] had shown (1927) that it was not possible to sterilize the testis of a rabbit by a single dose of radiation that would cause necrosis of the scrotal integuments, whereas a smaller total dose divided into several irradiations over several days would do so without causing permanent damage to the skin. This experiment had reaffirmed Regaud's concept and contributed to the universal adoption of fractional roentgentherapy in the treatment of patients with cancer. Benefiting by Aebersold's technical solution of the collimation of neutrons, Lampe was able to irradiate small animals. He found that it was possible by a single irradiation with neutrons to sterilize the rabbit's testis without damage to the scrotum and pondered whether or not further fractionation would enhance the selective effects.[8]

In the summer of 1943, Lampe was visiting a relative in Windsor, Canada; there he met a charming young lady of more than external beauty (Figure 4) who

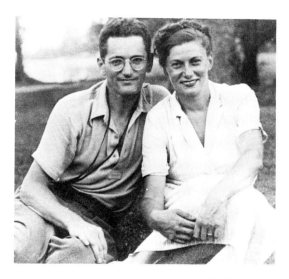

Fig. 4. Isadore and Rae Lampe enjoying a vacation (1943).

worked as an occupational therapist. Rae Ethel White (1912-) also of Eastern European ancestry and Isadore Lampe were married in Windsor in October 1943; They had a very congenial and lasting union, which in time brought them two sons: Wiliams Howard Lampe (1945-) and Matthew Mark (1951-) (Figure 5).

In 1944 an editorial appeared in Radiology under the signature of Isadore Lampe; it revealed his acquired stature and maturity as a therapeutic radiologist.[9] Radiotherapy, he wrote, has developed beyond the phase when the primary indication for it was inoperability. He emphasized the pre-eminent position of the radiotherapist in the treatment of tumors and his obligations in verifying diagnoses as well as in the administration of treatments. In collaboration with Hodges, he developed an index and cross filing system for radiodiagnostic data which was widely used in department of radiology for years.[10] He also reasoned that the clinical experience embodied in therapeutic records would be of little value for research and teaching purposes unless it was easily retrieved through a system simple enough not to require special clerical effort. He devised such a system that was carefully maintained in his department on a daily basis.[11] Thus, his rich resources were easily recalled.

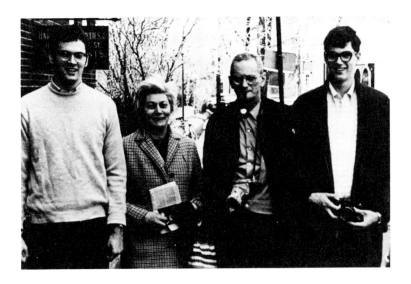

Fig. 5. The Lampe family: William Howard, Rae, Isadore and Matthew Mark (circa 1968). (Courtesy of Mrs. Isadore Lampe)

At the end of the Second World War, the Radiological Society of North America initiated a program of refresher courses that proved very successful. At the request of Charles Edgar Virden (1895-1958), the author undertook to recruit speakers in therapeutic radiology. Lampe volunteered a course of 90 minutes on the Biological Foundations of Radiotherapy: it was a capable summary of radiobiology for physicians that he delivered repeatedly to appreciative audiences.

Ever since Bailey and Cushing had segregated medulloblastomas from other gliomas,[12] the average survival of patients diagnosed with this tumor was reported to be seven months; various reports claimed an increase in the average survival with the use of post-operative radiotherapy. Lampe decided to attempt a course of radiotherapy with an aim to cure. Conscious of the fact that a frequent cause of failure was the metastatic spread of the tumor hrough the intermediate cerebrospinal fluid, he devised a plan to irradiate the entire central nervous system; initially, his course of treatment lasted five weeks. In 1949 Lampe and MacIntyre reported the results of these treatments on 25 patients:[13] 7 were living from three to eight years after radiotherapy. The evidence showed that medulloblastomas were curable and curable only by means of radiotherapy. Three years later, the authors recapitulated their experience and concluded that in order to minimize untoward radiation effects, they had to fractionate their course of treatments over longer periods.[14] This piece of work alone signals Lampe as an original researcher and an outstanding contributor to original radiotherapeutic literature.

Lampe's dedication to the demanding details of everyday clinical practice have seldom been equaled: he questioned and examined every patient brought to his care; he verified the positioning of every patient receiving treatment; he even checked the time of exposure. He read every note entered in the records and frequently made additions and corrections. He was an avid reader and spent evening hours in methodical review of the world literature. He wrote succinctly and only if there was something to be shown or said. He adopted the ethical reporting of results in 5-year absolute survival in which all patients who died, regardless of cause, or were lost to view before five years were considered failures, a procedure that discouraged the self-serving salesmen. These time-consuming activities did not interfere with his contributing a chapter on therapeutic radiology in a charming book, Radiology for Medical Students, which he co-authored with Fred Hodges and Jack Holt

(Figure 6).[15] With these same enthusiastic and congenial co-authors, he embarked on the demanding and arduous task of continuously reviewing and excerpting worthy works as his contribution to the radiation therapy portion of The Yearbook of Radiology,[16] a task that he faced for years.

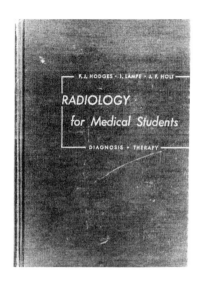

Fig. 6. Front cover of a handbook for medical students (1954).

As radioactive isotopes became available for clinical trials, Lampe collaborated in a number of tests for the study of uptake and dosimetry in human tissues of radioiodine.[17] He warned against the indiscriminate use of beta emitters for the treatment of adenoids in young children.[18] With Walter MacIntyre Whitehouse (1916-), he reported on the risk of asymmetrical bone growth, which could result from the irradiation of children with Wilms' tumors.[19] With Howard Bennett Latourette (1918-), he was among the first in the United States to discourage the aggressive irradiation of hemangiomas of the skin of children since the majority of them disappeared spontaneously without sequelae or could be easily stopped in their early development by inconsequential mild irradiation.

It was not generally understood that the prognosis of carcinomas of the meso- and hypopharynx depended greatly upon their point of departure under equal circumstances of treatment; he wrote on the results of radiotherapy of these tumors.[20] It was also generally believed that carcinomas of the oral cavity that invaded the mandible were not likely to be cured by means of radiation; Lampe provided objective and long-standing proof that adequate radiotherapy could be successful, despite bone involvement.[21]

Intracavitary pre-operative radium therapy was and is accepted as the procedure of choice in the treatment of most patients with adenocarcinoma of the endometrium. At the Second National Cancer Conference, held in Cincinnati in 1952, Lampe provided statistical evidence that external pelvic irradiation was by far preferable as a pre-operative procedure, reducing the occurrence of post-operative vaginal recurrences and yielding unprecedented 5-year survivals.[22,23]

The generosity of its alumni brought to the University of Michigan a handsome gift, the Alice Crocker Lloyd Radiation Therapy Center, named in the memory of an outstanding alumna (1954). The long sought facilities greatly enhanced the work of the Division of Radiotherapy.

Under a contract with the Atomic Energy Commission in collaboration with his faithful associate, Howard Latourette and his physicist, Charles S. Simons, Ph.D., Lampe undertook an exhaustive study of the value of Cesium 137 as an external source for clinical teletherapy. They concluded that Cesium could not replace Cobalt 60 but that it could become a valuable adjunct for the treatment of certain conditions, replacing conventional roentgentherapy units.[24]

The faculty and house staff of the University of Michigan Hospital were beneficiaries of a series of well conducted Pathology-Radiation Therapy Symposia, presenting a responsible approach to the diagnosis and treatment of malignant tumors. These conferences were capably carried out by Murray Richardson Abell (1920-), Professor of Pathology, by Lampe and by his longtime associate, Juan Vallvey Fayos (1929-). Ovarian tumors, multiple myeloma, retroperitoneal seminomas[25] were successively and comprehensively discussed.

A long-standing cordial relationship that Lampe had with Norman Fritz Miller (1894-), Professor of Gynecology, resulted in great benefit to the patients and remarkable experience for residents in the departments of gynecology and radiology. Lampe attended the weekly combined clinic and examined every patient presented. Lampe was not so fortunate with his colleagues in otolaryngology. Nevertheless, he made great efforts on behalf of patients with cancer of the tonsil, tongue, and floor of the mouth and published his results in a number of articles in co-authorship with Fayos (Figure 7).[26,27]

12

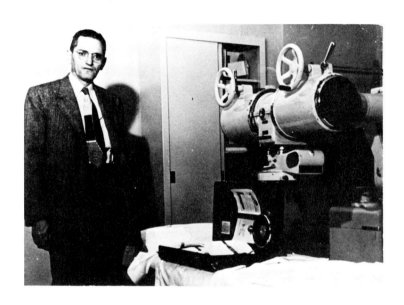

Fig. 7. Lampe in front of a conventional roentgentherapy unit provided with a light localizer and, over the couch, a set of specula for transvaginal roentgentherapy (circa 1948).

Before the Second World War, few institutions in the United States offered an opportunity for exclusive training in therapeutic radiology, and none offered a comprehensive program of training.[28] Most patients received radiotherapy administered by a variety of surgical specialists or by general radiologists whose heart was often behind the light boxes. The few available therapeutic radiologists often had their training abroad or spoke with a variety of accents. Lampe, foremost among the American radiotherapists, possessed the facilities and was endowed with the skill to undertake training of therapeutic radiologists. However, the Department of Radiology at the University of Michigan was committed to offer training in general radiology. Residents in training were assigned to Lampe for periods of six to nine months. The astonishing fact is that because of this short exposure, most of the Ann Arbor trainees acquired greater respect for radiotherapy and many of them were creditable therapists in their general practice of radiology. Moreover, several of them decided to make radiotherapy their specialty; abandoning the practice of radiodiagnosis, they sought additional training and qualifications in radiotherapy. Among these were Malcolm Bagshaw (1925-),

Howard Latourette, Robert W. Gillies (1933-), Irving Horowitz (1925-), Robert G. Parker, G. Ray Ridings (1918-), Phillip Rubin (1927), Gordon Lloyd Verity (1929-). In addition, Lampe contributed to the formation of others who had already qualified as therapeutic radiologists but sought his inspiring guidance. Among these were Jose Luis Campos (1934-), Patrick Joseph Michael Cavanaugh (1924-), Basil Considine (1921-), Juan Fayos, Alvin J. Greenberg (1923-), Seymour Herbert Levitt (1928-), Ruheri Perez-Tamayo (1926-). Latourette, Fayos, Levitt, Campos, and Perez-Tamayo became his trusted associates for variable periods of time with Latourette (1952-1959) and Fayos (1961-1974) having the longest tenure.

For most residents in radiology at the University of Michigan, their tour of duty in the Division of Radiotherapy became a memorable succession of mixed feelings. Their chief was a tall, stoop shouldered, craggy, prematurely edentulous man looking older than his age, who wore dark suits and ties and frequently, unnecessary rubber overshoes. He smoked a pipe and like most pipe smokers, smoked more matches than tobacco (Figure 8). The chief insisted on doing or checking everything himself; nothing was done without his approval.

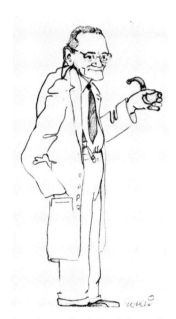

Fig. 8. Caricature of Isadore Lampe by Ruheri Perez-Tamayo, M.D. (1957).

Lampe's attitude merely reflected his extreme devotion to the best interests of the patients and his unwillingness to have them dealt with lightly or irresponsibly. "Before entering into any consideration of treatment," said Latourette, "he spent his intellect and energy, extracting meaningful details of history, evaluating the available information, then proceeded to do a very thorough clinical examination." "We learned never to act on information obtained from secondary sources," said Walter Whitehouse. "Above all else," wrote Irving Horowitz, "he maintained a superb clinical sense. With him, the residents learned to examine a larynx as well as a pelvis." "He taught us how to describe a lesion, how to evaluate the pathology, how to summarize our findings," said Herbert Rudolph Zatzkin (1915-). "He promoted the view that each resident should research his own answers with a minimum of spoon-feeding," wrote Donald Burnett Fletcher (1913-). "His fastidiousness was reflected in his extremely careful recordkeeping," wrote Melvin Morgan Figley (1920-). "He seldom spoke," said Edward Bivens Singleton (1920-), "except to comment unfavorably or critically." "He was a strict but kindly disciplinarian, in every sense a dedicated teacher," wrote Arthur Claussen Kittleson (1925-). Gradually, the residents felt in themselves the growing strength of the acquired experience.

In the discussions on treatment planning and therapeutic alternatives, they became amazed by the wealth of his knowledge and vast acquaintance with past and current literature: they felt enriched by the shared wealth. Soon the residents learned the names of fake authorities who were not to be invoked. "He did not tolerate 'phoniness' or intellectual deceit," wrote Robert Paker. He was weary of those with "high-powered equipment and low powered minds," recalled Stanley Anderson Moore (1919-). Throughout, he remained a physician concerned with his patients' care. "From him I learned what it meant to be a good doctor," affirmed Zatzkin. "He taught me to write articles with honesty and proper perspective," said Fayos. "He was precise, succinct, dry," wrote Guillermo Santin. "Lampe did nothing to put himself in the limelight and made no claims for himself," said Cavanaugh. Residents could draw him easily into discussions of medical ethics. As their tour of duty progressed, they became highly respectful of the generous man who gave them everything he had. They noted that senior members of the faculty as well as house staff from other departments came constantly to seek Lampe's opinion and advice; he was the most highly respected academician in the department. "An outstanding, intelligent and highly qualified member of our faculty," said professor Miller. During the evenings at his home, the residents and their wives would spend hours philosophizing and discussing a variety of subjects. In their political discussions, they were surprised to find that he was rather liberal in his own views, yet conservative about the nation's liberal traditions. Gradually, respect turned to reverence and affection. "He was the epitome of personal and scientific integrity," wrote Benjamin Reyer van Zwallenberg (1912-), "the most respected and indeed revered of all those who gave me my medical education." "His gentle manner, his demand for excellence, his thoroughness as well as his inspiration will always be with us," mourned Phillip Rubin (Figure 9 and 9a).

To the casual observer, Lampe appeared reserved, introverted, taciturn. In the intimacy of his family and close friends, he was warm, affable, cordial. In any light, his modesty and honesty were resplendent. Campos described him as "a man of extreme frugality and spartan tastes." These qualities and his drive for perfection were characteristic of his hardworking and devoted parents.

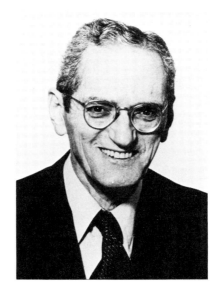

Fig. 9. Professor Isadore Lampe (1958) and Fig. 9a. his signature.

Everyone who came to know Lampe well was pleased to find that he was a fine photographer who owned some expensive gadgets, and that he liked to take snapshots of his dogs and other pets, and to make portraits of his friends' children. They were surprised to learn of his interest in athletic records which he carefully revised. They were also amazed at what some termed "contradictory" or "incongruous": his lavish interest in a succession of imported and sports automobiles, which, for the benefit of his guests, he drove at vertiginous speeds. Photography, athletics, speed were also avocations of his admired mentor, Dr. John Murphy.

In 1953, in Copenhagen, Lampe was elected one of the American members of the newly created International Club of Radiotherapists. In 1958 he was one of the founding members of the American Club of Therapeutic Radiologists. This organization (in its maturity, as the American Society of Therapeutic Radiologists) granted him its outstanding recognition with its Gold Medal in 1979. That same year, he was also awarded the Distinguished Teaching Service and Research Award of the University of Michigan Medical Alumni Society.

For years Lampe suffered from a peculiar sensitivity to certain foods. For the last 15 to 18 years of his life, he was known to have chronic lymphogenous leukemia. After his retirement, he developed myelofibrosis and had to receive occasional transfusions. While being driven on icy streets in order to receive one of these transfusions, he suffered an automobile accident and fractures which his spent system could not overcome. On January 25th, 1982 he expired.

"As a mentor and as a role model, I could have found no better," wrote Latourette. "A man is fortunate to be exposed to excellence and to pattern himself after someone he admires: Lampe was that model for me," said Zatzkin. "Only a few of us are fortunate enough to be exposed to someone of his caliber, as a person and as a teacher," wrote Kittleson. "I wonder if this awkward man ever realized how much we admired him," said Parker. "Lampe had few peers," stated Figley considerately. I say Iz had none. He was by far the outstanding academic radiotherapist in the United States in his lifetime.

NOTES

A. JOHN THOMAS MURPHY (1885-1944) received his M.D. degree from the University of Toledo (1906). He worked in radiology at Cook County Hospital of Chicago, then went to Toledo. Very active in organized radiology, he was the first secretary of the A.M.A. Section of Radiology. He was also secretary of the Executive Council of the A.R.R.S., of which he became president in 1933. He was an early member of the Commission on Safety Standards of the A.R.R.S. (1924), which was chaired by HENRY KUNRATH PANCOAST (1875-1939) and other members including, WILLIAM DUANE (1892-1935), WILLIAM DAVID COOLIDGE (1873-1976), BERNARD HENRY NICHOLS (1876-1964), PRESTON MENASSEH HICKEY (1865-1930), and JAMES LLOYD WEATHERWAX (1874-1965). He was elected president of the American College of Radiology (1935); his memorable presidential address launched an ambitious program that transformed the College.[29] Dr. Murphy was an excellent ice skater; he had great interest in track events, piloted his own airplane, and was a speedboat enthusiast as well as an excellent photographer.

B. PRESTON MENASSEH HICKEY (1865-1930) received his M.D. degree from the Detroit College of Medicine and Surgery (1892). He was a practicing otolaryngologist until 1900, when he became interested in x-rays. He became a member of the A.R.R.S. (1901) and was its president in 1907; he was the first editor of the American Journal of Roentgenology. A prolific writer, he had many early publications to his credit. A fine teacher, he was among the first to concern himself with the methods of instruction and the organization of training in radiology. He was appointed professor of roentgenology at the Detroit College of Medicine in 1910 and was chief of the Department of Radiology of Harpers Hospital until 1922, when he was appointed professor and chairman of the Department of Roentgenology at the University of Michigan. More than any other of his contemporaries, Hickey seems to have understood the need for exclusively trained therapeutic radiologists in academic centers in order to provide equitable training in general radiology. He went to France as a radiologist in the U.S. Army during the First World War. Upon his return, he enticed TRAIAN LEUCUTIA to join him at Harpers (Note C). He enticed to Ann Arbor another European trained radiotherapist, ERNST ALBERT POHLE (note D). Hickey fashioned an early tube-head applicator for radiotherapy that he called a "cone": the designation was generally adopted thereafter for any tube-head applicator, regardless of shape.

C. TRAIAN LEUCUTIA (1892-1977) was born in Calacea, Transylvania. He received his M.D. degree from the University of Vienna in 1916. He served as Romanian liaison officer to the French army during the First World War. He received post-graduate training and obtained the Certificat d'Electroradiologie (1920) from the University of Paris; he also qualified for the Diploma of Medical Radiology and Electrology in Cambridge, England. He was working at the St. Thomas Hospital of London before he was invited to join the firm of PRESTON M. HICKEY, WILLIAM A. EVANS AND LAWRENCE REYNOLDS at Harpers Hospital of Detroit, where he spent the rest of his professional life. He became president of the A.R.R.S. in 1961 and received the Gold Medal of the American College of Radiology in 1967. He was editor of the American Journal of Roentgenology from 1961 to 1974, when he retired. He was the victim of criminal violence and died of its consequences in 1977. He was one of the few and a highly respected American therapeutic radiologist for several decades.

D.  ERNST ALBERT POHLE (1895-1965) was born in Wiesbaden, Germany. He received his M.D. degree from the University of Frankfurt-on-Main in 1921 and did postgraduate work under FRIEDRICH DESSAUER (1881-1963) at the Institut fur Physikalische Grundlagen der Medizin in Frankfurt. In 1923 he came to the United States and was first an assistant roentgenologist at the Mount Sinai Hospital of Cleveland. At the invitation of PRESTON M. HICKEY, he became an assistant professor of roentgenology at the University of Michigan Medical School ((1925). While in Ann Arbor, he completed the requirements for a Ph.D. in biophysics, and shortly afterward, he was appointed the first professor and chairman of the Department of Roentgenology at the University of Wisconsin. He installed a radium emanation plant for the production of radon seeds and established Madison as a radiation therapy center. In 1938 he published a book, Theoretical principles of roentgentherapy, and edited a text, Clinical Roentgentherapy, containing a variety of chapters by American and European authors: these were among the few available authoritative works in English and were reference books for years. In 1951 he installed in his department one of the few one-million volt units. He retired in 1961; he died in 1965 as a result of an accident in his Shorewood Hills home.

E.  PAUL CLARENCE AEBERSOLD (1907-1967) was born in Fresno, California; he received his B.A. degree from Stanford University (1932) and an M.A. degree from the University of California (1934). He went to Berkeley seeking to qualify for the track team of the Olympic games and instead, casually met ERNEST ORLANDO LAWRENCE (1901-1958), who agreed to take him as his graduate student. He participated in the perfecting and testing of the cyclotron and collaborated with Lawrence and his brother, JOHN HINDALE LAWRENCE (1904-) in early biophysical testing of the effectiveness of neutrons.[4] With ROBERT SPENCER STONE (1895-1966), he worked on a clinical comparison of the effects of 200 kV roentgen rays (1937). "The Collimation of Fast Neutrons," his original solution to the problem of using neutrons for biological and clinical irradiations[5] was presented as his dissertation towards a Ph.D. degree from the Graduate Division of the University of California. He worked at Los Alamos and was one of those involved in the assembly of the plutonium bomb tested at Alamo Gordo, June 1945. After the war, he was put in charge of the production of radioactive isotopes at Oak Ridge; he lectured extensively throughout Latin America, then was transferred to the headquarters of the Atomic Energy Commission. Although a charming convivialist and a gregarious extrovert, he developed bouts of depression, and after several serious attempts, he finally ended his life on May 29, 1967. A Paul C. Aebersold Memorial Lecture was delivered by GLENN THEODORE SEABORG (1912-), Nobel Prize winner and chairman of the U.S. Atomic Energy Commission, in San Francisco on December 2and, 1969. The Society of Nuclear Medicine established (1973) an annual Paul Aebersold Award "for outstanding achievement in basic science applied to nuclear medicine."

F.  HAROLD WILLIAM JACOX (1904-) received his M.D. degree from the University of Michigan in 1928. After one year of internship at the Naval Hospital of Boston, he served another year of internship at the University Hospital in Ann Arbor. In 1930 he was appointed assistant resident in roentgenology under Profesor Hickey, who died that year. He continued his residency under Hodges. In 1932 he was put in charge of the Division of Radiotherapy and held the position until 1936, when he left to become head of radiation and physical therapy at the West Pennsylvania Hospital of Pittsburgh. During the Second World War, he served in the U.S. Navy, rising to the rank of commander. In 1947 he was appointed professor of radiology at Columbia

University and was for years in charge of radiotherapy at the Harkness Pavillion of the Columbia-Presbyterian complex. In 1969 he was elected Professor Emeritus and retired from active practice. He continues to serve as consultant in radiotherapy and lives in Englewood, New Jersey.

## ACKNOWLEDGEMENT

In composing this biographical sketch, I have become indebted to numerous persons. I am especially thankful to Mrs. Isadore Lampe and to Miss Helen Lampe for details and illustrations. Dr. Rodriguez-Antunez and Dr. Judah Rubenstein of Cleveland were very helpful. Dr. Lampe's former associates and residents who are briefly quoted in the text, contributed greatly to the composition of this portrait.

## REFERENCES

1.  Hodges, F.J. and Lampe, I. A comparison of oral cholecystographic findings and proven evidence of gallbladder disease. Am J Roentgenol 37:145-152, 1937.
2.  Peirce, C.B. and Lampe, I. Giant-cell bone tumor. Further observations on treatment. JAMA 107:1867-1871, 1936.
3.  Hodges, F.J. and Lampe, I. Organized clinical investigation of cancer. Second Report Univ Hosp Bull (U-Mich) 4:51-54, 1938.
4.  Lawrence, J.H., Aebersold, P.C. and Lawrence, E.O. Comparative effects of neutrons and x-rays on normal and tumor tissue. Proc Natl Acad Sci 22:543-557, 1936.
5.  Aebersold, P.C. The collimation of fast neutrons. Ph.D. Thesis, Graduate Division, University of California (Berkeley), May 11, 1939.
6.  Zirkle, R.E. and Lampe, I. Differences in the relative action of neutrons and roentgen rays on closely related tissues. Am J Roentgenol 39:613-627, 1938.
7.  Regaud, C. and Ferroux, R. Discordance des effects des rayons X, d'une part dans la peau, d'autre par dans le testicule, par le fractionement de la dose: diminution de l'efficacite dans la peau maintain de l'efficacite dans le testicule. Compt rend Soc Biol (Paris) 97:431-434, 1927.
8.  Lampe, I. Hodges, F.J. Differential tissue response to neutron and roentgen radiations. Radiology 41:344-349, 1943.
9.  Lampe, I. The radiation therapist in contemporary medicine (editorial). Radiology 43:181-183, 1944.
10. Hodges, F.J. and Lampe, I. Filing and cross-indexing roentgen ray records. Demonstration of a simple and efficient method. Am J Roentgenol 41:1007-1018, 1939.
11. Lampe, I. Filing and cross-indexing of radiation therapy records. Radiology 45:168-175, 1945.
12. Bailey, P. and Cushing, H. Medulloblastoma cerebelli. Arch Neurol Psych 14:192-224, 1925.
13. Lampe, I. and MacIntyre, R.S. Roentgen treatment of medulloblastomas of the cerebellum. Arch Neurol Psych 62:322-329, 1949.
14. Lampe, I. and MacIntyre, R.S. Experiences in radiation therapy of medulloblastoma of the cerebellum. Am J Roentgenol 71:659-668, 1954.
15. Hodges, F.J., Lampe, I. and Holt, J.F. Radiology for Medical Students. Yearbook Publisher, Chicago, 1947.

16. Hodges, F.J., Lampe, I. and Holt, J.F. (eds) Year Book of Radiology. Yearbook Publishers, Chicago, 1949.
17. Bierwalters, W.H., Lampe, I., Gomberg, H., Peelor, R.A., and Brown, P.W. Radioiodine uptake curves in humans. Univ Hosp Bull (U-Mich) 14:73-75, 1948.
18. Lampe, I. Potential biologic danger of nasopharyngeal beta irradiation. Trans Am Acad Opthal Otolaryngol 54:502-507, 1950.
19. Whitehouse, W.M. and Lampe, I. Osseous damage in irradiation of renal tumors in infancy and childhood. Am J Roentgenol 70:721-729, 1953.
20. Lampe, I. Malignant neoplasms of the tongue, tonsil and hypopharynx; evaluation of radiation therapy. Trans Am Acad Opthal Otolaryngol 55:231-243, 1951.
21. Lampe, I. Radiation therapy of cancer of the buccal mucosa and lower gingiva. Am J Roentgenol 73:528-538, 1955.
22. Lampe, I. Combined surgical and radiological treatment of endometrial carcinoma. Proc Second Natl Cancer Conf (Cincinnati) 1:754-764, 1952.
23. Lampe, I. Endometrial carcinoma. Am J Roentgenol 90:1011-1015, 1963.
24. Lampe, I., Simons, C.S. and Latourette, H.B. The physical aspects of a Cesium teletherapy source. Am J Roentgenol 82:587-596, 1959.
25. Abell, M.R., Fayos, J.V., and Lampe, I. Retroperitoneal germinomas (seminomas) without evidence of testicular involvement. Cancer 18:587-596, 1959.
26. Fayos, J. and Lampe, I. The therapeutic problem of metastatic neck adenopathy. Am J Roentgenol 114:=65-75, 1972.
27. Lampe, I., Fayos, J., Hendrix, R. and McDonald, V. Hodgkin's disease. A review of radiotherapeutic experience. Am J Roentgenol 93:557-567, 1965.
28. del Regato, J.A. Training centers in therapeutic radiology. Post-Graduate Med 14:161-162, 1953.
29. del Regato, J.A. The American College of Radiology Fiftieth Anniversary. Radiology 107:1-13, 1973.

RADICAL RADIATION THERAPY IN THE TREATMENT OF
LAPAROTOMY STAGED HODGKIN'S DISEASE PATIENTS*

SEYMOUR H. LEVITT, M.D. AND CHUNG K. K. LEE, M.D.

INTRODUCTION

Since 1970, Hodgkin's disease patients at the University of Minnesota have
been evaluated with the complete staging procedure, including laparotomy and
splenectomy, recommended by the Ann Arbor Conference.[1] Patients with
limited disease (Stage IA to IIIA) were treated with curative radiotherapy.
From 1970 to mid-1974, patients were treated with extended nodal fields
(mantle and periaortic fields or inverted "Y" and modified mantle) for Stage I
and II Hodgkin's disease, and total nodal fields (mantle and inverted "Y"
fields) for Stage IIIA. In 1975, analysis of treatment results led to a
re-evaluation of our treatment approach. High recurrence rates were found in
Stage IIIA and IIB patients and those Stage I and II patients with large
mediastinal masses and/or hilar disease.[2] Because of the poor results in
these patients, low dose whole lung irradiation for the patients with a large
mediastinal mass and/or hilar disease, and low dose hepatic irradiation to the
spleen positive Stage IIIA patients, were initiated as treatment
modifications. This paper will review the results of this treatment
modification.

WHOLE LUNG RADICAL RADIATION[2]

Materials and methods

From 1970 to 1980, 144 patients with Hodgkin's disease were treated in the
Department of Therapeutic Radiology at the University of Minnesota Hospitals
with curative radiotherapy following surgical staging. Of these 144 patients,
92 had mediastinal and/or hilar disease, and 52 did not. To have an objective
measure of the size of the mediastinal mass and to observe prognosis according
to size of the mass, we developed the concept of the MT ratio, which is

---

* Presented as the Third Annual Isadore Lampe Lecture at the University of
Michigan, Ann Arbor, April 15, 1983.

Recent Trends in Radiation Oncology and Related Fields, Amendola and Amendola, Editors

calculated as follows:

$$\text{MT ratio} = \frac{\text{largest transverse diameter of mediastinal mass}}{\text{transverse diameter of thorax at the level of T5-6}}$$

The 92 patients with mediastinal and/or hilar disease were divided into two groups depending on the MT ratio. Those with an MT ratio 0.35 were considered to have large mediastinal masses, and those with an MT ratio 0.35 were considered to have small mediastinal masses. Forty-one of the 92 patients had large mediastinal masses. One stage IIIB patient was eliminated. Twenty of these 40 patients were treated with regular mantle field irradiation before 1975. The 20 patients treated since mid-1974 received low dose whole or unilateral lung irradiation as part of the regular mantle field irradiation.

Twenty-six of the 144 patients with Hodgkin's disease showed evidence of hilar disease. Fifteen of these patients had large mediastinal masses and 11

TABLE 1.    PATIENT CHARACTERISTICS:   LARGE MEDIASTINAL MASS

|  | Lung Irradiation | No Lung Irradiation |
|---|---|---|
| Number of Patients | 20 | 20 |
| Year Treated | 1974 - 1980 | 1970 - 1974 |
| Age (in years): | | |
| Median | 23 | 24 |
| Range | 7 - 37 | 14 - 47 |
| Gender: | | |
| Male | 10 | 9 |
| Female | 10 | 11 |
| Stage and histopathology: | | |
| $I_{EA}$ nodular sclerosis | 0 | 1 |
| $II_A$ nodular sclerosis | 10 | 6 |
| mixed cellularity | 1 | 1 |
| others | 0 | 3* |
| $II_{EA}$ nodular sclerosis | 2 | 1 |
| $II_B$ nodular sclerosis | 3 | 2 |
| mixed cellularity | 1 | 2 |
| $III_A$ nodular sclerosis | 3 | 2 |
| mixed cellularity | 0 | 1 |
| $III_B$ mixed cellularity | 0 | 1 |
| Size of mediastinal mass (MT ratio): | | |
| 0.35 - 0.44 | 9 | 11 |
| 0.45 - 0.54 | 7 | 7 |
| greater or equal to 0.55 | 4 | 2 |
| Mean ratio | 0.45 | 0.46 |
| Median ratio | 0.44 | 0.43 |

* 1-undifferentiated,   2-LD

had small mediastinal masses. Only one patient had definite hilar disease, with no evidence of mediastinal mass on chest roentgenography. Thirteen of these 26 patients (7 with large masses, 6 with small) were treated since 1975 and received lung irradiation. The 13 patients treated before 1975 (8 with large masses, 5 with small) did not receive lung irradiation.

As shown in Table 1, for patients with large mediastinal masses in the two time periods, the distribution by stage and histopathologic subclassification, the male to female ratio, and the median age were comparable. The mean and median MT ratios were approximately 0.45 in both groups.

The characteristics of patients with hilar disease are shown in Table 2. Age, sex, and distribution by stage and histopathology were comparable in the two groups. Patients who had questionable involvement of the hilar region were eliminated from evaluation.

TABLE 2.      PATIENT CHARACTERISTICS:   HILAR DISEASE

| | Lung Irradiation | No Lung Irradiation |
|---|---|---|
| Number of Patients | 13 | 13 |
| Hilar Disease + large med. mass | 7* | 8** |
| Hilar Disease + small med. mass | 6 | 5 |
| Age (in years): | | |
|   Median | 23 | 23 |
|   Range | 8 - 33 | 6 - 47 |
| Gender: | | |
|   Male | 6 | 6 |
|   Female | 7 | 7 |
| Stage and histopathology: | | |
|   $II_A$ nodular sclerosis | 5*** | 6 |
|   $II_{EA}$ nodular sclerosis | 2 | 0 |
|   $II_A$ lymphocytic depletion | 0 | 1 |
|   $II_B$ nodular sclerosis | 3 | 1 |
|     mixed cellularity | 0 | 1 |
|   $III_A$ nodular sclerosis | 3 | 2 |
|     mixed cellularity | 0 | 1 |

\*   4 questionable patients were eliminated.
\*\* 3 questionable patients were eliminated.
\*\*\*1 patient died from generalized histoplasmosis during treatment.

TREATMENT

All patients were treated with radiotherapy as the primary curative modality. Radiotherapy was administered by a 10 MeV linear accelerator, except for a few patients who were treated with Cobalt 60. Stage I and II patients who did not receive whole or unilateral lung irradiation were treated with mantle and periaortic fields, as previously reported.[3-5]

The patients who received irradiation to one or both lungs had the treatment to the lung as part of the initial course of treatment of the mantle field. These patients' mantle area treatment was started without lung blocks, and they were treated with a daily midline dose of 75 to 100 rads (without lung correction). When the total dose to the lung reached 1000-2000 rads, depending on the response of the mediastinal mass, adequate lung blocking was added and treatment continued according to the routine mantle technique. Patients with unilateral disease, or with a large mass protruding to one side of the thoracic cavity, received ipsilateral lung irradiation in a similar manner with the one involved lung unblocked.

All patients tolerated whole or unilateral lung irradiation without problems. Only one patient had apical infiltration of unknown cause during the course of lung irradiation which was confirmed as an atypical infectious process by biopsy.

The total dose of radiation to the lung varied (Table 3) and was influenced by the age of the patient and by the speed of the regression of the masses on serial chest x-rays.

TABLE 3.       RADIATION DOSE TO THE LUNGS
IN PATIENTS WITH LARGE MEDIASTINAL MASSES*

| Dose (rad) | Number of patients |
|---|---|
| 1000 | 1 |
| 1200 | 2 |
| 1500 | 5 (3)** |
| 1700 | 1 |
| 1800 | 6 |
| 2000 | 4 (1)** |

* Daily dose of 75-100 rad at midplane without lung correction.
** 1 side of the lung was treated.

STATISTICS

Recurrence-free survival was calculated from the first day of treatment. Overall survival was calculated from the date of the diagnosis. Actuarial computation of both survival curves was performed by the method of Kaplan and Meier.[6] The statistical difference of each group was assessed by the method of Breslow.[7]

RESULTS:   RESPONSE TO TREATMENT

Response to treatment was classified as either complete remission or treatment failure.   Remission was assessed after the completion of radiotherapy. Complete remission was defined as the total disappearance of all symptoms and clinically measurable disease which persisted for at least one month, or continuous regression of measurable disease to eventual disappearance of mass.   Some of the larger masses took several months to completely regress.

Median follow up of patients who did not receive lung irradiation was 128 months (range from 106-140).   In this group, one patient out of the 20 failed to achieve complete remission and of the 19 patients who achieved complete remission, 15 (79%) relapsed.   The median time to disease recurrence was 18 months (range: 3 to 72).   Most patients (10 of 15) relapsed within 24 months.

Patients who received lung irradiation were followed for a median of 73 months (range from 24-103).   All patients in this group achieved complete remission.   There were three recurrences (19%), at 4, 32 and 48 months.

Figure 1 shows the recurrence-free survival in the two groups of patients with large mediastinal masses who achieved complete remissions.   Patients who

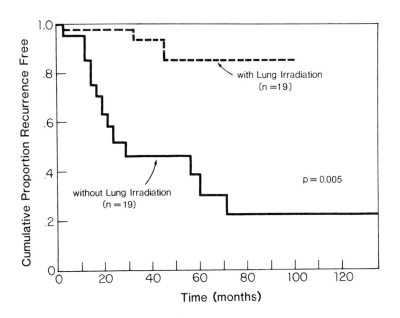

Fig. 1. Recurrence-free survival in the two groups of patients with large mediastinal masses.

26

were treated with regular mantle fields had a statistically significant
shorter remission duration (15/19 - 79%) and a higher relapse rate (P=0.005)
than the patients treated with lung irradiation (3/19 - 19%). Figure 2 shows
that the overall actuarial survival in the two groups did not show a
statistically significant difference.

In patients with the mediastinal masses and hilar disease treated with
whole or unilateral lung irradiation, only one of 13 recurred (1/13 - 8%). In
the non-lung irradiation group, eight patients recurred (8/13 - 62%).

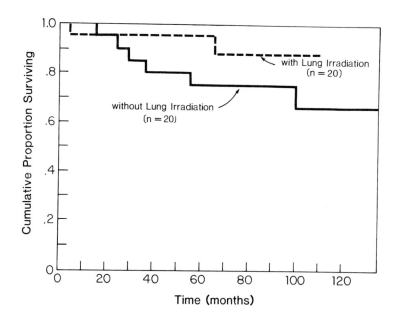

Fig. 2. Overall actuarial survival in the two groups of patients with large
mediastinal masses.

SITES OF DISEASE RECURRENCE IN PATIENTS WITH LARGE MEDIASTINAL MASSES

Mantle group. In these patients, there were 26 sites of recurrence above
the diaphragm and only five below the diaphragm (Table 4). The most common
sites of recurrence were the lung, pleura, and mediastinum adjacent to the
original mass. Nineteen of 28 sites (68%) were in the thorax. Nine of the 28
sites of recurrence (32%) were in the peripheral lymph nodes.

Lung irradiated group. There were only two recurrences of disease among
the patients in this group. One Stage IIIA patient relapsed in a right iliac

lymph node and the right ureter, which was a site of original disease found during staging laparotomy. This patient had a large mediastinal mass and had received 1500 rads to the left lung. He was alive and receiving chemotherapy at 72+ months. The other patient had Stage IIA nodular sclerosing Hodgkin's disease of the thymus and received 1800 rads to both lung fields as part of the initial course of supradiaphragmatic treatment; she relapsed in the right lung and mediastinum at 32 months. The patient had been in clinical remission following chemotherapy; however, she died from massive aspergillosis of the lung at 60 months from diagnosis.

TABLE 4. INITIAL SITES OF RECURRENCE IN PATIENTS WITH LARGE MEDIASTINAL MASSES

| | Lung irradiation (19 patients)* | No lung irradiation (19 patients)** |
|---|---|---|
| Above diaphragm: | 2 | 26 |
| Lung | 1 | 5 |
| Hilum | 0 | 2 |
| Pleura | 0 | 3 |
| Pericardium | 0 | 2 (1?)*** |
| Mediastinum | 2 | 3 |
| Chest wall | 0 | 3**** |
| Cervical lymph nodes | 0 | 2 |
| Supraclavicular nodes | 0 | 3 |
| Axillary nodes | 0 | 3 |
| Waldeyer's ring | 0 | 1 |
| Below diaphragm: | 1 | 5 |
| Retroperitoneal nodes | 1 | 1 |
| Inguinal nodes | 0 | 2 |
| Extradural mass | 0 | 1 |
| Bone (spine) | 0 | 1 |
| Bone marrow | 0 | 1 |

*1 patient died of generalized histoplasmosis during treatment.
**1 patient failed to achieve C.R.
***(1?) Clinical but not biopsy proven.
****Subcutaneous node.

SIGNIFICANT SIDE EFFECTS AND COMPLICATIONS

Low dose whole lung irradiation was well tolerated in general. A major concern with whole or unilateral lung irradiation is radiation pneumonitis and/or post-irradiation pulmonary damage.

There were 2 patients who showed significant paramediastinal fibrosis on chest x-ray, which could also have developed from mantle irradiation. One patient developed fatal generalized histoplasmosis, including generalized lung parenchymal infiltration. It is not clear whether lung irradiation triggered generalized spread of infection or not. One other recent patient died with pulmonary infiltration one week after lung irradiation which could have been fulminating radiation pneumonitis, although it is not clear whether his problem was due to low dose lung irradiation or wide width of the mediastinal field.

The pulmonary function test has been evaluated and followed in more recent patients. Usually lung function tests show a more significant drop and delayed recovery of diffusion lung carbon monoxide (DLCO) in the lung treated group. A review of DLCO in a limited number of regular mantle field irradiated patients (without large mediastinal mass) showed recovery within 6 months to 1 year, while lung treated patients showed recovery in 2 years or more.

## LIVER IRRADIATION

From 1970 to 1980, 36 laparotomy staged Stage IIIA Hodgkin's disease patients were treated with curative radiotherapy at the University of Minnesota Hospitals. Among these 36 patients were 33 who were found to have splenic involvement with or without other disease in the abdomen. Prior to 1975, the patients with splenic involvement were treated with routine total nodal irradiation (TNI), including the splenic pedicle. Evaluation of the treatment results in 1975 showed need for improvement. Subsequently, patients with splenic involvement received liver irradiation. This section will detail our results with this technique change.

## TREATMENT

All patients were treated with radiotherapy as the primary curative modality. Patients not receiving liver irradiation were treated with TNI (including splenic pedicle). The daily dose was 150 rads at midplane. A rest period of 4 weeks was given between treatments to the mantle and inverted Y fields.

Those patients who had liver irradiation received 2000 rads to the midplane of a field encompassing the liver and remainder of the inverted Y at the daily dose rate of 100 rads. After 2000 rads to the liver and inverted Y field (including splenic pedicle), the liver was shielded and radiation was continued to the regular inverted Y field with dose escalation of 150 rads daily to the appropriate dose. Patients in the liver treated group who had a large mediastinal mass or hilar disease also received whole or hemi lung irradiation. Treatment was initially given to that side of the diaphragm with the most extensive disease.

PATIENT CHARATERISTICS (Table 5)

Sixteen patients ($13-A_1$, $3-A_2$) did not receive liver irradiation; 17 patients ($14-A_1$, $3-A_2$) did. The median age was 27 and 25 years respectively in the two groups. There was a preponderance of males in the group that received liver irradiation, while the male to female ratio was equal in the untreated liver group. Distribution of patients by age, histology, and extent of disease as determined by anatomic substage was similar in the two groups. Median followup intervals were 143 months (range from 123-163) in the untreated liver group, and 79 months (range from 36 to 109) in the liver treated group.

Patients were subgrouped retrospectively according to the total number of primary sites as well as the number of disease sites below the diaphragm according to the criteria of Dresser, et al.[8] The liver treated group had a

---

TABLE 5.   PATIENT CHARACTERISTICS:   HODGKIN'S DISEASE STAGE IIIA

|  | Liver not treated | Liver treated |
|---|---|---|
| No. of patients | 16 | 17 |
| Age (in years): | | |
| Median | 27 | 24 |
| Range | 14 - 56 | 13 - 42 |
| Gender: | | |
| Male | 8 (50)* | 13 (76) |
| Female | 8 (50) | 4 (24) |
| Histopathology: | | |
| Nodular sclerosis | 9 (56) | 11 (ᴜ5) |
| Mixed cellularity | 5 (31) | 6 (35) |
| Lymphocytic predominant | 2 (13) | 0 (0) |
| Anatomic substage:** | | |
| IIIA1 | 13 (81) | 14 (82) |
| IIIA2 | 3 (19) | 3 (18) |
| No. of primary sites:*** | | |
| less than 5 | 9 (56) | 7 (41) |
| 5 or more | 7 (44) | 10 (59) |
| No. of sites below the diaphragm: | | |
| Spleen only | 7 (44) | 5 (29) |
| Spleen & hilar node | 6 (38) | 10 (59) |
| more than 2 sites | 3 (19) | 2 (12) |
| Extent cf splenic involvement: | | |
| S+ extensive | 8 (50) | 12 (71) |
| S+ minimal | 8 (50) | 5 (29) |
| Median follow-up (in months) | 143 (123-163) | 79 (35-111) |

*Number in parentheses is the percent by row totals.
**According to criteria suggested by Dresser, et al.[8]
***Recommendation by Hoppe, et al.[22]

---

slightly higher proportion of patients with more than five primary sites. The patients in the liver treated group also had more sites involved below the diaphragm. The extent of splenic involvement was also retrospectively grouped according to the Stanford recommendation. In the untreated liver group, the number of patients in the S+ minimal versus S+ extensive was equal, while there were more patients in the S+ extensive category in the liver treated group.

STATISTICAL METHODS

Survival and recurrence-free survival curves were calculated by the Kaplan and Meier technique.[6] Differences between patient groups were tested by using the method of Lee and Desu in the Statistical Package for the Social Sciences (SPSS).[9] Differences in percentage for discrete variables were tested using Fisher's exact test.[10]

None of the patients were lost to follow up.

RESULTS

All patients finished radiation treatment and achieved a complete remission. In the untreated liver group, 12 of 16 patients (75%) recurred. The median follow up time of the 16 patients was 120 months (range from 95-135); the median time of recurrence was 18 months (range from 11-77). In contrast, only 4 of 17 (23%) of the patients recurred in the liver treated group. Median follow up of the liver treated group was 59+ months (range from 39-81).

The five year recurrence free survival of the untreated liver patients was 41% as compared to 78% in the liver treated group. This difference is statistically significant (P=0.014). Overall survival also shows a slightly more favorable result for the liver treated group, although it is not statistically significant (80% vs. 90%). However, the follow up periods are quite different (the untreated liver group has been followed longer).

There were five deaths in the untreated liver group. Four died of Hodgkin's disease despite extensive chemotherapy, and one developed leukemia and died. There was one death in the liver treated group, from precocious myocardial infarction at the age of 30. The four recurrences after total nodal and liver irradiation have been salvaged with a combination of chemotherapy with or without local irradiation.

OTHER PROGNOSTIC FACTORS

A variety of possible prognostic factors were evaluated. Each prognostic factor was examined separately (by row) using the multivariate regression techniques of Desu.[9] In this analysis, no specific prognostic factor was found to be crucial in adversely affecting recurrence-free survival in either group. We failed to show a difference in the recurrence-free survival between anatomic substage III$_1$ and III$_2$ of Dresser.[8] The extent of splenic involvement was not found to be an unfavorable prognostic feature in our study. However, it may have some significance as a prognostic factor in the liver treated group because patients who had S+ extensive disease had a 25% (3/12) recurrence rate whereas none of the 5 patients with S+ minimal disease recurred.

The effect of liver irradiation was examined for each prognostic factor and was found to produce a significant trend of improvement in recurrence free survival for most of the factors (Table 6).

TABLE 6.          RECURRENCE:   HODGKIN'S DISEASE STAGE IIIA

|  | Liver not treated | Liver treated | P value* |
|---|---|---|---|
| Number of patients | 16 |  | 17 |
| Age (in years): |  |  |  |
|   Less than 40 | 10/13 (77)** | 4/16 (25) | 0.007 |
|   40 or older | 2/3 (67) | 0/1 (0) | 0.500 |
| Gender: |  |  |  |
|   Male | 7/8 (88) | 4/13 (31) | 0.017 |
|   Female | 5/8 (63) | 0/4 (0) | 0.071 |
| Histopathology: |  |  |  |
|   Nodular sclerosis | 8/9 (89) | 2/11 (18) | 0.003 |
|   Mixed cellularity | 2/5 (40) | 2/6 (33) | 0.652 |
|   Lymphocyte predominant | 2/2 (100) | 0 (0) | - |
| Anatomic substage: |  |  |  |
|   IIIA1 | 9/13 (69) | 3/14 (21) | 0.035 |
|   IIIA2 | 3/3 (100) | 1/3 (33) | 0.020 |
| No. of primary sites: |  |  |  |
|   less than 5 | 6/9 (67) | 2/7 (29) | 0.157 |
|   5 or more | 6/7 (86) | 1/10 (10) | 0.134 |
| No. of sites below the diaphragm: |  |  |  |
|   Spleen only | 4/7 (57) | 1/5 (20) | 0.247 |
|   Spleen & hilar node | 5/6 (83) | 2/10 (20) | 0.024 |
|   more than 2 sites | 3/3 (100) | 1/2 (50) | 0.400 |
| Extent of splenic involvement: |  |  |  |
|   S+ extensive | 5/8 (63) | 4/12 (33) | 0.200 |
|   S+ minimal | 7/8 (86) | 0/5 (0) | 0.005 |
| Total | 12/16 (75) | 3/17 (18) | 0.004 |

* The P value is the result of Fisher's exact test comparing recurrence rates by whether or nor the patient received liver treatment.
** ( ) denotes percentage.

SITES OF RECURRENCE (TABLE 7)

The most common sites of initial recurrence in both groups were lymph nodes. In the untreated liver group, 4 patients definitely recurred in the abdominal cavity and 2 of these recurred in the liver. An additional 2 patients most likely recurred in the liver since they had abnormal liver function studies at the time of relapse but did not have biopsy proof. Six of the 10 patients who recurred in this group had evidence of intra-abdominal disease. The 2 patients who recurred in the retroperitoneal lymph nodes were thought to be in-field recurrences. The only liver treated recurrence in the abdomen was in a lymph node. All peripheral lymph node recurrences were thought to be marginal.

TABLE 7.   INITIAL SITES OF RECURRENCE:   HODGKIN'S DISEASE STAGE IIIA

|  | Liver not treated | | Liver treated | |
|---|---|---|---|---|
|  | A1 | A2 | A1 | A2 |
| Intra abd. LN (retroperitoneal) | 2 | 0 | 1 | 1 |
| Liver | 2 | 0 | 0 | 0 |
| Peripheral LN | 4* | 3 | 2 | 0 |
| Lung & Hilum | 2** | 1 | 0 | 0 |
| Pericardium | 1 | 0 | 0 | 0 |
| Bone Marrow | 1 | 0 | 0 | 0 |
| Bone | 0 | 0 | 1 | 0 |
| Abnormal Liver Function*** | 4 | 0 | 0 | 0 |

\* 2 patients recurred in peripheral lymph node and extranodal sites.
\** 1 patient had large mediastinal mass.
\***Liver function tests were abnormal in two patients with liver involvement and two patients with peripheral lymph node involvement.

We analyzed patients with and without liver irradiation to determine the effect of treatment on mediastinal masses. Of the Stage IIIA patients with liver untreated, 13 had a small mediastinal mass and 9 of them recurred. Three of the untreated group had a large mediastinal mass which was not treated with whole lung irradiation. All three recurred.

Of the 17 stage IIIA patients with liver treated, 15 had a small mediastinal mass and did not receive whole lung irradiation. Four of the 11 recurred. Two patients had a large mediastinal mass and received whole lung irradiation in addition to the liver irradiation. Neither patient recurred.

## SIGNIFICANT SIDE EFFECTS AND COMPLICATIONS

All patients were able to finish treatment without significant problems compared with patients who received inverted Y field with hepatic field. On serial blood counts, 17% of the patients experienced white counts of less than $2000/m^3$ and 33% had platelet counts of less than $100,000/mm^3$ at one point during treatment, which usually happened after 3000 rads or so to the field below the diaphragm. The counts eventually recovered to normal range.

Serial liver function studies were performed on most of the patients (14 patients available with adequate evaluable follow up values). Out of 14 patients, 50% (7/14) showed a mild elevation of alkaline phosphatase ( 300 IU/L), and 21% (3/14) developed marked elevation of alkaline phosphatase ( 300 IU/L). Of the two patients, one developed possible radiation hepatitis on biopsy with transient ascites. This problem had developed during the course of treatment and was resolved later without special treatment. Liver function usually returns to normal 3 to 18 months post treatment.

## DISCUSSION

Although curative radiotherapy has been the accepted treatment of choice for Stage I and IIA Hodgkin's disease for many years, the treatment of choice for other stages of Hodgkin's disease remains controversial. There are a number of reports regarding the use of curative irradiation in the treatment of surgically staged Stage IIIA Hodgkin's patients.[11-21] However, the recurrence free survival has generally not been considered satisfactory in these patients. The Stanford group reported a five-year disease free survival rate of 86%.[22] These results included patients who received low dose prophylactic irradiation of the liver if the spleen was involved, or the lung if the pulmonary hilum was involved. The British National Lymphoma Investigation reported similar results.[23] Other centers have shown less favorable results with a five year disease-free survival rate of 35% to 64% with total nodal irradiation, although the five year survivals are about the same as the Stanford results.[12,15,24] Our results are the first to our knowledge, to report concomitant lung and liver irradiation as the only treatment for Hodgkin's disease in patients with large mediastinal masses or hilar disease and splenic involvement, and to demonstrate the excellent results with this approach.

The combined modality approach using chemotherapy and radiotherapy has become the treatment of choice for Stage IIIA Hodgkin's disease patients. Five year disease-free survivals, from 75% to 85%, have been reported with five year overall survival averaging 90%.[19,21,25] When compared to our results of 82% recurrence-free survival and 90% overall survival, it is clear that there is no significant advantage to chemotherapy plus total nodal irradiation.[16,17] Also, the addition of chemotherapy to extensive radiotherapy unnecessarily increases risk of long term complications (such as acute myelogenous leukemia and other tumors) for the whole population of Stage IIIA patients instead of exposing a minority of the recurrent group of patients to the risk.[23,26-29]

We have noted that surgically staged Hodgkin's disease patients with large mediastinal masses have a statistically significant higher relapse rate and shorter overall survival rate than patients with small mediastinal masses or no mediastinal disease. Several recent studies are confirmatory.[30-38] A possible reason for this might be the underestimation of the extent of the disease. Radiation ports are designed to cover all the grossly apparent disease with adequate margins, however it is possible that one could underestimate pulmonary extension even with the use of lung tomography and/or computerized tomographic scan. This problem becomes even more difficult when there is extensive mediastinal disease since it is difficult to spare the lung tissue and still treat with an adequate margin. Thus, a proportion of the recurrences may have been due to inadequate coverage of the disease by the radiation field. To alleviate this recurrence problem, we have advocated prophylactic low dose whole lung irradiation, which has considerably reduced lung parenchymal and intrathoracic recurrences in our patients.

Palos, et al.[39] have also recommended irradiating the lung parenchyma during mantle field treatment for Hodgkin's disease patients with large mediastinal masses and/or hilar disease. They advocated the use of the thin lung block technique (TLBT). The TLBT gives 37% of the midline mediastinal dose, with total dose to the lung of 1650 rads in 20 fractions over 4 weeks. Symptomatic pulmonary radiation reaction (SPRR) has been reduced using the TLBT, and the incidence of SPRR is reported to be approximately the same in the regular mantle field group and the TLBT group (2.2% vs. 3.7%).

Early and late pulmonary complications following lung irradiation have been a major concern. It is well known that lung tissue is more sensitive to radiation than surrounding tissue and the sequelae of the treatment could be very serious. However, there are several reports indicating that lung tissue can tolerate low dose irradiation.[30,34,40,41] We have not seen serious acute or subacute pulmonary or cardiac complications after low dose lung irradiation although the follow up period should be longer for the study of late complications.

Chemotherapy has been used successfully for patients with advanced Hodgkin's disease and it has been suggested that patients with large mediastinal masses should be treated with combined modality therapy rather than with radiation therapy alone. Recent results from the Southwest Oncology Group showed that mediastinal involvement is not as well controlled with radiation plus chemotherapy (MOPP), although there was no advantage in survival.[42] Levi, et al.[32,36] also suggested a combination of chemotherapy and radiotherapy for large mediastinal masses and/or hilar disease in patients with Hodgkin's disease. His group reported an improved recurrence-free survival in patients treated with combined treatment compared to those treated with radiation alone. More recently, Mauch, et al.[37] suggested that a combination of radiotherapy and chemotherapy be used for patients who have a large mediastinal mass.

In 1975, the Stanford group recommended the use of liver radiation in Hodgkin's disease patients with involved spleens.[43,22] We adopted this program in the hope of improving recurrence-free survival in Stage IIIA spleen positive patients, by using curative radiotherapy and thus avoiding the risks associated with combined modality therapy. Our results are thus of major interest because of the excellent results using radiation treatment alone. None of the patients received chemotherapy in conjunction with the radiation therapy nor had they received chemotherapy prior to radiation. Our current results show an encouraging improvement in recurrence-free survival in laparotomy staged Stage IIIA Hodgkin's disease patients. Our results support the findings of the Stanford group in that they show improvement of recurrence free survival with hepatic irradiation in S+ Hodgkin's disease stage IIIA.[18]

There are several recent reports which discuss prognostic factors in stage IIIA Hodgkin's disease.[8,14,15,21,22] Dresser, et al.[8] noted the need for substaging of Stage IIIA Hodgkin's disease because of the difference in prognosis, depending on the extent of intra-abdominal disease. He suggested that anatomic substage $IIIA_1$ patients should have only radiotherapy as their primary treatment. The addition of combination chemotherapy was recommended for anatomic substage $IIIA_2$ patients. This suggestion was supported by the results of a retrospective four institution collaborative study.[15] These results, however, have been challenged by others.[14,22] In our study, we were not able to show significant differences in recurrence free survival between $IIIA_1$ and $IIIA_2$ patients treated with TNI without hepatic irradiation. Moreover, patients treated with TNI plus hepatic irradiation had excellent long term results in both $IIIA_1$ and $IIIA_2$, so that we cannot

36

justify chemotherapy in either subgroup although the number of patients in
category $IIIA_2$ is too small to make a definitive statement.

Hoppe, et al.[22] found the extent of splenic disease to be an important
prognostic factor. In our series, the extent of splenic disease was not an
important prognostic factor, although there is some suggestion that it might
be a prognostic factor in the liver treated group. However, the numbers are
still too small to demonstrate this.

We have not noted a serious increase in the complication rate in this
series of liver irradiated patients as compared to our previous group of
patients treated in the usual manner.

In view of the fact that combination chemotherapy and chemotherapy alone do
not demonstrate improved results compared to radically irradiated patients and
in view of the lesser morbidity and possibility of carcinogenesis, we
recommend radical radiation therapy as the treatment of choice for IA, IIA,
and $IIIA_{S+}$ patients whether they have hilar disease or large mediastinal
masses. Commitment to this approach requires meticulous treatment planning,
observation, and care of these patients. The rewards are very much worth the
effort.

REFERENCES
1.  Carbone, P.P., Kaplan, H.S., Musshoff, K., et al. Report of the committee on Hodgkin's disease staging classification. Cancer Res 31:1860-1861, 1971.
2.  Lee, C.K.K., Bloomfield, C.D., Levitt, S.H. Results of lung irradiation for Hodgkin's disease patients with large mediastinal masses and/or hilar disease. Cancer Treat Rep 66:819-825, 1982.
3.  Lee, C.K.K., Bloomfield, C.D., Goldman, A.I., et al. Prognostic significance of mediastinal involvement in Hodgkin's disease treated with curative radiotherapy. Cancer 46:2403-2409, 1980.
4.  Lee, C.K.K., Bloomfield, C.D., Goldman, A.I., et al. The therapeutic utility of lung irradiation for Hodgkin's disease patients with large mediastinal masses. Int J Radiat Oncol Biol Phys, 7:151-154, 1981.
5.  Lee, C.K.K., Bloomfield, C.D., Nesbit, M.E., et al. Int J Radiat Oncol Biol Phys, 5:136-137, 1979.
6.  Kaplan, E.L., Meier, P. (1958) J Am Stat Assoc, 53:457-481, 1958.
7.  Breslow, N. Generalized Kruskal-Wallis test for comparing K samples subject to unequal patterns of censorship. Biometrika, 57:579-594, 1970.
8.  Dresser, R.K., Golomb, H.M., Ultmann, J.E., et al. Prognostic classification of Hodgkin's disease in pathologic Stage III, based on anatomic considerations. Blood, 49:883-893, 1977.
9.  Lee, E., Desu, M. A computer program for comparing K samples with right-censored data. Computer Programs in Biomedicine, 2:315-321, 1972.
10. Lindgren, B.W. in Statistical Theory, MacMillan, New York, pp. 440-441, 1976.

11. Hellman, S., Mauch, P., Goodman, R.L., et al. The place of radiation therapy in the treatment of Hodgkin's disease. Cancer, 42:971-978, 1978.
12. Mauch, P., Goodman, R., Rosenthal, D.S., et al. An evaluation of total nodal irradiation as treatment for Stage IIIA Hodgkin's disease. Cancer, 43:1255-1261, 1979.
13. Glatstein, E. Radiotherapy in Hodgkin's disease: past achievements and future progress. Cancer, 39:837-842, 1977.
14. Rodgers, R.W., Fuller, L.M. et al. Reassessment of prognostic factors in stage IIIA and IIIB Hodgkin's disease treated with MOPP and radiotherapy. Cancer, 47:2196-2203, 1981.
15. Stein, R.S., Golomb, H.M., et al. Anatomic substages of Stage IIIA Hodgkin's disease. Ann Intern Med, 92:159-175, 1980.
16. Rosenberg, S.A., Kaplan, H.S., Glatstein, E.J., et al. Combined modality therapy of Hodgkin's disease. Cancer (Suppl), 42:991-1000, 1978.
17. British National Lymphoma Investigation. Initial treatment of Stage IIIA Hodgkin's disease, comparison of radiotherapy with combined chemotherapy. Lancet, 2:991-995, 1976.
18. Rosenberg, S.A., Kaplan, H.S. The Management of Stages I, II and III Hodgkin's disease with combined radiotherapy and chemotherapy. Cancer 35:55-63, 1975.
19. Rosenberg, S.A. The management of Hodgkin's disease. N Engl J Med, 299:1246-1247, 1978.
20. Aienberg, A.C. Current concepts in cancer, the staging and treatment of Hodgkin's disease. New Engl J Med 299:1228-1232, 1978.
21. Neely, S.N., Golomb, H.M. Treatment of Stage IIIA Hodgkin's disease. Cancer Treat Rep, 66:827-834, 1982.
22. Hoppe, R.T., Rosenberg, S.A., Kaplan, H.S., et al. Prognostic factors in pathological stage IIIA Hodgkin's disease. Cancer, 46:1240-1246, 1980.
23. Krikerian, J.C., Burke, J.S., et al. Occurrence of non-Hodgkin's lymphoma after therapy for Hodgkin's disease. N Engl J Med, 300:452-458, 1979.
24. Prosnitz, L.R., Montalvo, R.I., Rischer, D.B., et al. Treatment of stage IIIA Hodgkin's disease is radiotherapy alone adequate. Int J Radiat Oncol Biol Phys, 4:4781-4787, 1978.
25. Farber, L.R., Prosnitz, L.R., Cadman, D.C., et al. Curative potential of combined modality therapy for advanced Hodgkin's disease. Cancer 46:1509-1517, 1980.
26. Coltman, C.A., Dixon, D.O. Second malignancies complicating Hodgkin's disease: a southwest oncology group 10-year followup. Cancer Treat Rep, 66:1023-1033, 1982.
27. Cadman, E.C., Capizzi, R.I., Bertino, J.R. Acute nonlymphocytic leukemia, a delay complication of Hodgkin's disease therapy: analysis of 109 cases. Cancer, 40:1280-1296, 1977.
28. Coleman, C.N., Williams, C.H., Flint, A., et al. Hematologic neoplasia in patients treated for Hodgkin's disease. N Engl J Med, 297:1249-1252, 1977.
29. Brody, R.S., Schottenfeld, D. Multiple primary cancers in Hodgkin's disease. Semin Oncol, 7:187-201, 1980.
30. Fuller, L.M., Jing, B.S., Shullenberger, C.C., et al. Radiotherapeutic management of localized Hodgkin's disease involving the mediastinum. Br J Radiol, 40:913-925, 1967.
31. Fuller, L.M., Madoc-Jones, H., Gamble, J.F., et al. New Assessment of the prognostic significance of histopathology in Hodgkin's disease for laparotomy-negative stage I and stage II patients. Cancer, 39:2174-2182, 1977.

32. Levi, J.A., Wiernik, P.H., O'Connell, M.J. Patterns of relapse in stages I, II, and IIIA Hodgkin's disease: influence of initial therapy and implicatins for the future. Int J Radiat Oncol Biol Phys, 2:853-862, 1977.

33. Lee, C.K.K., Bloomfield, C.D., Levitt, S.H. Prophylactic whole lung irradiation for extensive mediastinal Hodgkin's disease: meeting. Proc Am Assoc Cancer Res and ASCO, 20:441, 1979.

34. Carmel, R.J., Kaplan, H.S. Mantle irradiation in Hodgkin's disease, an analysis of technique, tumor eradication and complications. Cancer, 37:2813-2825, 1976.

35. Hoppe, R.T., Coleman, C.N., Kaplan H.S., et al. Hodgkin's disease, pathologic stage I-II, the prognostic importance of initial sites of disease and extent of mediastinal involvement. Proc Am Assoc Cancer Res and ASCO, 21:471, 1980.

36. Levi, J.A., Wiernik, P.H. Limited extranodal Hodgkin's disease, unfavorable prognosis and therapeutic implications. Am J Med, 63:365-372, 1977.

37. Mauch, P., Goodman, R., Hellman, S. The significance of mediastinal involvement in early stage Hodgkin's disease. Cancer, 42:1039-1045, 1978.

38. Thar, T.L., Million, R.R., Hausner, R.J., et al. Hodgkin's disease, stages I and II relationship of recurrence to size of disease, radiation dose and number of sites involved. Cancer, 43:1101-1105, 1979.

39. Palos, B., Kaplan, H.S., Karzmark, C.J. The useof thin lung shields to deliver limited whole-lung irradiation during mantle field treatment of Hodgkin's disease. Radiology, 101:441-442, 1971.

40. Newton, K.A., Spittle, M.F. An analysis of 40 cases treated by total thoracic irradiation. Clin Radiol, 20:19-22, 1969.

41. Gross, N.J. Pulmonary effects of radiation therapy. Ann Intern Med, 86:81-92, 1977.

42. Coltman, C.A., Fuller, L.M. Patterns of relapse in localized (stage I and II) Hodgkin's disease following extended field radiotherapy vs. involved field radiotherapy plus MOPP. Blood (Suppl), 50:188, 1977.

43. Schultz, H.P., Glatstein, E., Kaplan, H.S. Management of presumptive or proven Hodgkin's disease of the liver: a new radiotherapy technique. Int J Radiat Oncol Biol Phys, 1:1-8, 1975.

CHEMOTHERAPEUTIC APPROACH TO NON-HODGKIN'S LYMPHOMAS

STEVEN G. ROSHON, M.D. AND KENNETH S. ZUCKERMAN, M.D.

INTRODUCTION

The purpose of this chapter is to provide an overview of the classification, natural history, and chemotherapeutic management of non-Hodgkin's lymphomas (NHL). Also we will discuss experimental approaches to the treatment of this varied group of malignancies.*

There are three to six new cases of NHL per 100,000 people every year in the United States. This represents 2% of all cancers.[1] NHL is more common in males than females, with a ratio of 1.5 to 1. The incidence increases with advancing age to a least 70 years of age.[1] The unfavorable, or high grade lymphomas tend to occur predominantly in patients less than 35 and over 60 years old, whereas the low grade lymphomas tend to occur most frequently in patients between 35 and 60 years old.[1,2]

Several host and environmental factors have been associated with excessive risk for NHL. Familial aggregations of cases of NHL have been identified, but this is rare. Patients with primary immunodeficiency have been reported to have an increased incidence of NHL. Renal transplant recipients have been shown to have an increased incidence of NHL, with the incidence of intermediate and high grade central nervous system lymphomas being particularly notable.[1] A variety of acquired diseases with known immune consequences also have been associated with an excessive incidence of NHL. These include rheumatoid arthritis, systemic lupus erythematosus, Sjogren's syndrome, sarcoidosis, celiac disease and dermatitis herpetiformis. Ionizing radiation has been associated with a small increased risk of NHL in patients irradiated for ankylosing spondylitis and in Japanese survivors of the atomic bomb receiving greater than 100 rads. Evidence of Epstein-Barr virus infection is highly associated with African Burkitt's lymphoma, but has not been demonstrated convincingly to be associated with American Burkitt's lymphoma.[1]

---

*A glossary of abreviations used in the tables and text appears in the Appendix.

Published 1983 by Elsevier Science Publishing Co., Inc.
Recent Trends in Radiation Oncology and Related Fields, Amendola and Amendola, Editors

Recently, some patients with T cell lymphoblastic lymphomas have been shown to have antibodies directed against a type C retrovirus. Furthermore, the malignant lymphoblasts from these patients have been shown to contain genomic material from the same virus. This virus, termed human T cell leukemia/ lymphoma virus (HTLV), appears to have an etiologic role in certain patients with T cell malignancies.[3,4]

Chromosomal rearrangements have been detected in at least half of NHL patients. The most consistent abnormality is an 8:14 translocation occurring in Burkitt's lymphoma.[1] Recently an oncogene has been identified as being translocated and activated near the Burkitt's lymphoma 8:14 translocation site[5]. However, the pathophysiologic role of this and other chromosome abnormalities in lymphomas is not clear at the present time.

CLASSIFICATION

Many schemes for the classification of non-Hodgkin's lymphomas have been devised, yet each has limitations. A useful classification should provide understandable and logical nomenclature, scientific accuracy and reproducibility, and clinical relevance with regard to treatment and prognosis.[3] Most modern clinical series are based on the system originally proposed by Rappaport in 1956 and modified several times since. The Rappaport classification is based upon nodal architecture as well as cellular morphology. Clinical experience has demonstrated that prognosis is related to the presence of a nodular (follicular) architecture or a diffuse effacement of the lymph node with the neoplastic lymphoid cells.[2,5,7] The morphology of the malignant cells also plays an important role in determining prognosis, especially in diffuse lymphomas. New concepts about lymphoid neoplasms, including immunologic characteristics and morphologic refinements, have been applied to the plethora of classifications in order to separate types of lymphomas based on prognosis.

The National Cancer Institute recently sponsored an international multi-institutional study of classifications which resulted in a new working formulation for clinical usage.[8] In this study the clinical and pathologic material from 1175 patients was evaluated. The reproducibility and usefulness of the six most widely used classification systems was examined by a panel of prominent pathologists. Although each classification was valuable and comparable in terms of reproducibility and clinical correlation, the working formulation was prefered as a "means of translation among systems."

The working formulation distinguishes three broad prognostic categories

TABLE 1.

| INTERNATIONAL CLASSIFICATION | RAPPAPORT CLASSIFICATION |
|---|---|

### Low Grade

| | |
|---|---|
| Small lymphocytic or plasmacytoid | Diffuse, well differentiated lymphocytic lymphoma (DWDLL) |
| Follicular, Predominantly small cleaved cell ( ± diffuse areas; ± sclerosis) | Nodular, poorly differentiated lymphocytic lymphoma (NPDLL) |
| Follicular, mixed, small cleaved and large cell ( ± diffuse areas; ± sclerosis) | Nodular, mixed lymphocytic and histiocytic lymphomas (NML) |

### Intermediate Grade

| | |
|---|---|
| Follicular, predominantly large cell ( ± diffuse areas; ± sclerosis) | Nodular, histiocytic lymphoma (NHL) |
| Diffuse, small cleaved cell ( ± sclerosis) | Diffuse, poorly differentiated lymphocytic lymphoma (DPDLL) |
| Diffuse, mixed small and large cell ( ± sclerosis; ± epithelioid cells) | Diffuse, mixed lymphocytic and histiocytic lymphoma (DML) |
| Diffuse, large cleaved or non-cleaved cell ( ± sclerosis) | Diffuse histiocytic lymphoma (DHL) |

### High Grade

| | |
|---|---|
| Diffuse, large cell, immunoblastic ( ± plasmacytoid, clear cell, polymorphous, and/or epithelioid cell components) | Diffuse, histiocytic lymphoma (DHL) |
| Diffuse, lymphoblastic (convoluted or non-convoluted cell; usually T cells) | Diffuse, lymphoblastic lymphoma (DLL) |
| Diffuse, small non-cleaved cell (Burkitt's; vacuolated cytoplasm; occasionally follicular areas) | Diffuse, undifferentiated lymphoma (Burkitt's and non-Burkitt's types) (DUL) |

### Miscellaneous Non-Hodgkin's Lymphoproliferative Disorders

Composite Lymphoma
Mycosis Fungoides
Sezary Lymphoma/Leukemia
True Histiocytic Lymphoma (Histiocytic Medullary Reticulosis)
Hairy Cell Leukemia
Waldenstrom's Macroglobulinemia
Chronic Lymphocytic Leukemia

based on the patient survival curves that were generated based on histologic type of lymphoma. This "International Formulation" is described and compared with the Rappaport classificaton in Table 1. Low grade tumors have a favorable prognosis and are subdivided into the following sub-types: malignant lymphomas (ML), small lymphocytic; ML, follicular, predominantly small cleaved cell; and ML, follicular, mixed small and large cell. Median survival in these three groups was 5.8, 7.2, and 5.1 years respectively.

The intermediate grade lymphomas include lymphomas generally thought to be unfavorable in prognosis, with median survival in the range of 1.5 to 3.5 years. These four types are termed: ML, follicular, predominantly large cell; ML, diffuse, small cleaved cell; ML, diffuse, mixed small and large cell; and ML, diffuse, large cell. Median survival in these patients was 3.0, 3.4, 2.7, and 1.5 years respectively.

Finally, the high grade lymphomas in this classification represent tumors with particularly unfavorable prognoses. These are described as follows: ML, large cell, immunoblastic; ML, diffuse, lymphoblastic; and ML, diffuse small non-cleaved (Burkitt's and non-Burkitt's types). The survival in this group of patients was 1.3, 2.0, and 0.7 years.

A miscellaneous group of non-Hodgkin's lymphoproliferative disorders include composite lymphomas, mycosis fungoides, Sezary syndrome, histiocytic medullary reticulosis, perhaps some cases of Waldenstrom's macroglobulinemia and chronic lymphocytic leukemia. Each of these represents a distinct clinical entity which will not be discussed in further detail here.

As one might expect, the proposed working formulation also has been the target of several criticisms.[8] These include lack of immunologic characterization, failure to recognize the origin of the malignant cell and the cumbersome terminology. New advances in lymphoma biology, immunology and therapy undoubtedly will make this system, or at least its terminology, relatively obsolete within the next few years. However, in the interim, it provides a useful common language for comparison among studies by different investigators. Most clinical series reported up to this time have used the Rappaport classification. Thus, for this discussion the Rappaport terminology and, to a certain extent, the three major categories from the working classification (low grade, intermediate grade and high grade) will be used.

CLINICAL CHARACTERISTICS

The diagnosis of non-Hodgkin's lymphoma should be suspected in patients with painless enlargement of lymph nodes which are rubbery, firm, and moveable. Most patients have palpably enlarged nodes in several node bearing regions at the time of initial presentation. Paradoxically, low grade NHL have disease confined to a single nodal area less than 10% of the time, whereas the higher grade tumors may present with limited disease 20%-40% of the time. The pattern of spread in NHL is to non-contiguous sites in 30%-40% of cases which contrasts with non-contiguous spread in only 2% to 5% of Hodgkin's disease patients.

Patients who present with primary extranodal disease generally have diffuse high grade lymphomas. In patients with NPDLL under the Rappaport classification there is a 50% to 70% incidence of bone marrow involvement and a 30% to 50% incidence of hepatic involvement at the time of initial presentation of their disease. Marrow involvement in the intermediate and high grade lymphomas ranges from 15% to 50%, depending on the particular type of lymphoma. For example, there is a very high incidence of bone marrow involvement in patients with diffuse lymphoblastic and diffuse undifferentiated lymphomas, but a relatively low incidence of marrow involvement in patients with diffuse large cell (histiocytic) lymphomas. Patients who present initially with primary extranodal NHL generally have high grade or, less commonly, intermediate grade lymphomas. Two common sites of primary extranodal lymphoma are the central nervous system (CNS) and the gastrointestinal tract. The incidence of gastrointestinal lymphoma is 10% to 20% of all diffuse intermediate and high grade lymphomas, and these patients have a poor prognosis. Primary CNS lymphomas present as intracranial masses or spinal cord tumors, tend to be diffuse high grade histology, and are the most common secondary tumor in renal transplant recipients. Risk factors for secondary CNS lymphoma include diffuse histology, especially with large cell, undifferentiated or T-lymphoblastic lymphoma, and intermediate or high grade lymphomas with bone marrow involvement.[1,2,7,8]

DIAGNOSTIC EVALUATION

The Ann Arbor staging classification developed for and used in the assessment of Hodgkin's disease has been applied to non-Hodgkin's lymphomas. The usefulness of this staging system in evaluating patients with non-Hodgkin's lymphomas is severely limited because of the early dissemination of NHL and the lack of contiguous spread of disease. However, a "staging" evaluation remains useful as a means of determining all the major sites of disease involvement in a given patient. Staging evaluation includes a search for extranodal disease. The most common sites of extranodal lymphoma, in approximately descending order of incidence, include the bone marrow, liver, gastrointestinal tract, lungs, skin, extradural space and CNS, orbit, paranasal sinuses, bone, testes, and thyroid.    Bone marrow involvement usually is accompanied by a normal peripheral blood picture and is diagnosed more often by unilateral or bilateral iliac crest biopsies than by marrow aspiration alone.    Intra-abdominal nodal disease is evaluated by physical examination (useful only for massive lymphadenopathy), lymphangiography and CT scanning.    Ultrasound examination and [67]Gallium citrate scanning have been employed but are less useful.    Splenic involvement is more common in the presence of splenomegaly and bone marrow involvement.    Liver involvement most often occurs in patients who have splenic involvement.    Staging laparotomy in patients who clinically have Stage I or II disease will demonstrate occult abdominal disease in 10%-30% of patients.[9,10,11]    Thus, if there is a role for "staging" laparotomy in non-Hodgkin's lymphoma, it would be primarily to rule out disseminated lymphoma in patients in whom local aggressive radiation therapy with curative intent is contemplated.

PROGNOSTIC FEATURES

Prognosis in non-Hodgkin's lymphoma is related to a variety of factors. Histologic grade and stage of disease have been discussed.    Extranodal disease in intermediate and high grade lymphomas is also a poor prognostic sign. Systemic "B" symptoms usually reflect bulky disease and parenchymal organ involvement and are associated with a worse prognosis.    Bulky disease with a predominant mass greater than 7 to 10 cm in its greatest diameter is also a poor prognostic sign.[2,7,8]    Finally, patients who fail to respond or relapse following initial chemotherapy are unlikely to respond to further curative attempts at therapy, although transient responses to a variety of therapeutic regimens are common.

RADIATION THERAPY

The role of radiotherapy in the treatment of NHL will not be discussed in detail in this chapter.    To summarize, involved field (regional) radiotherapy is curative in 30% to 60% of pathologic Stage I and II lymphomas.    Localized radiation therapy may be a useful palliative measure in some patients with advanced disease, large masses or upper airway obstruction.    Total lymphoid irradiation may be useful in selected patients without extranodal involvement. Total body irradiation (TBI) used in advanced stages may result in long term remission, however, this treatment is rarely if ever curative.[12,13,14]

The combination of radiotherapy and chemotherapy needs further exploration and may find usefulness in selected patients, particularly those without known extranodal disease, and those with very large masses.[15]

THERAPY OF LOW GRADE LYMPHOMAS

The management of low grade lymphomas is influenced by their tendency to be widespread at presentation. Despite their advanced stages, the median survival of these patients is quite long. This group of diseases includes small lymphocytic - (WDLL by Rappaport), follicular predominantly small cleaved cell (NPDLL) and follicular, mixed small cleaved and large cell (nodular mixed lymphocytic and histiocytic; NMLH).[8] The rare patient in these groups who presents with stage I and II disease may experience prolonged disease free survival following involved field radiation therapy.[12,13] A recent trial from M.D. Anderson Hospital[16] evaluated Stage II low grade lymphomas treated with cyclophosphamide, adriamycin, vincristine, prednisone, and bleomycin (CHOP-Bleo) sandwiched between total nodal irradiation. Although this regimen was well tolerated and provided a 5 year survival of 87%, there appear to be relapses continuing to occur at least until 48 months. Continuing late relapse has been the major problem associated with aggresive therapy for this group of lymphomas with the possible exception of the nodular mixed lymphocytic and histiocytic type.

Single agent chlorambucil versus combination therapy (cyclophosphamide, vincristine and prednisone; COP) versus whole body irradiation (WBI) has been evaluated prospectively by the Stanford group.[17] Their findings are that each modality has a similar response rate, similar disease free survival and a similar overall survival. Early toxicity was greatest with COP. WBI provided the quickest response. Given the indolent nature of this group of diseases, Portlock and Rosenberg evaluated whether delaying therapy in relatively asymptomatic patients would alter their outcome.[18] They analyzed and compared 44 patients whose initial therapy was deferred with 112 patients treated at Stanford in the randomized prospective trial mentioned above. Initial therapy was withheld until these patients developed bulky lymphade- nopathy (18 patients), progressive extranodal disease (3 patients), hyper- calcemia (1 patient), early epidural compression (1 patient) and at the patients' request (2 patients). They found that the median time to initiation of therapy was 8+ years for WDLL, 32 months in NPDLL and 9.3 months in NMLH. Furthermore, delayed therapy was as effective in palliation as early therapy; and actuarial survival for both populations was identical. On retrospecive evaluation of their 112 protocol patients, they found that 60% would have been candidates for delayed therapy.

TABLE 2.

SINGLE CHEMOTHERAPEUTIC AGENTS WITH ACTIVITY IN THE TREATMENT OF LYMPHOMAS

| Drug | % Complete or Partial Remissions | |
|---|---|---|
| | "Lymphocytic" | "Histiocytic" |
| Prednisone | 60 - 80 | 20 - 30 |
| Mechlorethamine | 50 - 70 | 30 - 50 |
| Cyclophosphamide | 50 - 70 | 50 - 70 |
| Chlorambucil | 40 - 60 | 20 - 40 |
| Procarbazine | 40 - 50 | 20 - 40 |
| Vinblastine | 15 - 25 | 20 - 35 |
| Vincristine | 40 - 65 | 40 - 80 |
| VP-16-213 | 25 - 30 | 10 - 20 |
| VM-26 | 40 - 60 | 20 - 35 |
| Adriamycin | 35 - 50 | 50 - 65 |
| Bleomycin | 30 - 60 | 30 - 60 |
| BCNU, CCNU, methyl-CCNU | 20 - 30 | 20 - 35 |
| Streptozoticin | 20 - 30 | 10 - 15 |
| Imadazole Carboxamide (DTIC) | 20 - 25 | 10 - 15 |
| Methotrexate (standard dose) | 15 - 25 | 15 - 25 |
| Methotrexate (high dose and rescue) | 30 - 60 | 20 - 50 |
| Cytosine Arabinoside | 20 - 25 | 15 - 20 |
| L-Asparaginase | 20 - 30 | 15 - 30 |
| Cis-Platinum | 15 - 30 | 15 - 30 |
| Methylglyoxal-bis(guanylhydrazone) (MGBG) | 30 - 50 | 20 - 40 |

Tables 2 and 3 enumerate the multiple agents and regimens available to treat the indolent lymphomas.[7] Delayed therapy is often possible, but at the expense of the necessary close follow-up, the psychological trauma of untreated neoplastic disease and the possiblity of a complication developing.[19]

TABLE 3.     COMBINATION CHEMOTHERAPY REGIMENS FOR PRIMARY THERAPY OF LOW GRADE LYMPHOMAS (Stages III and IV)

| Drug Regimen | % Complete Remissions | Median Duration of Remission (months) | Median Duration of Survival (months) |
|---|---|---|---|
| Single Alkylating Agent | 40 - 60% | 24 - 36 | 48 - 96+ |
| COP | 50 - 80% | 24 - 36 | 48 - 96+ |
| COPP | 50 - 80% | 18 - 90+ | 48 - 100+ |
| ACOP | 60 - 70% | ? | ? |
| BACOP | 80 - 90% | ? | ? |

Nontheless, for the vast majority of patients with low grade NHL, the benefits of delaying therapy for as long as possible outweigh these potential problems; the risks and complications of early therapy outweigh the risks of delaying therapy. It is hoped that new developments will provide curative rather than palliative results.

THERAPY OF INTERMEDIATE AND HIGH GRADE LYMPHOMAS

The intermediate and high grade lymphomas include follicular predominantly large cell, diffuse small cleaved cell, diffuse mixed small and large cell, diffuse large cleaved or non-cleaved, diffuse large cell immunoblastic, diffuse lymphoblastic and diffuse small non-cleaved cell. The corresponding Rappaport classes are listed in Table 1. Perhaps the greatest advances in the therapy of NHL have been made in this group of diseases, as aggressive therapy has been shown to lead to prolonged disease free survival and relatively high cure rates.

Stage I and II aggressive lymphomas are more radioresistant than indolent lymphomas and require higher amounts of irradiation to effect cures.[2] Aggressive lymphomas presenting with limited disease also have been success-fully treated with systemic chemotherapy.[20] As opposed to the low grade lymphomas, single agent therapy and whole body irradiation generally are ineffective in achieving long term survival in patients with intermediate and high grade lymphomas. COP therapy results in a 20% to 40% remission rate, but relapse free survival is short.[21] COP plus procarbazine therapy results in a portion of patients with prolonged disease-free survival; in these cases, relapse is rarely seen after two years.[2] The addition of doxorubicin to chemotherapy regimens has been associated with higher complete response rates (50%) and a higher rate of long term disease-free survival, which generally corresponds to cure (about 40%).[22] The success of these treatment regimens depends on such pretreatment factors as limited versus disseminated disease, presence of "B" symptoms, performance status, bulk of lymphoma, and extranodal sites of involvement. The addition of high dose methotrexate to regimens utilizing an alkylating agent and an anthracycline appears to have enhanced efficacy, although this has never been tested in a prospective randomized trial.[2] A compilation of regimens used in high grade lymphomas is given in Table 4.

Although aggressive therapy holds promise for prolonged disease free survival in 40% to 50% of patients with intermediate and high grade lymphomas, the prognosis of the other 50% to 60% of patients has been poor. Salvage

TABLE 4.    COMBINATION CHEMOTHERAPY REGIMENS FOR PRIMARY THERAPY
            OF HIGH GRADE LYMPHOMAS (Stages II to IV)

| Drug Regimen | % Complete Remissions | % Disease-Free Survival at 2 Years |
|---|---|---|
| CP | 15 - 25% | 15 - 20% |
| COP | 20 - 40% | 15 - 20% |
| COPP | 20 - 40% | 15 - 30% |
| BCOP | 50 - 60% | 40 - 50% |
| ACOP | 40 - 70% | 30 - 50% |
| BACOP | 50 - 70% | 40 - 50% |
| M-BACOD | 85% | 75% |
| COMA/COMLA | 50 - 80% | 50 - 60% |
| ProMACE-MOPP | 74% | 56% |
| COP-BLAM | 73% | 55% |
| AOP/C Ara-C | 90% | 73% |
| CHOP, HOAP-Bleo IMVP-16 | 82% | 60% |

regimens given to heavily pretreated patients have a 20% to 60% response rate
but responses generally are not long lasting (Table 5).  One recently
developed concept to improve upon these results involves the use of sequential
multiple non-cross-resistant agents.[1,2]  This approach has theoretic appeal
based on the Goldie hypothesis[23] that the sequential use of multiple agents
with different mechanisms of action will not allow resistant clones of malignant cells to emerge.  The early success of the MOPP alternating with ABVD
regimen of Bonnadona in Hodgkin's disease is one example.  Similar approaches
include COP alternating with ABP proposed by Bonnadona.  Fisher et al. at the
NCI have published early results of ProMACE followed by MOPP therapy.[24]
Median survival is expected to exceed 4 years, and as many as 65% of patients
are projected to have at least a four year disease-free survival.[25]
Cabanillas, et al. from M.D. Anderson have experienced encouraging results
using sequential CHOP, HOAP-Bleo and IMVP-16.[26]  This regimen also includes

TABLE 5.    "SALVAGE" THERAPY FOR RELAPSED OR THERAPY RESISTANT LYMPHOMAS

| Drug Regimen | % Response |
|---|---|
| IMVP-16 | 37 - 62 |
| B-V-Pl | 30 - 50 |
| PL-VF16-MGBG | 40 - 60 |
| MGBG-DFMO | ? |
| Continuous infusion Vincristine | 20 - 40 |
| New Antracyclines | 10 - 20 |

late intensification chemotherapy in patients achieving a complete remission. The Southwest Oncology Group is evaluating the usefulness of CHOP alternating with CVB.

At the University of Michigan, we have treated patients with intermediate and high grade lymphomas with a regimen employing a very high dose of adriamycin (120 mg/m$^2$ every three weeks for three courses) in combination with Vincristine and Prednisone. This is followed by three courses of cyclophosphamide and high dose (3 gm/m$^2$) Ara-C. Our early results are encouraging, with an overall 90% remission rate and a 73% disease free survival at 2 years, and a 100% remission rate and 87% disease free survival at 2 years in patients with diffuse large cell ("histiocytic") lymphoma.

Other advances in the therapy of NHL of the aggressive type involve therapy directed at specific sub-types of lymphomas. For instance, the most successful therapy of diffuse, small non-cleaved cell (Burkitt-like) lymphoma has been reported using CHOP with high dose methotrexate and CNS prophylaxis.[27,28] Diffuse lymphoblastic (convoluted cell) lymphoma is usually a T-cell disorder and is most common in childhood or young adulthood. It has been reported that these tumors are best treated with regimens similar to those used for treatment of childhood acute lymphoblastic leukemia, including aggressive chemotherapy CNS prophylaxis. Mycosis fungoides and Sezary syndrome are T-cell neoplasms which have been reported to respond to the relatively T-cell specific agent 2-deoxycoformycin.[29]

## NEW APPROACHES TO THERAPY

It is apparent that further advances in the therapy of both indolent and aggressive lymphomas are needed. Several innovative approaches based on new technology already are undergoing limited clinical trials. Patients with syngeneic and HLA identical allogenic siblings have been treated successfully with high dose chemotherapy and radiation followed by bone marrow transplantation. Treatment with high dose radiation and chemotherapy followed by transplantation of frozen stored autologous bone marrow also is being explored. The development of specific monoclonal antibodies may allow normal marrow to be separated from malignant cells in vitro, allowing subsequent high dose therapy of rescue with the autologous marrow depleted of any residual malignant cells. Miller et al. from Stanford have developed an in vivo monoclonal antibody therapy for low grade lymphomas.[30] Their technique uses the patients' B-cell lymphoma tissue which is known to express monoclonal surface immunoglobin. This surface immunoglobin has a unique variable region termed an idiotype. Lymphoma cells are fused with myeloma cells which then secrete the specific surface immunoglobin. The immunoglobin is harvested and used to immunize mice. Then anti-idiotpye antibodies are mass produced by hybridoma techniques. Miller et al. have reported on one patient with NPDLL who has responded to treatment with monoclonal anti-idiotype antibody.

CONCLUSIONS

NHL represents a heterogeneous group of diseases. Advances in the understanding of the histology, biology and analysis of the clinical course of these disorders has allowed increasingly sophisticated classification schemas. Prognosis and therapy can be planned based on classification, stage and the other prognostic features. Therapy of advanced low grade lymphomas generally has been based on palliation. Curability is an unrealized potential in the low grade lymphomas. A progressively increasing proportion of patients with intermediate and high grade lymphomas are being cured as a result of advances in chemotherapy. New approaches involving such technologies as bone marrow transplantation and specific anti-lymphoma cell monoclonal antibodies also hold promise for further advancement in the management of non-Hodgkin's lymphomas in the next few years.

APPENDIX

| | |
|---|---|
| CP: | Cyclophosphamide, Prednisone |
| COP: | Cyclophosphamide, Vincristine (Oncovin), Prednisone |
| COPP: | Cyclophosphamide, Vincristine, Procarbazine, Prednisone |
| BCOP: | Bleomycin, Cyclophosphamide, Vincristine, Prednisone |
| ACOP: | Adriamycin/Daunamycin, Cyclophosphamide, Vincristine, Prednisone |
| BACOP: | Bleomycin, Adriamycin/Daunamycin, Cyclophosphamide, Vincristine, Prednisone |
| M-BACOD: | High dose Methotrexate, Bleomycin, Adriamycin, Cyclophosphamide, Vincristine, Dexamethasone |
| IMVP-16: | Ifosfamide, Methotrexate, and VP-16 |
| COMA/COMLA: | Cyclophosphamide, Vincristine, moderate dose Methotrexate, Leucovorin rescue, Ara-C |
| ProMACE-MOPP: | Prednisone, moderate dose Methotrexate, Adriamycin, Cyclophosphamide, VP-16; consolidations with Nitrogen Mustard, Vincristine, Procarbazine, Prednisone |
| CHOP, HOAP-Bleo, IMVP-16: | Cyclophosphamide, Adriamycin, Vincristine, Prednisone, if PR, then Adriamycin, Vincristine, Cytarabine, Prednisone, Bleomycin, intensify with Ifosfamide, Methotrexate, VP-16. |
| COP-BLAM: | Cyclophosphamide, Vincristine, Prednisone, Bleomycin, Adriamycin, Procarbazine (Matulane). |
| AOP-C Ara-C: | High dose Adriamycin, Vincristine, Prednisone, Cyclophosphamide, high dose Ara-C |

REFERENCES

1.  Berard, C.W., Greene, M.H., Jaffe, E.S., et al. A Multidisciplinary Approach to Non-Hodgkin's Lymphomas. Annals of Internal Medicine 94:218-235, 1981.
2.  Horwich, A., Peckham, M. "Bad-Risk" Non-Hodgkin's Lymphomas. Seminars in Hematology 20:35-56, 1983.
3.  Posner, L.E., Robert-Gurof, M., Kalyanaramon, V.S., et al. Natural Antibodies to Human T-cell Lymphoma Virus in Patients with Cutaneous T-cell Lymphomas. Journal of Experimental Medicine 154:333-346, 1981.
4.  Popovic, M., Sarin, P.S., Robert-Gurroff, M., et al. Isolation and Transmission of Human Retrovirus (Human T-cell Leukemia Virus). Science 219:856-859, 1983.
5.  Marcus, K.B., Harris, L.J., Stanton, L.W., et al. Transcriptionally Active C-myc Oncogene Is Contained Within NIARD, a DNA Sequence Associated With Chromosome Translocation In B-cell Neoplasia. Proceedings of the National Academy of Sciences. 80:519-523, 1983.
6.  Garvin, A.J., Simon R, Young, R.C., et al. The Rappaport Classification of Non-Hodgkin's Lymphoma: A closer look using other proposed classifications. Seminars in Oncology 7:234-243, 1980.
7.  Potlock, C.S. "Good Risk" Non-Hodgkin's Lymphomas: Approaches to Management. Seminars in Hematology 20:25-34, 1983.
8.  Rosenberg, S.A., Berard, C.W., Brown, B.W., et al. National Cancer Institute Sponsored Study of Classifications of Non-Hodgkin's Lymphomas. Cancer 49:2112-35, 1982.
9.  Lotz, M.J., Chabner, B., DeVita, V.T., et al. Pathologic Staging of 100 Consecutive Untreated Patients With Non-Hodgkin's Lymphomas. Cancer 37:266-270, 1976.
10. Chabner, B.A., Johnson, R.E., Young, R.L., et al. Sequential Nonsurgical and Surgical Staging of Non-Hodgkin's Lymphoma. Annals of Internal Medicine. 85:149-154, 1976.
11. Veronesi, U., Musumeci, R., Pizetti, F., et al. The Value of Staging Laparotomy in Non-Hodgkin's Lymphomas. Cancer 33:446-458, 1974.
12. Bush, R.S., Gospodarowicz, M., Sturgeon, J., et al. Radiation Therapy of Localized Non-Hodgkin's Lymphoma. Cancer Treatment Reports 61:1129-1136, 1977.
13. Jones, S.E., Furs, Z., Kaplan, H.D., et al. Non-Hodgkin's Lymphomas, Results of Radiotherapy. Cancer 32:682-691, 1973.
14. Brereton, H.D., Young, R.C., Longo, D.L., et al. A Comparison Between Chemotherapy and Total Body Irradiation Plus Compunction Chemotherapy in Non-Hodgkin's Lymphoma. Cancer 43:2227-2231, 1979.
15. Kinsella, T.J., Role of Combined Modality Therapy in the Curative Management of Advanced Stage "Favorable" Non-Hodgkin's Lymphomas. Cancer Treatment Reports 66:421-425, 1982.
16. Flippin, T., McLaughlin, P, Conrad, F.G., et al. Stage III Nodular Lymphomas, Preliminary Results of a Combined Chemotherapy/Radiotherapy Program. Cancer 51:987-993, 1983.
17. Hoppe, R.T., Kushlan, P., Kaplan, H.S. The Treatment of Advanced Stage Favorable Histology in Non-Hodgkin's Lymphoma: A Preliminary Report of a Randomized Trial Comparing Single Agent Chemotherapy, Combination Chemotherapy and Whole Body Irradiation. Blood 58:592-598, 1981.
18. Portlock, C.S., Rosenberg, S.A. No Initial Therapy for Stage III and Stage IV Non-Hodgkin's Lymphomas of Favorable Histiologic Types. Annals of Internal Medicine 90:10-13, 1979.
19. Portlock, C.S., Deferral of Initial Therapy for Advanced Indolent Lymphomas, Cancer Treatment Reports 66:417-419, 1982.

20. Miller, T.P., Jones, S.E. Chemotherapy of Localized Histiocytic Lymphoma. Lancet 358-360, 1979.

21. Armitage, J.O., Dick, F.R., Cordner, M.P., et al. A Comparison Between Chemotherapy and Total Body Irradiation Plus Combination Chemotherapy in Non-Hodgkin's Lymphoma. Cancer 43:2227-22231., 1979.

22. Schein, P.S., DeVita, V.T., Hubbard, S., et al. Bleomycin, Adriamycin, Cyclophosphamide, Vincristine, and Prednisone (BACOP) Combination Chemotherapy in the Treatment of Advanced Diffuse Lymphoma. Annals of Internal Medicine 85:417-422, 1976.

23. Goldie, J.H., Coldman, A.J., Gudauskas, G.A., Rationale for the Use of Alternating Non-Crossresistant Chemotherapy. Cancer Treatment Reports 66:439-449, 1982.

24. Fisher, R.J., Vincent, D.T., Hubbard, S.M., et al. Diffuse Aggressive Lymphomas: Increased Survival After Alternating Flexible Sequences of ProMace and MOPP Chemotherapy. Annals of Internal Medicine 98:304-309, 1983.

25. Cabanillas, F., Burgess, M.A., Bodez, G.P., et al. Sequential Chemotherapy and Late Intensification for Malignant Lymphomas of Aggressive Histologic Type. American Journal of Medicine 74:382-388. 1983.

26. Cabanillas, F., Hagemeister, F.B., Bodey, G.P. IMVP-16: An Effective Regimen for Patients with Lymphoma Who Have Relapsed After Initial Combination Chemotherapy. Blood 60:693-697.

27. Ziegler, J.L. Burkitt's Lymphoma. New England Journal of Medicine 305:735-746, 1981.

28. Ziegler, J.L. Treatment Results of 54 American Patients With Burkitt's Lymphoma Are Similar To The African Experience. New England Journal of Medicine. 297:75-80, 1977.

29. Grever, M.R., Bisaccia, R., Scarborough D.A., et al. An Investigation of 2'-Deoxycoformycin in the Treatment of Cutaneous T-cell Lymphoma. Blood 61:279-289, 1983.

30. Miller, R.A., Maloney, D.G., Warnke, R., et al. Treatment of B-cell Lymphoma With Monoclonal Anti-Idiotype Antibody. New England Journal of Medicine. 306:517-522, 1982.

COMPUTED TOMOGRAPHY IN LYMPHOMA

MARCO A. AMENDOLA, M.D. AND BEATRIZ E. AMENDOLA, M.D.

INTRODUCTION

In the study of patients with lymphoma an ideal imaging procedure should assist in: 1) the staging and detection of disease and definition of the anatomic extent; 2) guiding biopsy either at laparotomy or at percutaneous needle biopsy, 3) outlining radiation therapy ports and 4) follow-up, monitoring completeness of response to treatment and detecting early relapse. At the moment of this writing such an ideal test has not been found, however computed tomography (CT) is the single imaging method closest to fulfilling such criteria.

TECHNICAL CONSIDERATIONS

Adequate body CT examination of patients with suspected or proven lymphoma requires meticulous attention to technique if optimal results are to be achieved. Our present protocol for abdominal examination calls for consecutive, 10 mm thick, CT sections from the level of the dome of the diaphagm to the symphysis pubis.

Opacification of the intestinal lumen is accomplished with the following routine: 16 oz of diluted oral contrast (3% Hypaque) 10-12 hours before scanning, the same dose 2 hours prior to the exam, plus 8 oz as the patient arrives for the exam. Nonopacified loops of bowel can be confused with mesenteric adenopathy or even periaortic or pericaval nodal enlargement especially when the lack of retroperitoneal fat permits bowel loops to rest directly on the aorta and inferior vena cava. Unless contraindicated, intravenous contrast material is routinely used to opacify vascular structures and separate them from adjacent nodes and also to evaluate hepatic, splenic and renal involvement.

When studying the thorax, 10 mm consecutive sections are obtained from the low cervical region to the lung bases, including the costophrenic angles. Again in the evaluation of mediastinal and hilar adenopathy the addition of intravenous contrast enhancement occasionally using dynamic scanning may at times signify the difference between a diagnostic study and an indeterminate one.

Recent Trends in Radiation Oncology and Related Fields, Amendola and Amendola, Editors

CT LYMPH NODE ANATOMY AND PATHOLOGY

Normal mediastinal nodes can be visualized at CT in up to 90% of patients including nodes in the pre- and paratracheal area, subcarinal region, anterior mediastinum and aortic-pulmonary window.[1] According to Schnyder and Gamsu, nodes larger than 10 mm in size should be viewed with suspicion of being abnormal, and if over 15 mm in size should be considered abnormally enlarged.[2] The cause of such enlargement can be either inflamatory or neoplastic and by the same token microscopic tumor may be found in nodes less than 1 cm in cross-sectional diameter. The same caveats are true in the case of intra-abdominal and pelvic adenopathy.

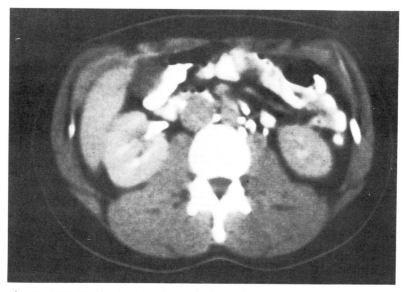

Fig. 1. CT scan at the level of the kidneys demonstrating normal retroperitoneal nodes surrounding the aorta and inferior vena cava opacified by previous lymphangiogram. Oral contrast has been administered to opacify the intestinal lumen. Both kidneys show excretion of intravenous contrast and a normal left ureter is seen lying on the anterior margin of the left psoas muscle.

In the retroperitoneal space normal lymph nodes are visualized as small oval or round densities less than 1 cm in size in the periaortic and pericaval regions (Figure 1). Any node greater than 2 cm in size is considered abnormal.[3-5] Most investigators consider nodes larger than 1.5 cm to be enlarged.[6-7] Similar parameters can be applied to pelvic adenopathy.[8-9]

Other criteria for abnormality include, the presence of numerous nodes larger than 1 cm, and the loss of margins of great vessels and or of psoas muscles.[10] In the particular case of nodes in the retrocrural space, they are thought to be pathologically enlarged when they measure more than 6 mm in size (Figure 2).[11] In the lymphoma patient with full blown retroperitoneal adenopathy, a rounded or multilobular mass of confluent enlarged nodes surrounds and obscures the margins of the aorta, cava and lateral contours of the psoas muscles which are normally well seen on CT (Figure 3).[12] Enlarged nodes may desplace and/or obstruct the ureters causing hydronephrosis and may displace the aorta and vena cava especially anteriorly producing the "floating-aorta" sign (Figure 3).[13] The coalescent mass may simulate a tumor in the head of the pancreas or may even displace the pancreas, kidneys, adrenals or bowel.[14] It must be realized that massive retroperitoneal adenopathy can be caused by other malignancies including leukemia, and metastases from other tumors notably carcinoma of the lung, breast, cervix and prostate, especially when they have poorly differentiated histology. CT is unable to separate malignant from benign retroperitoneal adenopathy seen on inflammatory, viral, or granulomatous disease like sarcoidosis. However the

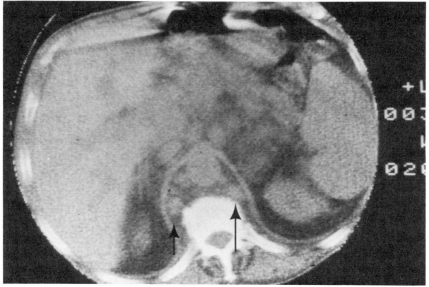

Fig. 2. Several enlarged nodes involved by lymphoma are present dorsal to the crura of the diaphragm (arrows).

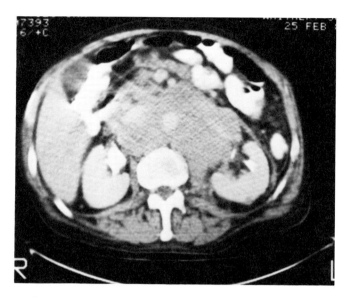

Fig. 3. Massive retroperitoneal adenopathy displacing bowel anteriorly and kidneys laterally. Note aorta and cava (outlined by IV contrast) surrounded by the mass and separated from the lumbar spine ("floating aorta sign").

conglomerate nodal mass, typical of lymphoma is very rarely seen in benign conditions.[15,16] Other pathological processes in the retroperitoneum can cause obscuration of the aortic contour by a soft tissue mass on CT, simulating adenopathy. These include retroperitoneal hematoma, retroperitoneal fibrosis, (Figure 4) leaking aortic aneurysm with perianeurysmal fibrosis, and primary retroperitoneal tumor.[17-19] The clinical setting as well as the ancillary CT findings will help to narrow the differential diagnosis in each situation. Normal anatomic structures or variants which may occasionally cause confusion with mild retroperitoneal adenopathy include duplication of the inferior vena cava, large gonadal veins and most frequently, as previously emphasized, unopacified loops of bowel.[20]

CT is a useful diagnostic technique for evaluation of pelvic adenopathy from lymphoma. In order to avoid redundancy, the reader is referred to the chapter on "Computed tomography of prostatic malignancy" for a detailed discussion of the CT anatomy and pathology of the pelvic nodes.

Prior to the advent of CT (and ultrasound) the diagnosis of mesenteric adenopathy could only be made from indirect findings on barium studies of the

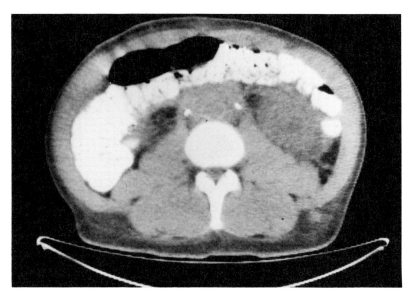

Fig. 4. Idiopathic retroperitoneal fibrosis mimicking retroperitoneal adenopathy: amorphous plaque of soft tissue surrounds the aorta (recognizable by
its calcified wall) and cava. Radiopaque stents indicate position of ureters
encased by the process.

stomach and small bowel. With CT scanning the diagnosis of mesenteric masses
can be made directly.[21,22] The superior mesenteric lymph nodes can be
divided in 3 principal groups: 1) the mesenteric nodes (100-150 in number)
lying between the layers of the mesentery, along the trunk of the superior
mesenteric artery and its primary and terminal branches; 2) the ileocolic
nodes (10-20) forming a chain around the ileocolic artery and its branches,
and 3) the mesocolic nodes, lying between the layers of the transverse
mesocolon, in close relation to the transverse colon.[23] The inferior
mesenteric nodes consist of a) small nodes along branches of left colic and
sigmoid arteries, b) a group around the superior rectal artery in the sigmoid
mesocolon and c) a pararectal group.[23] CT criteria of normality regarding
size of mesenteric nodes are not well established and it is obvious that minor
degress of enlargement will be unrecognizable by CT. However lymphomatous
involvement of mesenteric nodes usually presents as bulky lesions.[6] Three
general CT patterns have been described: rounded masses, cake-like masses and
ill-defined masses.[24] By far the most common CT appearance of mesenteric

lymphoma is as rounded masses (Figure 5A). In the series of Whitley et al., of 130 patients with non-Hodgkin's lymphoma studied with CT, 41 (30%) had mesenteric involvement.[24] In 33 patients this manifested as rounded masses, in 7 there were ill-defined masses and in only one did the CT show a cake-like mass. By contrast in the same series of 60 patients with Hodgkin's disease undergoing CT examination mesenteric involvement was found in only one patient (presenting as an ill-defined mass).

In the rounded mass category a peculiar "sandwich-like" appearance has been described as highly characteristic of lymphomatous involvement of the mesentery.[25] This is caused by a lobulated, confluent mass infiltrating the leaves of the mesentery and encasing the superior mesenteric vessels (Figure 5B). In the experience of Mueller et al.,[25] as well as in our own, this is much more commonly seen in non-Hodgkin's than in Hodgkin's lymphoma.

CT LYMPH NODE IMAGING: COMPARISON WITH LYMPHANGIOGRAPHY

In the twenty years prior to the development of CT scanning, bipedal lymphangiography (LAG) was the only useful modality to evaluate the status of the abdominal and pelvic nodes in patients with lymphoma. In expert hands LAG has achieved high levels of overall accuracy: 92% in Hodgkin's and 88% in non-Hodgkin's lymphoma.[26] Why then use CT for imaging adenopathy? Aside from the fact that LAG cannot evaluate extralymphatic sites of involvement like CT does, there are several important drawbacks to LAG. It is a rather invasive study requiring a small surgical procedure; it is uncomfortable for the patient, and tedious to the operator. Due to the constant microembolization of the oily contrast material into the lungs the procedure should be used selectively and is even contraindicated in patients with impaired pulmonary function. Also, LAG only opacifies a limited number of nodal groups, mainly those surrounding the middle and lower portion of the abdominal aorta, inferior vena cava, and common and external iliac vessels. The upper para-aortic lymph nodes above the renal pedicle are inconsistently opacified at LAG.[27] Celiac, porta hepatis, mesenteric and splenic hilar nodes are not seen at LAG, however they are clearly depicted by CT when they are enlarged (Figure 6).[6] The retrocrural lymph nodes, part of the high para-aortic group, and located dorsal to the crura of the diaphagm, are easily seen at CT, surrounded by retrocrural fat (Figure 2). These nodes are visualized in conventional radiography only when markedly enlarged. In the pelvis, pedal lymphangiography seldom visualizes internal iliac (hypogastric) nodes.[28]

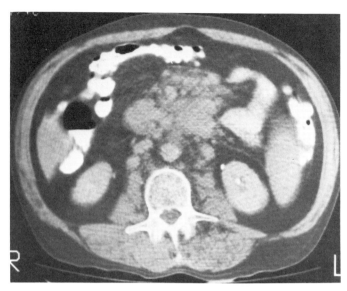

Fig. 5A (Above) Mesenteric lymphadenopathy presenting as multiple rounded masses = non-Hodgkin's lymphoma.

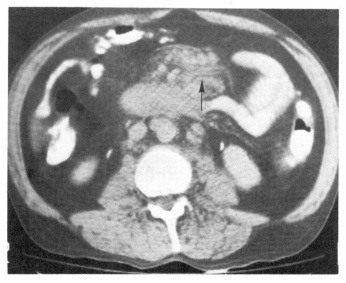

Fig. 5B. CT in the same patient at a slightly lower level = lobulated confluent masses encasing mesenteric vessels (arrow) creating a "sandwich-like" appearance.

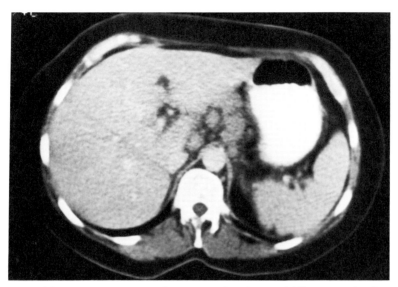

Fig. 6. Celiac and porta hepatis adenopathy in a middle aged female with non-Hodgkin's lymphoma.

The most frequently opacified node of the entire internal iliac group is the lateral sacral node of the parietal subgroup and that is seen only in approximately 50% of the cases.[29] When there is lymphomatous enlargement of the internal iliac nodes, CT is able to demonstrate the abnormality (Figures 7A and B).

Even in the nodal groups routinely opacified at LAG, CT usually shows that many involved bulky nodes and entire nodal chains are only partially filled with lymphographic contrast.[7,30] This is especially true in those patients in which there is no opacification of intraabdominal nodes either due to lymphatic obstruction or to consumption of all the opaque LAG contrast by markedly enlarged pelvic nodes (Figures 8A and B). Thus it is not rare that CT demonstrates that LAG abnormality represents only the "tip of the iceberg."[31] In view of the facts described above, the potential for LAG underestimation (especially superior and lateral extent) in outlining radiation therapy treatment portals should be easily understood. In a comparative study of 23 patients with biopsy proven lymphoma which were studied with bipedal LAG and CT within one week; Schaner et al. found that in 13 of the 23, LAG underestimated the true cephalad extent and in 11 of the 23 patients, LAG underestimated the lateral extent of the adenopathy when compared to CT.[32]

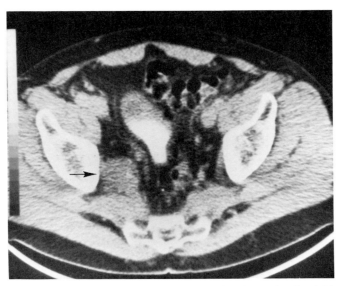

Fig. 7A. CT scan at midpelvis: lymphomatous involvement of right internal iliac nodes which are asymmetrically enlarged (arrow).

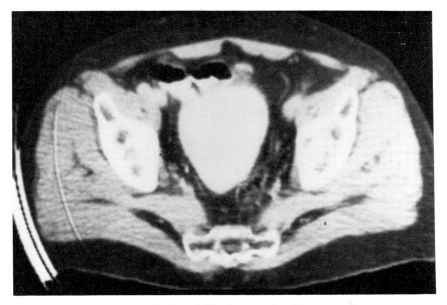

Fig. 7B. Marked reduction in size following treatment.

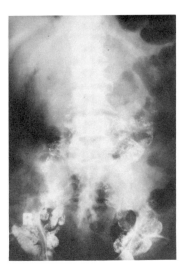

Fig. 8A. Nodal phase of bipedal lymphangiogram: grossly abnormal pelvic and low retroperitoneal nodes bilaterally. The high periaortic, and pericaval nodes are not opacified.

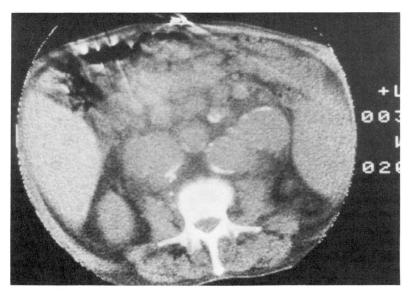

Fig. 8B. CT scan in the same patient shows the true lateral extent of the retroperitoneal adenopathy. Figure 2 shows evidence of retrocrural adenopathy in the same patient.

TABLE 1.    DISEASE SITES BELOW THE DIAPHRAGM FOUND AT LAPAROTOMY

PREVIOUSLY UNTREATED PATIENTS[33,34]

| ORGAN | Hodgkin's | Non-Hodgkin's |
|-------|-----------|---------------|
| Para-aortic nodes | 25% | 49% |
| Mesenteric nodes | 4% | 51% |
| Liver | 8% | 14% |
| Spleen | 37% | 41% |

When comparing the value of CT versus LAG in lymphoma is important to differentiate the group of Hodgkin's from the non-Hodgkin's lymphoma patients (Table 1). Due to the tendency of the non-Hodgkin's lymphomas to exhibit bulky adenopathy in multiple sites, with high incidence of mesenteric lymph node disease not demonstrable at LAG, and the frequency of extranodal intra-abdominal involvement, CT is generally accepted as the radiologic examination of choice in the staging of abdominal non-Hodgkin lymphoma.[27,35,36] This has been additionally stressed in the recent literature regarding the histologic subtypes of histiocytic lymphoma and Burkitt's lymphoma.[37,38] Regarding the initial evaluation of patients with Hodgkin's disease, there has been no unanimous agreement in the literature. The major disadvantage of CT versus LAG in evaluating lymph node disease is the inability of CT to detect architectural abnormalities in normal size nodes which would account for most false negative exams at CT. Indeed in a recent study from the Stanford group, LAG showed an overall accuracy of 95% versus 83% of CT in evaluating retro-peritoneal and pelvic nodes.[27] However the potential advantage of LAG in detecting disease in normal sized nodes as judged from architectural changes within the nodes was not demonstrated in a large series from the Manchester lymphoma group.[39] In 60 patients with Hodgkin's disease in whom LAG was also performed, CT detected all disease shown by LAG and showed additional disease in 13 other cases (3 within the LAG area). On the basis of these findings Blackledge et al. recommended the routine use of CT when available as the primary non-invasive staging exam of the abdomen in Hodgkin's disease. Our own experience is in agreement with this statement, leaving LAG as a backup procedure for instances in which CT is technically unsatisfactory (i.e. the emaciated patient without retroperitoneal fat), equivocal or if CT is negative in a patient highly suspected of harboring infradiaphagmatic lymphoma and a staging laparotomy is not feasible or planned.

We have not found the use of surveillance abdominal films following LAG to be reliable for evaluation of treatment response and relapse. This has also been the experience of other groups.[39,41]

Ultrasound is another useful method for the detection of abdominal lymphadenopathy.[42-45] Several studies have shown comparable accuracies to CT in the evaluation of upper retroperitoneal lymph node involvement, although with a lower sensitivity for ultrasound,[43] partly due to interference of intestinal gas in the study of the low para-aortic and iliac regions.[45] However, ultrasound represents a valuable supplement to CT in the examination of thin patients and for guidance in the performance of percutaneous needle biopsies.

CT OF HEPATIC LYMPHOMA

Involvement of the liver by lymphoma is not rare. It is present in at least 14% of patients with non-Hodgkin's lymphoma and 8% of patients with Hodgkin's disease on initial presentation at staging laparatomy (Table 1), and in over 50% of patients dying with both types of lymphoma.

In CT of the liver, lymphomatous lesions usually appear as single or multiple focal areas of low density or rarely as diffuse areas of diminished attenuation.[46] These findings are not specific and similar CT abnormalities can be seen for example with metastatic cancer to the liver or hepatoma. Liver enlargement is a poor indicator of liver involvement by lymphoma.

In the series of 58 patients studied by Zornoza and Ginaldi with an 18-second scanner, only 4 out of 7 patients with liver lymphoma were detected by CT for a disappointing sensitivity of only 57%.[46] This limited usefulnes of CT in detecting hepatic lymphoma has also been documented in other large series.[7,47]

This may be explained by the inability of CT to show either microscopic or small macroscopic lesions and/or to the low CT contrast differences between the tumor and normal liver tissue, even after intravenous contrast enhancement.

The cause of jaundice in patients with lymphoma may not be apparent. It may be caused by involvement of the liver or extrahepatic bile ducts or by iatrogenic hepatitis among other causes.[48] Adenopathy in the porta hepatis or peripancreatic region causing biliary obstruction can be easily demonstrated by CT although small lesions may be overlooked.[41] Direct lymphomatous infiltration of the liver parenchyma by adjacent nodal masses can be also depicted by CT.

As it is the case with CT, ultrasound is able to demonstrate liver abnormalities in lymphoma,[49] however, the low rate of positive studies, 23 of 443 patients (5.2%) in a recent series studied at M.D. Anderson Hospital would indicate that gross disease must be present before it is detectable by ultrasound.[50]

CT OF SPLENIC LYMPHOMA

Splenic involvement at initial presentation is a frequent occurrence in both Hodgkin's (37%), and non-Hodgkin's lymphoma (41%), Table 1. Furthermore, the spleen may be the only diseased intraabdominal organ at staging laparotomy, especially in patients with Hodgkin's disease.[51] Conventional radiographic studies including angiography have given disappointing results concerning the spread of lymphoma to the spleen.[52] Although, CT gives accurate indication of splenomegaly the value of this observation is somewhat relative: 1) in non-Hodgkin lymphoma it indicates high probability of splenic disease, 2) one third of Hodgkin's patients with splenomegaly will have negative pathology, and 3) one third of normal size spleens will harbor disease in unselected, untreated patients with either type of lymphoma.[51]

In the assessment of focal deposits of lymphoma in the spleen, current CT technology has proven unreliable, detecting only one of 11 diseased spleens in the series of Earl et al.[53] and only 4 out of 18 in the series of Zornoza and Ginaldi.[46] In several other series CT failed to image splenic nodules of less than 1 cm[3,12] and attenuation values were found to be unreliable indicators of lymphomatous involvement.[54] Regarding other imaging modalities: 1) Gallium citrate scans have an unacceptable low diagnostic accuracy below the diaphragm,[55,56] 2) 99mTc Sulfur colloid scans have significant false negative and false positive rates,[57] 3) the overall accuracy of a positive sonographic diagnosis is only 50%.[49] Based on the above it is clear that until new diagnostic methods can reliably detect small (less than 1 cm diameter) foci of splenic involvement, staging laparotomy with splenectomy will be needed to exclude it.

Active research is being conducted looking for new contrast agents capable of increasing the CT diagnostic accuracy in splenic imaging.[58,59] Preliminary clinical results with a new organ-specific agent: Ethiodol-Oil-Emulsion-13 (EOE-13) are highly encouraging. The detection rate in patients with splenic lymphoma increased from 8% before EOE-13 infusion to 92% after EOE-13 infusion.[60] Lesions greater than 0.5 cm were consistently imaged.[60] This contrast material is still an investigational agent, not yet approved by the Food and Drug Administration for general use.

CT OF GASTROINTESTINAL LYMPHOMA

Gastric lymphoma represents 3% to 5% of all gastric neoplasms. Its incidence appears to be rising while the rate of gastric cancer is declining.[61] The most common gastrointestinal site for lymphoma is the stomach (48-50%) followed by the small intestine (30-37%) and the ileocecal region (12-13%).[62] Gastric lymphoma may be part of the systemic disease or be primary in the stomach (10%). Non-Hodgkin's lymphoma accounts for 80% of all gastric lymphomas.[61]

Because of its submucosal pattern of spread, barium studies in gastric lymphoma may only show thickening of gastric wall and rugal folds without mucosal abnormalities. Endoscopy and mucosal biopsy are often nondiagnostic. The ability of CT to directly image the entire thickness of the gastric wall makes it especially attractive to study lymphomatous involvement of the stomach (Figure 9). In a series of 12 patients with gastric lymphoma studied by Buy and Moss,[63] CT scans were abnormal in all cases, clearly demonstrating the thickened gastric wall, and intramural location of the tumor. CT provided information regarding concomitant lymphadenopathy (92%) and direct extension to adjacent organs (42%), not obtainable by any other imaging technique. It appears that CT may accurately stage gastric lymphoma.

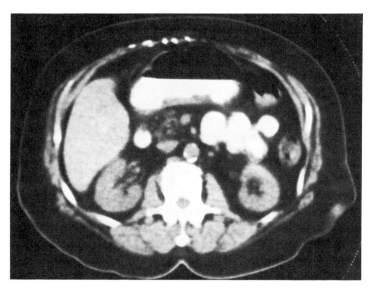

Fig. 9. Gastric lymphoma = note localized thickening of the posterior wall of the stomach.

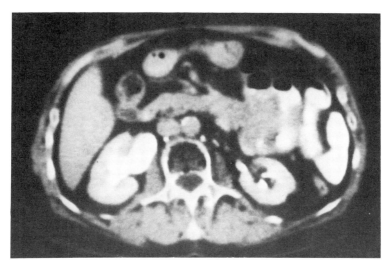

Fig. 10. Histiocytic lymphoma involving the small bowel.

This has potential therapeutic implications, since Stage I and II gastric lymphoma may be surgically removed while radiation and/or chemotherapy are usually preferred for Stages III and IV.[37,63]

CT is useful in the recognition of intestinal pathology when the bowel lumen is adequately opacified with oral or rectal contrast. CT can directly image the bowel wall and the adjacent mesentery. Lymphoma may affect primarily the bowel wall rather than the mesentery.[64] Bowel position, bowel wall thickness, bowel contour and the integrity of the perivisceral fat planes should be systematically studied.[65]

Lymphomas account for 20% of all small bowel tumors with non-Hodgkin's lymphomas being the most common type. The small bowel may be the single site of involvement or part of the systemic disease. Although barium studies remain the preferred modality for diagnosis of small bowel lymphomas, CT helps to stage the disease and demonstrate the relation of the tumor to the bowel and adjacent organs (Figure 10). Benign causes of bowel wall thickening such as intramural hematomas, granulomatous or radiation enteritis may be difficult to differentiate from isolated small bowel lymphoma on the basis of the CT findings. However clinical features can help in the differential diagnosis.[66]

Primary lymphoma of the colon constitutes only 0.5% of all malignant tumors of the colon, most commonly affecting the cecum or the rectum. Secondary colon involvement is uncommon. Of all patients with gastrointestinal lymphoma only 10% will have colonic involvement.[61]

Large mesenteric masses easily diagnosed by CT are commonly associated with colonic involvement. Only a handful of cases demonstrated by CT have been reported. However, CT findings have included abnormal thickening of the colonic wall and mass effects on the bowel.[65,67]

## CT OF PANCREATIC LYMPHOMA

Primary pancreatic lymphoma is extremely rare in Hodgkin's disease but it is reported to occur in 1% of patients with non-Hodgkin's lymphoma at initial staging.[33,68] Direct extension to the pancreas from peripancreatic adenopathy is more common than primary involvement, however, it may be difficult to distinguish between the two because the pancreas has no readily definable capsule.

At CT, pancreatic lymphoma is usually depicted as diffuse or localized enlargement of the gland. The CT picture is not characteristic of lymphoma and localized enlargement has been reported to mimic pancreatic arcinoma in patients with histocytic lymphoma[37] while diffuse pancreatic enlargement has simulated acute pancreatitis in patients with Burkitt's lymphoma.[69] Since pancreatic or peripancreatic involvement may represent the first manifestation of lymphoma, differentiation between these different processes has important therapeutic implications. Percutaneous pancreatic biopsy under CT guidance may help resolve this important diagnostic dilemma (Figure 11A, B).

## CT OF RENAL AND ADRENAL LYMPHOMA

Although the urinary tract is a frequent site of lymphoma outside the hematopoietic system, involvement of the kidneys and adrenals has been uncommonly detected before autopsy.[70,71] With the advent of CT and ultrasound these lesions are being identified more commonly and at an earlier state.[72-76]

Renal involvement by lymphoma is thought to occur from hematogenous spread or from direct extension of retroperitoneal adenopathy. Hematogenous spread manifests itself by single or multiple renal masses or nodules with or without renal enlargement. Direct extension may present as focal or diffuse renal infiltration with occasional engulfment of the kidney by contiguous retroperitoneal disease.[73-75]

Renal and adrenal involvement in our experience is much more common in non-Hodgkin's lymphoma than in Hodgkin's disease. Histologically diffuse forms are more frequent than nodular types.[75]

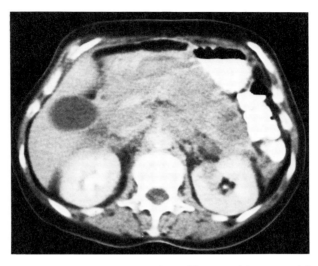

Fig. 11A. Diffusely enlarged pancreas in a 59 year old woman with a clinical picture of pancreatitis in previous clinical remission from Burkitt's lymphoma.

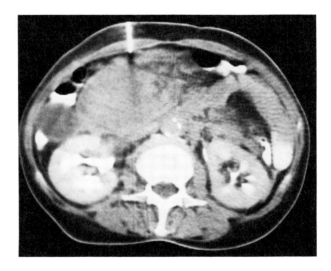

Fig. 11B. More caudal scan at the level of the pancreatic head for localization of needle biopsy which was positive for Burkitt's lymphoma. (Courtesy of I.R. Francis, G.M. Glazer, and Raven Press.[69])

70

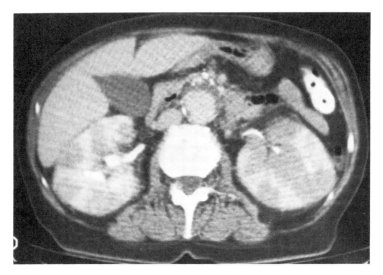

Fig. 12A. Multiple intrarenal nodules and bilateral renal enlargement in a patient during relapse of non-Hodgkin's lymphoma. Retroperitoneal adenopathy was present at other levels.

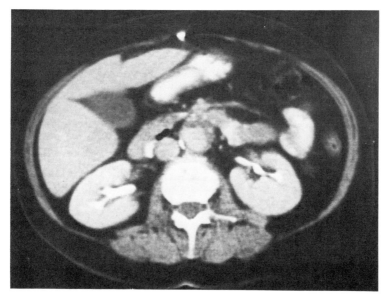

Fig. 12B. Resolution of the abnormalities on follow-up CT scans after successful chemotherapy.

Renal, perirenal and adrenal involvement by lymphoma rarely detected using conventional radiography, can be imaged noninvasively by CT scanning. Using CT, the most common appearance of GU tract lymphoma is that of bilateral multiple intrarenal nodules and enlarged kidneys with associated retroperitoneal adenopathy (Figure 12). Adenopathy was associated with renal lymphoma in 24 of the 25 patients we studied with CT.

Adrenal involvement by lymphoma is fairly common pathologically.[77] Radiologic detection has been rarely reported. CT is capable of visualizing adrenal lymphoma if the glands are enlarged and deformed; the shape of the enlarged gland may be oval round or triangular (Figure 13). In our material, retroperitoneal adenopathy was associated with the involved adrenals in 7 out of 8 patients.[70] However, we have recently encountered an additional patient in which the right adrenal was the only intraabdominal site of disease (Figure 13).

Although the CT findings of renal, perirenal and adrenal lymphoma are not specific, the presence of multiple intrarenal nodules with associated retroperitoneal adenopathy and perirenal or adrenal abnormality should suggest a possible diagnosis of GU tract lymphoma. Clinical work-up can then be directed so unnecessary nephrectomy can be avoided.

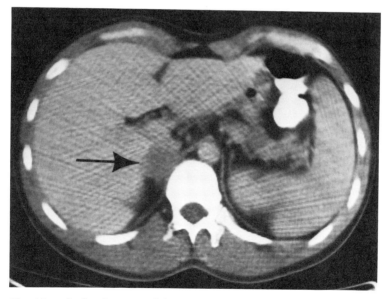

Fig. 13. Adrenal lymphoma = right adrenal mass (arrow) in a patient with T-cell lymphoma was the only area of intraabdominal involvement at laparatomy.

CT OF INTRATHORACIC LYMPHOMA

CT is the most valuable radiologic method for the evaluation of mediastinal masses.[78] Mediastinal lymphadenopathy is only detectable on plain chest radiography or conventional tomography, when the nodes have reached sufficient size to distort relationships of adjacent pleural reflections with aereated lung.[79] Because of its superior contrast resolution and ability to display cross sectional anatomy, CT is the modality of choice to diagnose subtle mediastinal adenopathy.

Based on CT attenuation coefficients typical of fatty tissue, mediastinal widening due to lipomatosis can be easily differentiated by CT from adenopathy, and pericardiac fat pads discerned from pericardial and paracardiac lymphomatous involvement.[78-80]

Subcarinal nodes are difficult to detect with plain films and esophagograms until they are large, however, on CT, filling of the normally concave azygoesophageal recess allows early recognition of subcarinal adenopathy (Figure 14).

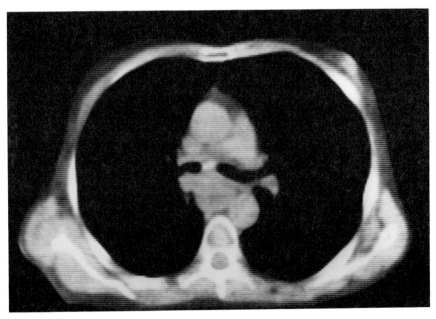

Fig. 14. Convex azygo-esophageal recess caused by subcarinal adenopathy (arrow).

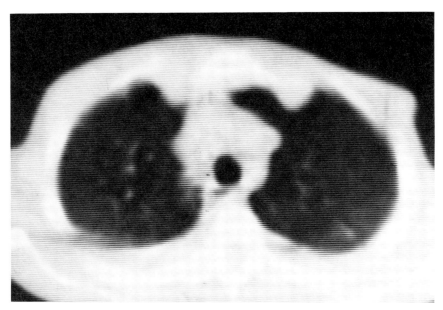

Fig. 15. Bilateral internal mammary adenopathy and right anterior chest wall involvement. Pleural effussions are also evident.

Paravertebral and posterior mediastinal nodes are commonly involved in lymphomatous disease. Abnormality in this area may influence selection of therapy and delineation of radiotherapy portals. When a displaced paraspinal line is noted on a chest radiograph, CT is most rewarding to confirm the presence and extent of adenopathy, being clearly superior to lymphangiography.[81]

The internal mammary nodes are more numerous in the upper hemithorax and when enlarged can be recognized in the lateral chest radiography as extrapleural masses lying anteriorly against the chest wall, or if they are prominent enough as an ill defined density lateral to the sternum on the PA film.[79] If the abnormality is questionable, CT scans can depict these nodes to advantage (Figure 15).[82,83]

One of the major contributions of CT to radiation therapy planning in thoracic lymphoma is the demonstration of extension of disease along the chest wall. Such was the case in the series of Pilepich et al.:[82] in 28 patients with mediastinal lymphoma, 15 had extension along the anterior chest wall. Appreciation of this abnormality resulted in significant alteration of treatment portals in nine patients.

Evaluation of the pulmonary hila is important in the work-up of patients with lymphoma since their involvement usually implies modification of treatment. Despite early reports considering CT of little value in the investigation of the pulmonary hila, detailed hilar anatomy and pathology can be routinely imaged with current scanners.[84,85] In addition, contrast enhanced dynamic CT with table incrementation between scans has been found superior to conventional CT because hilar vascular structures can be clearly opacified.[86] Kaplan has indicated the importance of detecting hilar adenopathy in Hodgkin's disease since it is commonly a precursor of pulmonary parenchymal involvement.[87]

Direct extension of lymphoma from mediastinum to lung does not alter staging but influences therapy (see chapter by Levitt et al.). In newly diagnosed patients with Hodgkin's or non-Hodgkin's lymphoma having normal chest x-rays, routine lung tomography is not warranted due to its low yield.[88] However, in those patients with questionable lung extension by conventional radiography, CT may be useful.

Recent studies suggest that the presence and extent of mediastinal disease at initial presentation is important in the outcome of patients with Hodgkin's disease. For this reason CT has been recommended for evaluation of patients with low neck or supraclavicular adenopathy, in whom there is no obvious mediastinal adenopathy in whom disease in nodal chains in continuity may be difficult to detect.[89] As previously discussed, patients with questionable mediastinal involvement may benefit from CT examinations of the chest.

Discrete parenchymal nodules either solitary or multiple, from less than 1 cm to several cm in size are a common radiographic finding in malignant lymphomas.[79] CT has been shown to be superior to conventional radiography for the detection of small pulmonary nodules.[90] In patients with lymphoma the radiographic finding of a large mediastinal mass frequently overshadows the presence of airway narrowing. In a recent series tracheobronchial compression ws observed in 55% of 20 consecutive newly diagnosed children with Hodgkin's lymphoma.[91] In doubtful cases CT can precisely assess the degree and length of the stenosis.

Pericardial lymphoma may occur at presentation or during relapse. A high index of suspicion is needed especially in patients with extensive mediastinal tmor. Underdosage of the pericardium or paracardiac region with subsequent relapse in this area may occur if lymphomatous involvement is not recognized.[89]

## CT ASSISTED BIOPSY IN LYMPHOMA

CT provides precise guidance for percutaneous needle biopsy of suspected lymphomatous nodes or masses. For the initial diagnosis in which the pattern of involvement is essential for histologic typing, a formal biopsy is needed. However, in patients with suspected recurrent or persistent disease with known lymphoma, a positive aspiration biopsy may obviate the need for exploratory surgery. An overall success rate of 64% was obtained by Zornoza et al.[92]

## CT IN EVALUATION OF TREATMENT RESPONSE AND FOLLOW-UP

Remission status at the end of the treatment is an important prognostic factor. CT has been useful as a non-invasive method in both Hodgkin's and non-Hodgkin's lymphoma to document response to treatment.

It must be noted that occasionally a CT scan will show residual adenopathy or mass in patients in which second look laparotomy or thoracotomy will find only fibrous tissue (Figure 16).[93-95] When there is doubt about complete remission, biopsy under CT or ultrasound guide may be helpful. However, a negative result is of no value because of possible technical or sampling error.

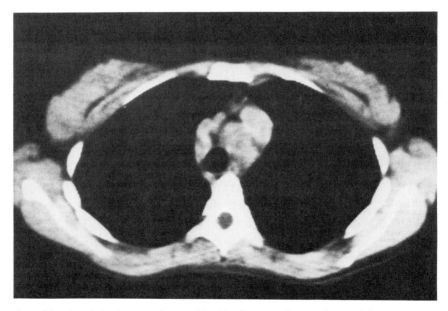

Fig. 16. Persistent anterior mediastinal mass in patient with Stage IIIB nodular sclerosing Hodgkin's after radiation and chemotherapy. Enlarged nodes found at thoracotomy. Histologic study only revealed fibrosis without residual tumor.

Obtention of CT scan for investigation of relapse following treatment of Hodgkin's disease has been advocated in the following situations: 1) when there is clinical evidence of either nodal or extranodal disease, 2) when other studies like for example, abnormal liver function tests, suggest relapse and 3) when a patient has "B" symptoms but no other clinical signs of relapse.[94]

Reduction in tumor bulk may be monitored satisfactorily by CT, which in this respect is clearly superior to LAG. Ability to detect otherwise unsuspected disease in patients in relapse or remission make CT an important investigation in the management of lymphoma.

CONCLUSION

We hope that this review shows with clarity the tremendous impact of CT in the evaluation of lymphomatous involvement of the body. There are areas like CT of bone lymphoma in which scant information is available. Unsuspected areas of bone involvement are occasionally found during CT examination of he chest and abdomen. Problems posed by some of these cases include the uncertainty about these lesions representing areas of healing after treatment, very early metastatic deposits or other non-lymphomatous lesions such as bone islands. Clearly more research is needed in this area. It should be emphasized that conventional radiographs and radionuclide bone scanning are the mainstay of the initial work-up of a suspected osseous lymphoma. It is already clear however that exquisite CT demonstration of anatomic relationships of soft tissue components of osseous lymphoma can be used to advantage in outlining radiation therapy ports for optimization of treatment planning.[96] In conclusion, CT has already proven to be an essential tool in the initial investigation, follow-up and guidance of treatment in the patient with lymphoma.

REFERENCES
1.  Sagel, S.S., Aromberg, D.J., Thoracic anatomy and mediastinum. Chapter 4 in Computed Body Tomography. Lee, J.K.T, Stanley, R.J., and Sagel, S.S., eds Raven Press, New York, pp 55-97, 1983.
2.  Schnyder, P.A., Gamsu, G. CT of the pretracheal retrocaval space. AJR 136:303-308, 1981
3.  Redman, H.D., Glatstein, E., Castellino, R. A., et al. Computed tomography as an adjunct in the staging of Hodgkin's disease and non-Hodgkins lymphomas. Radiology, 124:381-385, 1977.
4.  Zelch, M., Haaga, J.R., Clinical comparison of computed tomography and lymphangiography for detection of retroperitoneal adenopathy. Radiol Clin N. Amer 17:157-168, 1979.

5. Korobkin, M., Callen, P., Fisch, A.E. Computed tomography of the pelvis and retroperitoneum. Radiol Clin N. Amer. 17:301-319, 1979.

6. Korobkin, M. Computed tomography of the retroperitoneal vasculature and lymph nodes. Semin Roentgenol 16:251-267, 1981

7. Ellert, J., Kreel, L. The role of computed tomography in the initial staging and subsequent management of lymphomas. J Comput Assist Tomogr 4:368-391, 1980

8. Lee, J.K.T., Stanley, R.J., Sagel, S.S., et al. Accuracy in CT detecting intraabdominal and pelvic lymph node metastases from pelvic cancers. AJR 131:675-679, 1978.

9. Walsh, J.W., Amendola, M.A., Konerding, K.F., et al. Computed tomographic detection of pelvic and inguinal lymph node metastases from primary and recurrent pelvic malignant disease. Radiology 137:157-166, 1980.

10. Glazer, G.M., Goldberg, H.I., Moss, A.A., Axel, L. Computed tomographic detection of retroperitoneal adenopathy. Radiology 143:147-149, 1982.

11. Callen, P.W., Korobkin, M, Isherwood, I. Computed tomographic evaluation of the retrocrural prevertebral space. AJR 129:907-910, 1977.

12. Breiman, R.S., Castellino, R.A , Harrel, G.S., et al. CT Pathologic corrections in Hodgkin's disease and non-Hodgkin's lymphoma. Radiology 126:159-166, 1978.

13. Havrilla, T.R,, Reich, N.E., Haaga, J.R. The floating aorta in computerized tomography: a sign of retroperitoneal pathology. Comp Axial Tomogr 1:107-111, 1977.

14. Carter, B.L., Wechsler, R.J. Computed tomography of the retroperitoneum and abdominal wall. Seminars Roentgenol 13:201-211, 1978.

15. Lee, J.K.T. Retroperitoneum. Chapter 10 in: Computed Body Tomography, Lee, J.K.T., Sagel, S.S., Stanley, R.J., eds, Raven Press, New York, pp 257-286, 1983.

16. Miller, K.L., Rochester, D., Miller, J.W. Extensive abdominal lymphadenopathy in sarcoidosis. Amer J Gastroenterol 75:367-369, 1981.

17. Amendola, M.A., Tisnado, J., Fields, W.R. et al. Evaluation of retroperitoneal hemorrhage by computed tomograph before and after translumbar aortography. Radiology 133:401-404, 1979.

18. Stephens, D.H., Sheedy, P.F., Hattery, R.R., et al. Diagnosis and evaluation of retroperitoneal tumors by computed tomography. AJR 129:395-402, 1977.

19. Feinstein, R.S., Gatewood, O.M.B., Goldman, S.M., Copeland, B., Walsh, P.C., Siegelman, S.S. Computerized tomography in the diagnosis of retroperitoneal fibrosis. J Urol 126:255-259, 1981.

20. Tisnado, J., Amendola, M.A., Vines, F.S., Beachley, M.D. Computed tomography of a double inferior vena cava. The "double cava" sign. Computerized Tomogr 3:195-199, 1979.

21. Levitt, R.G., Sagel, S.S., Stanely, R.J. Detection of neoplastic involvement of the mesentery and omentum by computed tomography. AJR 131:835-838, 1978.

22. Bernardino, M.E., Jing, B.S., Wallace, S. Computed tomography diagnosis of mesenteric masses. AJR 132:33-36, 1979.

23. Gray, H. Anatomy of the human body. Philadelphia, Lea and Febiger, 29th edition pp 764-766, 1973.

24. Whitley, N.O., Bohlman, M.E., Baker, L.P. CT Patterns of mesenteric disease. J Comput Assist Tomogr, 6:490-496, 1982.

25. Mueller, P.R., Ferrucci, J.T., Harbin, W.P., Kirkpatrick, R.H., Simeone, J.F., Wittenberg, J. Appearance of lymphomatous involvement of the mesentery by ultrasonography and computed tomography: the "sandwich sign." Radiology 134:467-473, 1980.

26. Marglin, S., Castellino, R.A.  Lymphographic accuracy in 623 consecutive previously untreated case of Hodgkin's disease and Non-Hodgkin's lymphoma Radiology 140:351-353, 1981.

27. Castellino, R.A., Marglin, S.I.  Imaging of abdominal and pelvic lymph nodes: Lymphography or computed tomography?  Invest Radiol 17:433-443, 1982.

28. Harrison, D.A.  Normal anatomy.  In Clouse, M.G. ed, Clinical Lymphography, Williams and Wilkins, Baltimore, pp 14-57, 1977.

29. Herman, P.G., Benninghof, D.L., Nelson, J.H., Mellins, H.Z.  Roentgen anatomy of the ilio-pelvic-aortic lymphatic system.  Radiology 80:182-193, 1963.

30. Marshall, W.H., Breiman, R.S., Harrel, G.S., Glastein, E., Kaplan, H.S. Computed tomography of abdominal, para-aortic lymph node disease: preliminary observations with a 6-second scanner.  AJR 128:759-764, 1977.

31. Lee, J.K.T., Stanely, R.J., Sagel, S.S., Levitt, R.E.  Accuracy of computed tomography in detecting intraabdominal and pelvic adenopathy in lymphoma.  AJR, 1318:311-315, 1978.

32. Schaner, E.G., Head, G.L, Doppman, J.L, Young, R.E.  Computed tomography in the diagnosis, staging and management of abdominal lymphoma.  J Comput Assist Tomogr 1:176-180, 1977.

33. Goffinet, D.R., Warnke, R., Dunnick, N.R., et al.  Clinical and surgical (laparotomy) evaluation of patients with non-Hodgkin's lymphomas.  Cancer Treat Rep 61:981-992, 1977.

34. Kadin, M.E., Glatstein, E.J., Dorfman, R.E.  Clinicopathology studies in 177 untreated patients subjected to laparotomy for the staging of Hogkin's disease.  Cancer 27:1277-1299, 1971.

35. Castellino, R.A., Marglin, S., Blank, N.  Hodgkins disease, the non-Hodgkin's lymphoma and the leukemias in the retroperitoneum.  Semin in Roentgenol 15:288, 1980.

36. Lee, J.K.T., Stanley, R.J., Sagel, S.S., Levitt, R.G.  Accuracy of computed tomography in detecting intraabdominal and pelvic adenopathy in lymphoma.  AJR 131:311-3, 1978.

37. Burgener, F.A., Hamlin, D.J.  Histiocytic lymphoma of the abdomen: Radiographic spectrum.  AJR 137:337-342, 1981.

38. Krudy, A.G., Dunnick, N.R., Magrath, I.T.  CT of American Burkitt's lymphoma.  AJR 136:747-754, 1981.

39. Blackledge, G., Best, J.J.K., Crowther, D., Isherwood, I.  Computed tomography (CT) in the staging of patients with Hodgkins' disease: a report on 136 patients.  Clin Radiol 31:143-147, 1980.

40. Lee, J.K.T, Stanley, R.J., Sagel, S.S., Melson, G.L., Koehler, R.E. Limitations of the post-lymphangiogram plain abdominal radiograph as an indicator of recurrent lymphoma: comparison to computed tomography. Radiology 134:155, 1980.

41. Best, J.J.K., Blackledge, G., Forbes, W.S.C, et al.  Computed tomography of abdomen in staging and clinical management of lymphoma.  Br Med J 2:1675-1677. 1978.

42. Brascho, D.J., Durant, J.R., Green, L.E.  The accuracy of retroperitoneal ultrasonography in Hodgkin's disease and non-Hodgkin's lymphoma. Radiology 125:485-487, 1977.

43. Rochester, D., Bowie, J.D., Kunzmann, A., Lester, E.  Ultrasound in the staging of lymphoma.  Radiology 124:483-487, 1977.

44. Ritchie, W.G.M.  Sonographic demonstration of abdominal visceral lymph node enlargement.  AJR 138:517-521, 1982.

45. Magnusson, A., Hagberg, H., Hemmingsson, A., Lindgren, P.G.  Computed tomography, ultrasound and lymphography in the diagnosis of malignant lymphoma.  Acta Radiol Diag, 23:29-35, 1982.

46. Zornoza J, Ginaldi S. Computed tomography in hepatic lymphoma. Radiology 138:405-410, 1981.
47. Jones, S.E., Tobias, D.A., Waldman, R.S. Computed tomographic scanning in patients with lymphoma. Cancer 41:480-486, 1978.
48. Severin, A., Bellomi, M., Cozzi, G., Pizzetti, P., Spinelli, P. Lymphomatous involvement of intrahepatic and extrahepatic biliary ducts. PTC and ERCP findings. Acta Radiol Diag 22:159-163, 1981.
49. Carroll, B.A., Ta, H.N. The ultrasonic appearance of extranodal abdominal lymphoma. Radiology 136:419-425, 1980.
50. Ginaldi, S., Bernardino, M.E., Jing, B.S., et al. Ultrasonographic patterns of hepatic lymphoma. Radiology 136:427-431, 1980.
51. Harrell, G.S., Breiman, R.S., Glatstein, E.S., Marshall, W.H., Castellino, R.A. Computed tomography of the abdomen in malignant lymphomas. Rad Clin North Am 15:391-400, 1977.
52. Jonsson, K., Lunderquist, A. Angiography of the liver and spleen in Hodgkin's disease. AJR 121:789-792, 1974.
53. Earl, H.M., Sutcliffe, S.B.J., Kelsey-Fry, I., et al. Computed tomogrpahy (CT) abdominal scanning in Hodgkin's disease. Clin Radiol 31:149-153, 1980.
54. Alcorn, F.S., Mategrano, V.C., Petasnick, J.P, Clark, J.W. Contributions of computed tomography in the staging and management of malignant lymphoma. Radiology 125:717-723, 1977.
55. Kaplan, H.S. Essentials of staging and management of the malignant lymphomas. Semin Roentgenol 15:219-226, 1980.
56. Johnston, G.S., Go, M.F., Benna, R.S., et al. Gallium-67 citrate imaging in Hodgkin's disease: final report of cooperative group. J Nucl Med 18:692, 1977.
57. Bernardino, M.E., Thomas, J.L., Barnes, P.A., Lewis, E. Diagnostic approaches to liver and spleen metastases. Radiol Clin N Amer 20:469-485, 1982.
58. Havron, A., Seltzer, S.E., Davis, M.A., Shulkin, P. Radio-opaque liposomes: A promising new contrast material for computed tomography of the spleen. Radiology 140:507-511, 1981.
59. Vermess, M., Bernardino, M.E., Doppman, J.L., et al. The use of intravenous liposoluble contrast material for the examination of the liver and spleen in lymphomas. Preliminary report. J Comp Assist Tomogr 5:709-713, 1981.
60. Thomas, J.L., Bernardino, M.E., Vermess, M., et al. EOE-13 in the detection of hepatosplenic lymphoma. Radiology 145:629-634, 1982.
61. Zornoza, J., Dodd, G.D. Lymphoma of the gastrointestinal tract. Semin Roentgenol 15:272-287, 1980.
62. Brady, L.W., Asbell, S.O. Malignant lymphoma of the gastrointestinal tract. Radiology 137:291-298, 1980.
63. Buy, J.N., Moss, A.A. Computed tomography of gastric lymphoma. AJR 138:859-865, 1982.
64. Gore, R.M., Goldberg, H.I. Computed tomographic evaluation of the gastrointestinal tract in diseases other than primary adenocarcinoma. Rad Clin N Amer 20:781-796, 1982.
65. Scanlon, M.H., Blumberg, M.L., Ostrum, B.J. Computed tomographic recognition of gastrointestinal pathology. Radiographics 3:201-227, 1983.
66. Pagani, J.J., Bernardino, M.E. CT radiographic correlation of ulcerating small bowel lymphomas. AJR 136:998-1000, 1981.
67. Fisher, J.K. Abnormal colonic wall thickening on computed tomography. J Comput Assist Tomogr 7:90-97, 1983.

68. Castellino, R.A., Marglin, S., Blank, N. Hodgkin's disease, non-Hodgkin's lymphomas, and the leukemias in the retroperitoneum. Semin Roentgenol 15:283-301, 1980.
69. Francis, I.R., Glazer, G.M. Burkitt's lymphoma of pancreas presenting as acute pancreatits. J Comput Assist Tomogr 6:395-397, 1982.
70. Richmond, J., Sherman, R.S., Diamond, H.D., Craver, L.F. Renal lesions associated with malignant lymphomas. Am J Med 32:184-207, 1962.
71. Martinez-Maldonado, M., Ramirez De Arellano, G.A. Renal involvement in malignant lymphomas. A survey of 49 cases. J Urol 95:485-488, 1966.
72. Rubin, B.E. Computed tomography in the evaluation of renal lymphoma. J Comput Assist Tomogr 3:759-764, 1979.
73. Hartman, D.S., Davis, C.J., Goldman, S.M., Friedman, A.C., Fritzsche, P. Renal lymphoma: radiologic-pathologic correlation of 21 cases. Radiology 144:759-766, 1982.
74. Jafri, S.Z.H., Bree, R.L., Amendola, M.A., et al. CT of renal and perirenal non-Hodgkin's lymphoma. AJR 138:1101-1105, 1982.
75. Amendola, M.A., Jafri, S.Z.H., Glazer, G.M., Bree, R.L., Tisnado, J., Hoskins PA. Imaging of renal and adrenal lymphoma. Scientific exhibit. Presented at the 68th Scientific Assembly and Annual Meeting of the Radiological Society of North America, Nov 28-Dec 3, 1982, Chicago, Ill
76. Jafri, S.Z.H., Francis, I.R., Glazer, G.M., Bree, R.L., Amendola, M.A. CT detection of adrenal lymphoma. J Comput Assist Tomogr 7:254-266, 1983.
77. Rosenberg, S.A., Diamond, H.D., Jaslowitz, B., Craver, L.F. Lymphosarcoma: a review of 1269 cases. Medicine 40:31-84, 1961.
78. Heitzman, E.R. Computed tomography of the thorax: current perspective. AJR 136:2-12, 1981.
79. Blank, N. Castellino, R.A. The intrathoracic manifestations of the malignant lymphomas and the leukemias. Semin Roentgenol 15:227-245, 1980.
80. Jochelson, M.S., Balikian, J.P., Mauch, P., Liebman, H. Peri and paracardial involvement in lymphoma: a radiographic study of 121 cases, AJR 140:483-488, 1983.
81. Efremidis, S.C., Dan, S.J., Cohen, B.A., Mitty, H.A., Rabinowitz, J.G. Displaced paraspinal line: role of CT and lymphography. AJR 136:505-509, 1981.
82. Pilepich, M.V., Rene, J.B., Munzenrider, J.E., Carter, B,L. Contribution of computed tomography to the treatment of lymphomas. AJR 131:69-73, 1978.
83. Meyer, J.E., Munzenrider, J.E. Computed tomographic demonstration of internal mammary lymph node metastasis in patients with locally recurrent breast carcinoma. Radiology 139:661-663, 1981.
84. Webb, W.R., Glazer, G.M., Gamsu, G. Computed tomography of the normal pulmonary hilum. J Comput Assist Tomogr 5:476-484, 1981.
85. Webb, W.R., Gamsu, G., Glazer, G.M., Computed tomography of the abnormal pulmonary hilum. J Comput Assist Tomogr 5:485-490, 1981.
86. Glazer, G.M., Francis, I.R., Gebarski, K., Samuels, B,I,, Sorensen, K.W. Dynamic incremental computed tomography in evaluation of the pulmonary hila. J Comput Assist Tomogr 7:59-64, 1983.
87. Kaplan, H.S. Hodgkin's disease. Second Edition, Harvard Press, Cambridge, 1980.
88. Castellino, R.A., Filly, R., Blank, N. Routine full lung tomography in the initial staging and treatment planning of patients with Hodgkin's disease and non-Hodgkin's lymphoma. Cancer 38:1130-1136, 1976.
89. North, L.B., Fuller, L.M., Hagemeister, F.B., Rodger, R.W., Butler, J.J., Schullenberger, C.C. Importance of initial mediastinal adenopathy in Hodgkin's ;disease. AJR 138:229-235, 1982.

90. Schaner, E.G., Chang, A.E., Doppman, J.L., et al. Comparison of computed and conventional whole lung tomography in detecting pulmonary nodules. A prospective radiologic and pathologic study. AJR 131:51-54,1978

91. Mandell, G.M., Lantieri, R., Goodman, L.R. Tracheobronchial compression in Hodgkin's lymphoma in children. AJR 139:1167-1170, 1982.

92. Zornoza, J., Cabanillas, F.F., Altoff, T.M., Ordonez, N., Cohen, M. Percutaneous needle biopsy in abdominal lymphoma. AJR 136:97-103, 1981.

93. Lewis, E., Bernardino, M.E., Salvador, P.G., Cabanillas, F., Barnes, P., Thomas, J.L. Post-therapy CT detected mass in lymphoma patients: is it viable tissue? J Comput Assist Tomogr 6:792-795, 1982.

94. Blackledge, G., Mamtora, H., Crowther, D., Isherwood, I., Best, J.J.K. The role of abdominal CT in lymphoma following treatment. Br J Radiol 54:955-960, 1981.

95. Baron, R.L., Sagel, S.S., Baglan, R.J. Thymic cysts following radiation therapy for Hodgkin's disease. Radiology 141:593-597, 1981.

96. Amendola, M.A., Shiraizi, K., Amendola, B.E., Kuhns, L.R., Tisnado, J., Yaghmai, I. Computed tomography of malignant tumors of the osseous pelvis. Computerized Radiol 7:107-111, 1983.

PROGRESS AND PROBLEMS OF THE TREATMENT OF BRAIN STEM GLIOMA,
MEDULLOBLASTOMA, AND CRANIOPHARYNGIOMA IN CHILDHOOD

J. ROBERT CASSADY, M.D., PATRICIA EIFEL, M.D., AND JAMES A. BELLI, M.D.

INTRODUCTION

Central nervous system (CNS) tumors represent the most common group of solid tumors seen in children. Brain stem gliomas, medulloblastomas, and craniopharyngiomas account for more than half of these pediatric neoplasms.[1] Although all three tumors occur in the CNS, they vary markedly in their biology and natural history, and striking differences are noted in their response to current therapy.

The purpose of this chapter is to discuss certain clinical features of these tumors, to assess the radiotherapeutic approaches in use at the Joint Center for Radiation Therapy (JCRT) and elsewhere, and to present the current results of that treatment. Sites and frequency of relapse will be noted and used to suggest potential improvements in current therapeutic management.

BRAIN STEM GLIOMA

Thalamic, midbrain, and brain stem (pons and medulla) gliomas are the most common pediatric CNS tumors seen at the JCRT, and three-fourths of the gliomas located in this region are diagnosed in children.[2] Two-thirds originate in the caudal brain stem (pons and medulla) and one-third in the thalamus and midbrain. A male-to-female ratio of approximately 2-to-1 is usually noted, and most patients are between 5 and 10 years of age at presentation. These tumors are rare before the age of 3 years.[2-5]

Children with these lesions nearly always present with symptoms of headache, nausea, and vomiting. Neurologic signs of cranial nerve or motor dysfunction predominate, and ataxia is also commonly demonstrated.

The diagnosis is usually made radiographically. The noninvasiveness and high yield of computed tomography has made it the diagnostic technique of choice, replacing pneumoencephalography, ventriculography, and arteriography, in most cases.

Biopsy is almost always contraindicated for the following reasons: 1) biopsy in these critical areas is associated with substantial morbidity, 2) when performed, biopsy almost always reveals an astrocytic neoplasm, usually

Published 1983 by Elsevier Science Publishing Co., Inc.
Recent Trends in Radiation Oncology and Related Fields, Amendola and Amendola, Editors

of high grade, 3) the known morphologic heterogeneity of gliomatous neoplasms decreases the value of information gained by biopsy, 4) because these tumors are invariably unresectable, radiation is almost always the treatment of choice, regardless of histologic appearance.

## Treatment techniques

Although spinal seeding has been noted, most commonly with the high-grade lesions at post mortem, this has rarely been a clinically symptomatic occurrence, and radiation fields have usually been designed to encompass the radiographically evident lesion with a wide margin.[6,7]

Using megavoltage equipment such as a 4-6 MeV linear accelerator or a [60]Co unit, most children are treated to a dose of 5000-5600 rads in 150-180 rad fractions over 6-7 weeks. Lateral fields may be supplemented by a stationary vertex or coronal arc field.

Most patients in both groups benefit from radiation therapy, with 70%-80% showing clinical improvement or stabilization. From 1970-1981 we have seen 80 children with these lesions at the Joint Center for Radiation Therapy and Children's Hospital in Boston. Twenty-seven lesions were located in the midbrain, thalamus, or floor of the third ventricle, and 53 were in the pons or medulla. Optic nerve gliomas and apparent dysgerminomas of the suprasellar area were excluded from this analysis. Figure 1A demonstrates 3, 5, and 10-year survival for these patients. The thalamic and midbrain tumors were considered "Group I" lesions, while the caudal brain stem tumors were considered "Group II". A significant difference in the outcome of the two groups is apparent. This difference in survival for similarly treated Group I and II patients has been noted by several authors.[2,4,5] In general, patients with midbrain/thalamic tumors have a 5-year survival which is about twice that of children with caudal brain stem lesions. Overall survival is about 50% (Figure 1B). The reason for these observed differences in prognosis is unclear, although some authors have suggested that they simply reflect varying proportions of high-grade neoplasms.[5]

Local recurrence is still the overwhelming cause of initial relapse and ultimately, death. Although treatment with steroids, cytotoxic chemotherapy regimens, and, on occasion, retreatment with radiation, have produced temporary improvement or stabilization, the ultimate outcome following relapse is invariably death.

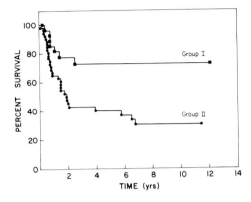

Fig. 1A. Actuarial survival for mid brain, thalamic and hypothalamic patients (Group I) compared to patients with caudal brain stem disease (pons, medulla), Group II.

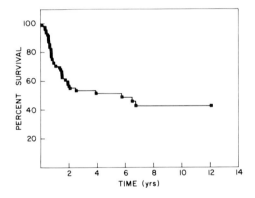

Fig. 1B. Actuarial survival for the entire group of 80 children with mid brain and brain stem tumors.

MEDULLOBLASTOMA

This malignant tumor of the cerebellum usually arises in young people (80% are less than 15 years of age), and it is one of the most common pediatric brain tumors. Males predominate by a 2-to-1 ratio. Most patients present with signs of increased intracranial pressure manifested by nausea, vomiting, and headache combined with ataxia and gait disturbance. Less commonly, visual symptoms and/or cranial nerve palsies are noted.[8]

These neoplasms are characterized by dense, homogeneous infiltrates of cells with dense staining cytoplasm and hyperchromatic nuclei. Occasionally, "pseudorosettes" are seen, as are areas of neuronal differentiation and ganglion cells. Although considerable effort has been made to relate certain pathologic features to prognosis, no convincing correlations have been demonstrated.

Medulloblastoma may spread by means of local extension, CSF dissemination, or by systemic spread to lymph nodes, bone, or bone marrow. The development of a TM staging system by Chang has made comparison between varying institutions and therapies possible (Table 1).[9] In addition to a CT scan,

---

Table 1          STAGING SYSTEM FOR MEDULLOBLASTOMA[9]

---

$T_1$    Tumor less than 3 cm diameter and limited to the classic midline position in the vermis, the roof of the fourth ventricle, and less frequently to the cerebellar hemispheres.

$T_2$    Tumor 3 cm or greater in diameter, further invading one adjacent structure or partially filling the fourth ventricle.

$T_3$    This stage is subdivided into $T_{3A}$ and $T_{3B}$.

       $T_{3A}$:   Tumor further invading two adjacent structures or completely filling the fourth ventricle with extension into the aqueduct of Sylvius, foramen of Magendie, or faramen of Luschka, thus producing marked internal hydrocephalus.

       $T_{3B}$:   Tumor arising from the floor of the fourth ventricle or brainstem and filling the fourth ventricle.

$T_4$    Tumor further spreading through the aqueduct of Sylvius to involve the third ventricle or midbrain, or tumor extending to the upper cervical cord.

$M_0$    No evidence of gross subarachnoid or hematogenous metastases.

$M_1$    Microscopic tumor cells found in cerebrospinal fluid.

$M_2$    Gross nodular seedings demonstrated in the cerebellar, cerebral subarachnoid space, or in the third or lateral ventricles.

$M_3$    Gross nodular seeding in spinal subarachnoid space.

$M_4$    Metastases outside the cerebrospinal axis.

---

the workup following an established diagnosis of medulloblastoma should include cytologic examination of cytocentrifuged cerebrospinal fluid (CSF), myelography, and bone marrow exam. Myelography reveals a significant number of unsuspected spinal canal lesions even in patients with negative CSF cytology.[10] Overt tumor spread beyond the primary site has generally been associated with larger primary lesions, usually measuring more than 3 cm.[11]

Treatment techniques

The purpose of initial surgery is to establish a histologic diagnosis, determine the local extent of tumor, and relieve elevated intracranial pressure. The value of extensive surgical "debulking" procedures has been debated. Most investigators have found a higher survival rate among patients having gross total removal of their tumors than among those having only biopsy prior to irradiation.[9,11] However, these reviews undoubtedly include hidden biases resulting from patient selection, and it is impossible to accurately assess the role of surgery per se in the improved survival of children who have tumor resection. Certainly, surgical procedures that are attended by a high risk of neurologic disability are to be decried.

In patients with known or suspected medulloblastoma, shunting procedures are contraindicated prior to the completion of definitive radiation therapy. Such procedures place the systemic circulation or peritoneal surfaces at unnecessary risk for tumor dissemination. Increased intracranial pressure may be relieved by external drainage or a tapable reservoir system, deferring more definitive decompressive surgery, should it be needed, until the completion of treatment.

Progressive improvements in survival rates have accompanied improvements in radiation therapy techniques. In addition to surgery, posterior fossa irradiation, treatment of the spine as well as the posterior fossa, irradiation of the entire CNS, and most recently, delivery of an increased posterior fossa tumor dose, have all accomplished improved results.[9,11-14]

The use of higher doses (5400-5600 rads) to the posterior fossa was accompanied by increases in radiation dose to the remainder of the CNS neuraxis. It is therefore unknown whether radiation doses greater than 3000 rads to the brain and 2500 rads to the spinal canal (in CSF and myelogram negative patients) have actually contributed to improved survival figures. The added toxicity can be substantial.

A number of authors have stressed the importance of using sophisticated techniques in order to optimize radiotherapeutic management of medullo- blastoma.[9,11-15] These include pretreatment simulation and the use of immobilization techniques that permit reproducibility and precision in treatment. Couch and gantry rotation and moving junction ("feathering") techniques eliminate geometric "hot" and "cold" regions in the treatment volume. Irradiation of the entire CNS neuraxis each day for a significant portion of the overall treatment period avoids recirculation of viable tumor cells into previously irradiated sites.

At the JCRT, patients who have negative CSF cytology and myelography receive a total radiation dose of 2500-2800 rads to the spinal canal, 3500-3750 rads to the cranial contents, and 5400-5500 rads to the posterior fossa. Treatment is delivered in 180-200 rad fractions. Initial irradiation is directed to the posterior fossa for 1500-2000 rads and is followed by treatment of the entire brain and its meninges for 1000-1500 rads. Following this, treatment to the entire neuraxis is commenced and continued until the desired cumulative cranial and spinal canal dose has been delivered. Craniospinal doses are increased for patients with positive cytology or other evidence of CNS spread. Myelographically positive areas are boosted to a total dose of 4500 rads.

To date there is no convincing evidence for the efficacy of adjuvant chemotherapy (vide infra), and chemotherapy has generally not been part of our initial treatment plan. Two randomized trials have yielded generally negative results in properly irradiated patients, and several non-randomized series also have not been encouraging.[16,17] In view of the toxicity of these regimens in intensively irradiated patients, the routine use of adjuvant chemotherapy is not indicated.

It has been our experience and that of other authors that nearly all patients who relapse have recurrence at the primary site, either alone or in combination with other sites.[8,11,12,14] Of 40 failures in one series of patients, 20 involved the posterior fossa alone or in combination with other sites, and 9 were described as "CNS dissemination"[18] Six patients in this series failed solely at the cribiform plate, a finding which suggests technical difficulties in delivering irradiaton to all meningeal sites. Five patients failed systemically. In a more typical series, 11 of the 13 failures occurred in the posterior fossa alone or in combination with other sites.[14]

### Results

In our most recent series, 30%-50% of patients treated for medulloblastoma survive five or more years following irradiation . Disease-free survival gains which accompanied improved radiotherapeutic techniques appear to have been stable with time. More recent increases in radiation dose, especially to the posterior fossa, have clearly improved short-term and intermediate disease-free survival. However, relatively few patients treated with these larger doses are at risk beyond five years, and the durability of these gains is still somewhat in question.

Patients with T1 and T2 lesions fare better than those wth T3 and T4 lesions, almost all of whom ultimately die of tumor.[11] Another consistent finding in our patients and in other series is the grave prognosis of children who present with medulloblastoma at less than two years of age.[19] Most have extensive primary disease at diagnosis and almost all die of rapid tumor regrowth and spread.

Careful examination of survival curves presented by Bloom, Harisiadis and Chang reveals the importance of relatively long term followup of these patients, especially for children who are older at the time of diagnosis.[9,11] Older children and adults initially appear to have better survival. However, between three and five years, survival curves cross for these two groups, and the younger patients (excluding those less than 2 years old) ultimately do better. For this reason, assessment of survival after a Collins risk period (age at diagnosis + 9 months) yields more secure results, as very few children in any series have recurred beyond the Collins interval. In this respect, the series of Kopelson et al. is encouraging for the older patients.[20]

CRANIOPHARYNGIOMA

This benign brain tumor is a relatively common childhood neoplasm and is thought to represent neoplastic growth of an embryologic rest. Symptoms result from growth by cell division and cyst formation and from reactive gliosis. Sixty to seventy-five percent of patients are less than 15 years of age at diagnosis.[21] Visual symptoms and signs are noted in about 75% of both pediatric and adult patients. Evidence of increased intracranial pressure (headache, vomiting, papilledema) is seen relatively commonly in children, as is growth or developmental delay. Dementia is a more frequent presenting symptom in adults. Evaluation should include a high resolution CT scan of the sella and suprasellar regions as well as a thorough eye examination including formal visual field testing, with mapping of results. Electrolytes, endocrine and growth parameters and psychologic and memory functions should be tested at presentation.

Radiographically evident calcification is nearly always seen in childhood cases, although its presence is less frequent in adult patients.[22]

Treatment techniques

For at least two decades there has been a major controversy over the optimal management of this lesion. Prior to the administration of exogenous steroids, operative mortality precluded surgical attempts to remove the tumor. Relatively primitive radiation therapy equipment also impeded the ability of the therapist to treat these lesions adequately. Kramer was the first to demonstrate the efficacy of high dose megavoltage irradiation in controlling these lesions after conservative surgery.[23] Matson subsequently published his results following radical excision in children, and the resulting controversy has continued.[24] However, even technically facile neurosurgeons are unable to remove all tumor in many patients. Furthermore, a review of the long-term followup of children in Matson's original series demonstrated an overall disease-free survival of only 54% (22/40).[25] These discouraging results, combined with the significant morbidity occasioned by radical surgical attempts, have increasingly focused attention on potentially more effective and less morbid treatment with conservative surgery and irradiation. The widespread availability of megavoltage radiation equipment with rotational capabilities and recent data regarding late neurologic and psychophysiologic sequelae of radical surgery have further encouraged this trend.[26]

Usually diagnosis can be obtained and decompression accomplished via a transphenoidal approach with biopsy and cyst aspiration. On occasion, shunting procedures are still required. On very rare occasions, in very young patients with limited lesions, a subfrontal complete removal of tumor can be accomplished with acceptable morbidity.

Following diagnosis, decompression and stabilization, radiation therapy should commence. We have routinely used a coronal rotational plan ("arc-wedge") which results in an excellent isodose distribution. Patients, regardless of age, receive 5400-5500 rads in 150-180 rad fractions over 6-7 weeks. We do not feel that higher doses are necessary for adults. Fields must be designed to incorporate the entire gross tumor volume plus an adequate margin within the 100% isodose. Surgical experience has demonstrated the ability of this tumor to spread microscopically beyond grossly uninvolved areas.[27] We have also noted rapid reaccummulation of cyst fluid and therefore, recommend treatment of the original (pre-cyst aspiration) volume with irradiation.

Several current series show prolonged disease-free survival and excellent functional results in nearly all children treated with adequate techniques and doses.[28-30]

At the JCRT we have seen and irradiated 40 children with craniopharyngioma. Twenty-five of these children were treated primarily with irradiation after conservative surgery, in all but one instance by the transphenoidal approach.

Four patients with a classic radiographic appearance for craniopharyngioma and no prominent cystic component or evidence of ventricular obstruction were treated solely with irradiation. All 25 children are living without evidence of disease activity (Figure 2). Several children required a second (or, rarely, third) cyst aspiration within the first 2-3 months after irradiation because of reaccumulation of fluid within the cyst. Following this period, all but one of the 25 have required no further intervention and have had progressive decrease of mass and cyst size. One patient with a massive tumor and cyst extending into the posterior fossa has required several cyst aspirations but has not had evidence of solid tumor progression. Intelligence and mental function in these children appear normal.[26]

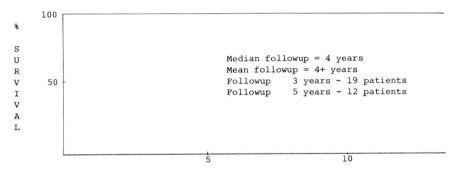

CRANIOPHARYNGIOMA SURVIVAL (1972-1981) 25 PATIENTS
Treated with Conservative Surgery/Radical Radiation Therapy at
Joint Center for Radiation Therapy/Children's Hospital

Median followup = 4 years
Mean followup = 4+ years
Followup    3 years - 19 patients
Followup    5 years - 12 patients

YEARS AFTER TREATMENT

Fig. 2. Actuarial survival for 25 patients treated with conservative (21) or no (4) surgery and definitive irradiation.

Fifteen children have been irradiated after prior "definitive" surgery, with documented recurrence (10) or immediately following an attempt at radical surgical removal, with known gross or microscopic residual tumor (5). All but 2 are currently living, without disease activity. One child died suddenly one year after treatment, without post mortem evidence of tumor, apparently of electrolyte imbalance which was secondary to hypothalamic and hypopituitary difficulties related to initial tumor extent. One Iranian child was treated here but has been lost to followup due to the current political situation. One of 13 children known to be living was treated elsewhere following incomplete surgery complicated by blindness. She received 5000 rads to a small field. She recurred locally a second time 3 years later and was retreated at the JCRT and is currently living 3+ years following re-irradiation. In general, the functional status of many of the children treated after radical surgery was considerably worse than that of those treated after conservative surgery.

DISCUSSION

These three brain tumors of children represent three very different clinical problems. Craniopharyngioma is a benign tumor and hence represents a purely local problem. With conservative surgery and high dose megavoltage irradiaton, the great majority of children obtain not only tumor control, but an excellent functional result as well. The major problem, therefore, appears to be one of educating physicians as to the advantages of using conservative surgery followed by definitive irradiation in the treatment of craniopharyngioma.

Unfortunately, therapy for both brain stem gliomas and medulloblastomas continues to be unsatisfactory. For both lesions, local control of the primary tumor continues to be the major obstacle to improved results. Anecdotal use of increased doses of radiation has not appeared to produce improved results for the brain stem group and may not warrant the attendant risk of brain necrosis. Similarly, use of concurrent or adjuvant chemotherapy regimens has not yet resulted in improved results. Because of the location of these gliomas, improvements in surgical technique do not appear to offer much hope. Hyperfractionated radiation schedules appear to improve somewhat the results for high-grade gliomas in adults and may provide a promising experimental approach to these resistant neoplasms.

It is important, however, to not allow pessimism to result in therapeutic nihilism. Nearly half of the thalamic and midbrain group have functionally excellent extended survival beyond 5-10 years, as do at least 25% of the brain stem group. Although treatment with irradiation is far from optimal, successfully treated patients testify to its value.

The treatment of medulloblastoma offers some interesting problems. Despite the use of progressively more radical and more toxic craniospinal treatment, primary tumor control continues to represent the major therapeutic challenge. Questions that should or are currently being addressed are:

What are the necessary and sufficient radiation doses to the spinal cord and brain (other than the posterior fossa) for patients with varying extents of disease?

Can an effective adjuvant chemotherapy program be developed in conjunction with neuraxis radiation therapy?[16,17]

Is there a place for "second-look" surgery, following a significant response to radiation and/or chemotherapy? (This is a particularly valid question for patients who present with T3 or T4 lesions, almost all of whom eventually succumb to their disease. This would be a promising approach if reports of improved success after total surgical removal can be substantiated after correction for tumor extent.)

Can adjuvant chemotherapy permit decreased radiation doses to the spinal canal and supratentorial brain without altering survival?
This might significantly decrease morbidity, particularly in very young children.

These and other questions can be answered only by carefully constructed clinical studies directed towards improving the therapeutic results in this relatively common and often devastating disease.

REFERENCES

1. Kornblith, P.L., Walker, M.D., Cassady, J.R. Neoplasms of the central nervous system in Cancer: Principles and Practice of Oncology, chapter 33:1181-1253. DeVita, V., Hellman, S., Rosenberg, S., ed., Lippincott, Philadelphia, 1982.
2. Greenberger, J.S., Cassady, J.R., Levene, M.B. Radiation therapy of thalamic, mid brain, and brain stem gliomas. Radiology 122:463-468, 1977.
3. Shin, K.H., Fisher, G., Webster, J.H. Brain stem tumors in children. J. Can Assoc Radiol 30:77-78, 1979.
4. Sheline, G.E., Phillips, T.L., Boldrey, E. The therapy of brain stem tumors. Radiology 93:664-670, 1965.
5. Marsa, G.W., Goffinet, D.R., Rubinstein, L.R., et al. Megavoltage irradiation in the treatment of gliomas of the brain and spinal cord. Cancer 36:1681-1689, 1975.
6. Bryan, P. CSF seeding of intracranial tumors: a study of 96 cases. Clin Radiol 25:355-360, 1974.
7. Gilles, F. Personal communication.
8. Bloom, H.J.G., Wallace, E.W.K., Heuk, J.M. The treatment and prognosis of medulloblastoma in children: A study of 82 verified cases. Am J Roentgenol Radium Ter Nucl Med 105:43-62, 1969.
9. Chang, C.H., Housepian, E.M., Herbert, C. Jr. An operative staging system and a megavoltage radiotherapeutic technique for cerebellar medulloblastoma. Radiology 93:1351-1359, 1969.
10. Deutsch, M.D, Reigel, D.H. The value of myelography in the management of childhood medulloblastoma. Cancer 45:2194-2197, 1980.
11. Harisiadis, L., Chang, C.H. Medulloblastoma in children: a correlation between staging and results of treatment. Int J Rad Oncol Biol Phys 2:833-841, 1977.

12. Landberg, T.G., Lingren, M.L., Cavalinn-Stahl, E.K., et al. Improvements in radiotherapy of medulloblastoma, 1946-1975. Cancer 45:670-678, 1980.

13. Smith, C.E., Long, D.M., Jones, T.K., et al. Medulloblastoma: an analysis of time-dose relationships and recurrence patterns. Cancer 32:722-728, 1973.

14. Cumberland, R.L. Medulloblastoma: treatment results and effects on normal tissues. Cancer 43:1014-1020, 1979.

15. Van Dyk, J. Medulloblastoma: treatment techniques and radiation dosimetry. Int J Rad Oncol Biol Phys 2:993-1005, 1977.

16. Bloom, H.J.G. Prospects for increasing survival in children with medulloblastoma: present and future studies. Multidisciplin Aspects Br Tum Ther 1:245-259, 1979.

17. Evans, A.E., Anderson, J., Chang, C, et al. Adjuvant chemotherapy for medulloblastoma and ependymoma. Multidisciplin Aspects Br Tum Ther 1:219-222, 1979.

18. Jereb, B. Patterns of failure in patients with medulloblastoma. Cancer 50:2941-2947, 1982.

19. Allen, J.C., Epstein, F. Medulloblastoma and other primary malignant neuroectodermal tumors of the CNS. J Neurosurg 57:446-451, 1982.

20. Kopelson, G., Linggood, R.M., Kleinman, G.M. Medulloblastoma: Identification and implications of prognostic subgroups. Cancer In press.

21. Bartlett, J.R. Craniopharyngiomas, a summary of 85 cases. J Neurol Neurosurg Psychiat 34:37-41, 1971.

22. Strand, R. Personal communication.

23. Kramer, S., McKissock, W., Concannon, J.P. Craniopharyngiomas: treatment by combined surgery and radiation therapy. J Neurosurg 17:217-226, 1961.

24. Matson, D.D., Crigler, J.R. Jr. Management of craniopharyngiomas in children. J Neurosurg 30:377-390,1969.

25. Katz, E.G. Late results of radical excision of craniopharyngiomas in children. J Neurosurg 42:86-93, 1975.

26. Cavazutti, V., Fischer, E.G., Welch, K., Belli, J.A. Neurological and psychophysiological sequelae following different treatments of cranio-pharyngiomas in children. J Neurosurg In press.

27. Sweet, W.H. Radical surgical treatment of craniopharyngioma Clin Neurosurg 23:52-79, 1975.

28. Bloom, H.J.G., Harmer, E. Craniopharyngiomas. Br Med J 1:288-289, 29 April, 1972.

29. Bloom, H.J.G., Combined modality therapy for intracranial tumors. Cancer 35:111-120, 1975.

30. Kramer, S. Southard, M., Mansfield, C.M. Radiotherapy in the treatment of craniopharyngiomas: further experiences and late results. Am J Roentgenol 103:44-52, 1968.

INTERMITTENT AND CONTINUOUS REGIONAL CHEMOTHERAPY FOR CNS TUMORS

WILLIAM F. CHANDLER, M.D., HARRY S. GREENBERG, M.D.,
AND WILLIAM D. ENSMINGER,M.D.

## INTRODUCTION

In this chapter we are reporting our experience in treating two types of malignant central nervous system neoplasms with intermittent and/or continuous regional chemotherapy. We have treated Grade III and IV malignant astrocytomas (glioblastoma multiforme) via the internal carotid artery with intermittent and continuous intra-arterial chemotherapy, and meningeal carcinomatosis via the ventricular system with continuous chemotherapy.

## MALIGNANT ASTROCYTOMAS

Grade III and IV malignant astrocytomas are uniformly and rapidly fatal with current medical and surgical management. The best results with maximum surgical resection followed by radiation therapy and systemic chemotherapy achieve only a median survival of 52 weeks.[1-3] These discouraging results warrant aggressive and innovative new approaches. There are several characteristics of malignant gliomas that make them particularly attractive for regional intra-arterial chemotherapy. First, they are tumors which in the majority of cases receive their blood supply via a single carotid artery. Secondly, they rarely metastasize and almost always cause brain destruction and ultimately death of the patient by continued growth within their primary location. Thirdly, malignant gliomas have been shown to have a steep dose-response curve for a variety of chemotherapeutic agents. This last point leads to the impression that if there were some way to deliver a greater concentration of drug to the tumor without inflicting toxicity, then perhaps a more significant response could be achieved. Crafts et al.[4] demonstrated that a fourfold increase in peak drug concentration in the brain could be achieved with intracarotid bichloroethylnitrosourea (BCNU) as opposed to intravenous BCNU.

Based on these observations we have initiated clinical trials to administer BCNU and other chemotherapeutic agents via the carotid artery in patients with malignant astrocytomas. In addition to the bolus administration of traditional

©1983 Elsevier Science Publishing Co., Inc.
Recent Trends in Radiation Oncology and Related Fields, Amendola and Amendola, Editors

cycle, non-specific, alkylating agents such as BCNU, we have, in a few selected instances, also given cycle specific antimetabolites on a continuous basis, using a new fully implantable pump system.

## Intermittent Carotid Infusions

Bolus infusions of BCNU have been infused directly into the internal carotid artery (ICA) on 73 occasions in 23 patients with primary malignant astrocytomas. Of these infusions, 59 have been given via a transfemoral selective catheterization of the ICA by our neuroradiologist, and 14 infusions have been accomplished via the side port of the implantable pump (see below). Doses of BCNU ranged from 200 to 300 $mg/m^2$ and these were administered over 12-20 minutes. Initially the drug was dissolved in ethanol, but due to eye toxicity the solvent was switched to a larger volume of water. Intra-arterial BCNU was given every 6 weeks, up to a maximum dose of 1500 mg.

One series of 10 patients received intra-arterial BCNU immediately following surgical biopsy with maximum resection and prior to radiation therapy. If the tumors did not respond or progressed, then radiation therapy was instituted. These patients responded to chemotherapy alone for an average of 6.5 months (range = 2-14 months) and to date have an average survival from the time of diagnosis of 12 months (range = 5-28 months).

A second series of 8 patients received intra-arterial BCNU to treat recurrent malignant astrocytomas after receiving a full course of radiation therapy. They have all died from their tumors, but responded for an average of 5 months (range = 3-6.5 months) to chemotherapy. Two additional patients with large unresectable tumors received radiation and chemotherapy concomitantly, but died at 5 and 8 months after diagnosis.

Three other patients with recurrent grade I and II astrocytomas were treated after failure of radiation therapy 7, 48, and 54 months after initial diagnosis. The patients have responded for an average of 11 months after initiation of chemotherapy.

Complications of intra-arterial BCNU chemotherapy have been limited to changes in the fundus of the eye, which were probably related to the concentration of the ethanol in the injected solution.[7] Nine patients were noted to have ipsilateral fundal hemorrhages and exudates, with four of these progressing to blindness. Patients demonstrated these symptoms 2 to 14 weeks after the second or third course of intra-arterial BCNU. These ocular complications have been essentially eliminated since the concentration of ethanol was reduced from 2 ml/100 mg BCNU to 0.75 ml/100 mg BCNU. More recently we have tried using sterile water as the solvent to further reduce this risk and possibly reduce the eye pain experienced during the infusion.

## Continuous Carotid Infusions

A fully implantable continuous internal carotid artery infusion system was placed in 6 patients.[6] In these patients the carotid bifurcation was exposed under general anesthesia and a silastic catheter introduced retrograde down the distally ligated external carotid artery to the carotid bifurcation. The catheter tip was left flush with the opening into the common carotid artery and secured in place with ties around the external carotid artery. The proximal catheter was then tunneled subcutaneously to an infraclavicular subcutaneous pocket and attached to the Infusaid Model 400 pump (Infusaid Corporation, Sharon, MA). The pump consists of two chambers separated by a mobile diaphragm (Figure 1). The lower charging fluid chamber contains Freon, which is in the gaseous state at body temperature. The upper chamber contains the drug to be infused and can be refilled percutaneously through a self-sealing septum. The pressure exerted in filling the drug chamber compresses the charging fluid chamber, causing the gas to go into a liquid state. Then, at body temperature, the liquid Freon slowly reverts back to a gas, exerting a constant pressure on the drug chamber. A small outlet

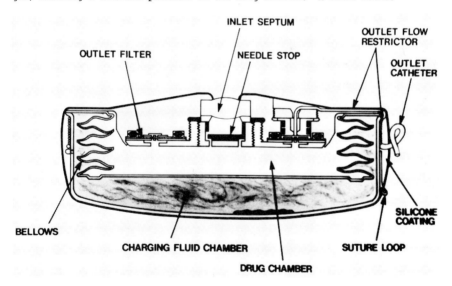

Fig. 1. Cross-section diagram of Model 100 Infusaid pump.

catheter leading from the drug chamber provides a constant resistance, thus discharging the drug solution at a specific constant rate, and at a presssure exceding systolic arterial pressure. The drug chamber holds 47 ml of fluid and flows constantly at approximately 2.5 ml per day. The Model 400 also contains a side port for bolus intra-arterial injections.

After initial testing in animals[6] this system has been placed without apparent complication, in 6 patients. The pumps have remained functional for over 22 months with no sign of infection or neurologic deficit from emboli or stenosis. Angiograms and autopsies have shown the bifurcation region to be free of thrombus formation. When drugs are not being infused the pump is refilled with heparinized saline.

All of the pump patients received from 1 to 4 doses of BCNU (200 mg/m$^2$) via the side port, and on three occasions either 2'-deoxy-5-fluorouridine (FUdR) or dichloromethotrexate (DCMTX) was continuously infused via the drug chamber. FUdR was infused in one patient at 6.5 mg/day for 70 days and in another for 14 days at 4.8 mg/day. One patient received DCMTX for 25 days at 3 mg/day. No side effects were noted with DCMTX infusion, and one of the patients receiving FUdR developed a dermatitis over the forehead region and so the drug was stopped at 14 days.

Of the 6 patients, 4 died at 6 to 19 months after diagnosis and 2 were still living at 20 and 22 months, for an average survival to date of 15 months. Although these numbers are far too small to comment on the therapeutic efficacy of this system, we have demonstrated that patients tolerate this internal carotid continuous infusion system quite well. This system provides a totally implantable, purely internal, carotid continuous infusion, and will provide an opportunity in the future for a variety of chemotherapeutic agents to be given, both by continuous and bolus infusion.

MENINGEAL CARCINOMATOSIS

The incidence of meningeal spread of malignant neoplasms has increased over the past few decades, due to better control of the primary site of involvement. This neoplastic involvement of the central nervous system carries a prognosis measured in only a few months.[7] The blood brain barrier limits many system-ically administered drugs from reaching therapeutic levels in the cerebral spinal fluid (CSF). Because of this, bolus injections into the CSF of chemo-therapeutic agents such as methotrexate (MTX) or cytosine arabinoside (Ara-C) have been used for lymphomas, leukemias and breast cancers.[8] Direct intra-ventricular injections may provide CSF drug concentrations that are 100 to 1000-fold greater than corresponding plasma levels.[9]

Because intermittent bolus drug injections do not provide a constant effective drug concentration in the CSF, we have used the implantable pump system described above to achieve a slow continuous infusion of drugs into the CSF via a ventricular catheter.[10] This system involves placement of a frontal ventricular catheter attached at the trephine site to a small reservoir, and via a side arm on the reservoir to an Infusaid Model 100 pump. The Model 100 has no side port since the reservoir serves as a port for bolus infusions as well as CSF sampling.

The pump system has been placed in 8 patients with meningeal carcinomatosis without infections or complications related to the system. Five of the patients had breast cancer as a primary, one a lung tumor, one leukemia, and one a lymphoma. The patients received one or more infusions of either MTX, Ara-C, or FUdR via the ventricular pump system. Six of the eight patients ultimately cleared their CSF and died of their systemic disease. Of interest is that there were 2 patients who did not respond to the traditional drugs MTX and Ara-C, but did clear their CSF with a continuous infusion of FUdR. Again this series is too small to allow comparison with intermittent intraventricular drug injections, but it apppears clear that this system is safe and reliable and that there are a number of patients who will fail to respond to traditional medications, but may respond to the continuous infusion of agents such as FUdR.

REFERENCES
1.  Walker, D., Green, S.B., Byar, D.P., et al. Randomized comparisons of radiotherapy and nitrosureas for the treatment of malignant glioma after surgery. N Engl J Med 303:1323-1329, 1980.
2.  Walker, M., Alexander, E., Hunt, V., et al. Evaluation of BCNU and/or radiotherapy in the treatment of anaplastic gliomas. J Neurosurg 49:333-343, 1978.
3.  Wilson, C.B. Brain tumors. N Engl J Med 300:1469-1570, 1979.
4.  Crafts D.C, Levin V.A., Nielson, S. Intracarotid BCNU: A toxicity study in six Rhesus monkeys. Cancer Treat Rep 60:541-545, 1976.
5.  Shingleton, B.H, Bienfang, D.C., Albert, D.M., et al. Ocular toxicity associated with BCNU. Arch Ophthalmol 100:1766-1772, 1982.
6.  Phillips, T.W., Chandler, W.F., Kindt, G.W., et al. A new implantable intracarotid drug deliver system for the treatment of malignant gliomas. Neurosurgery 11:213-2189, 1982.
7.  Shapiro, W.R., Posner,J.B., Ushio, Y., et al. Treatment of meningeal neoplasms. Cancer Treat Rep 61:733-743, 1977.
8.  Bleyer W.A. Current status of intrathecal chemotherapy for human meningeal neoplasms. Nat Cancer Inst Monogr 46:171-178, 1977.
9.  Shapiro, W.R., Young, E., Mehta, B.M. Methotrexate: Distribution in cerebrospinal fluid after intravenous, ventricular and lumbar injections. N Eng J Med 293:161-166, 1975.
10. Dakhil, S., Ensminger W.D., Kindt G.W., et al. An implanted system for intraventricular drug infusion in central nervous system tumors. Cancer Treat Rep 65:401-411, 1981.

MANAGEMENT OF CNS TUMORS IN CHILDREN:    SURGERY


JOAN L. VENES, M.D.


INTRODUCTION

Tumors of the central nervous system account for a significant percentage of all pediatric tumors, nevertheless, only 1400 new cases are reported annually,[1] and about 70% of these are gliomas. Fifty-five percent of all pediatric brain tumors occur in the posterior fossa with an equal incidence of cerebellar astrocytoma, medulloblastoma and brainstem glioma. Only the more common tumors will be discussed in this chapter. Earlier diagnosis, improved surgical techniques and the increased utilization of radiation therapy and chemotherapy have combined to significantly improve the duration and quality of survival in this age group.

PREOPERATIVE EVALUATION AND MANAGEMENT

In the infant and young child, tumors are frequently very large at the time of diagnosis. History is often nonspecific. In tumors of the posterior fossa, hydrocephalus leads to irritability and/or lethargy, gait disturbance and in the young child an increase in head circumference. Vomiting may be a prominent symptom. Tumors in and about the optic chiasm may cause severe loss of visual acuity before they are recognized in the pre-schooler. Tumors of the cerebral hemisphere may cause minimal dysfunction until large enough to cause significant increased intracranial pressure at which time clinical differentiation from posterior fossa lesions may be difficult. Not infrequently, these tumors may present with seizures. Deep thalamic gliomas may present with focal motor deficit as the sole complaint. The infant and young child cannot cooperate in examinations of fine motor function and often a high index of suspicion is necessary to interpret subtle findings on examination.

The relatively non-invasive nature of CT scanning and its wide availability has led to earlier diagnosis of many lesions. The impact of earlier surgical intervention has been particularly noteworthy in medulloblastoma where diagnosis prior to invasion of the brainstem permits total gross tumor removal using magnification techniques. Radical tumor excision in medulloblastoma is

Published 1983 by Elsevier Science Publishing Co., Inc.
Recent Trends in Radiation Oncology and Related Fields, Amendola and Amendola, Editors

reported to be associated with increased length of survival.[2] Angiography is now reserved for the atypical posterior fossa lesion and tumors of the cerebral hemispheres.

Preoperative identification of intracranial neoplasms of germ cell origin is possible using highly sensitive radioimmunoassay techniques for the detection of specific markers in serum and cerebrospinal fluid. Embryonal cell tumors (endodermal sinus tumors) produce alpha feto protein (AFP) and the beta subunit of human chorionic gonadotropin (HCG), choriocarcinoma (found in some intra-cranial teratomas) produces HCG.[3] High levels of HCG have also been reported in a girl with an ectopic pinealoma and precocious puberty.[4] The polyamines, putrescine and spermatadine, have proven useful in the early detection of recurrent medulloblastoma.[5]

Initiation of preoperative corticosteroid therapy improves brain compliance, lessens intracranial pressure and protects the brain against surgical insult.[6] The dynamics of these beneficial effects are widely accepted, but remain poorly understood. The efficacy of corticosteroids in cerebral gliomas is similar to that seen in adults and the usefulness of corticosteroids in tumors of the hypo-thalamo-pituitary axis is well documented. In children with posterior fossa tumors and hydrocephalus, administration of cortico-steroids preoperatively is associated with a fall in intracranial pressure and marked symptomatic improvement.[7]

Preoperative shunting has been used rather extensively in the management of children with hydrocephalus secondary to cerebellar medulloblastoma and appeared to significantly improve operative mortality and postoperative morbidity.[8] Reports of systemic metastases[9] and upward herniation[10] have led some surgeons to abandon this approach except in the severely ill child. Earlier dianosis and the efficacy of preoperative corticosteroids have combined to decrease the need for this procedure.

External ventricular drainage begun either preoperatively or intraopera-tively is generally used in patients without a shunt. In these patients monitoring of cerebrospinal fluid drainage in the early postoperative period allows one to make a reliable decision concerning, the need for a postoperative shunt. The patient for whom postoperative radiation and/or chemotherapy is indicated, every effort should be made to avoid shunt placement during periods of immune suppression.

INTRAOPERATIVE MANAGEMENT

Significant advances in anesthesia techniques and the understanding of intracranial pressure/cerebral blood flow relationships have contributed to improving the safety of intracranial surgery in the pediatric age group. Hyperventilation to decrease intracranial pressure is a standard technique. Intravenous induction with a rapid acting barbiturate is extremely valuable in patients with intracranial hypertension. The use of cerebrospinal fluid and osmotic diuretics allows for maximum surgical exposure with reduced need for traction. Although the sitting position is still quite popular with most general neurosurgeons for tumors of the posterior fossa, it has been largely abandoned in the pediatric population. The prone position has several distinct advantages in pediatrics, chiefly improved cardiovascular reserve and easier temperature control.

Improved or innovative instrumentation has also facilitated intracranial surgery. Increased illumination in the depth of the field, the ability to visualize small perforating vessels and ease of differentiation between normal brain tissue and the leading edge of tumor have made the operating microscope indispensable to the pediatric neurosurgeon. The Cavitron Ultrasound Aspirator (CUSA) allows for reduction of tumor mass without retraction of surrounding brain.[12] It is of particular value in the tougher, non-suckable tumors in which attempts at resection have, in the past, caused significant edema in the underlying brain due, in part, to manipulation of the tumor.

Identification of deep gliomas by intraoperative ultrasonography has proven invaluable for safe biopsy of these surgically inaccessible lesions. Ultrasound can also be used for accurate catheter placement when drainage of a cyst is indicated and for the localization of subcortical lesions which have not altered the surface anatomy.[13]

Hall and coworkers in 1971 described bloodless incisions of tissue using the $CO_2$ laser.[14] In this country the $CO_2$ laser is the most widely used of the available lasers. (The YAG and argon lasers have certain specific advantages which make them a useful addition to the $CO_2$ laser, but their restricted applicability and expense have limited their utilization.) The $CO_2$ laser facilitates resection along critical neural structures and clearly makes feasible procedures which, with other instrumentation, would be impossible. It has been estimated that 10-15% of all patients undergoing neurosurgical procedures would benefit from the use of the laser at some point in the operative procedure.

Technical problems and difficulty with interpretation of data have limited the widespread use of evoked responses. However, improved averaging techniques and computer assisted data analysis are prompting reinvestigation of their clinical usefulness. Visual evoked responses are valuable aids in the surgery of craniopharyngioma and other lesions near or involving the optochiasmatic tract. Brainstem evoked responses may be helpful in surgery involving the brainstem or adjacent structures.[15]

The use of the stereotactic head holder and CT scanner allows the accurate determination of coordinates for the biopsy of deep gliomas.[16] When appropriate, this can be followed by implantation of radioactive seeds.[17] It remains to be proven whether or not brachytherapy for certain lesions affords significant improvement over results obtained with conventional radiotherapy.

SURGICAL CONSIDERATIONS

Medulloblastoma. A midline surgical plane is easily developed in children in whom the brainstem is not invaded and protection of structures lying beneath the floor of the fourth ventricle is readily accomplished. Invasion of the brainstem, however, limits the dissection in this area and an attempt to totally resect the tumor under these conditions is inadvisable. Re-establishment of cerebrospinal fluid circulation is almost always possible, although development of basilar arachnoiditis and symptomatic communicating hydrocephalus make shunting a necessity in 20-30% of children. Resection under magnification can be done laterally and superiorly with minimal morbidity usually limited to gait dysfunction, nystagmus and occasional diplopia. As noted, the ability to achieve a gross total tumor removal appears to correlate well with the length of survival.

Brainstem Glioma. Computed tomography has made the diagnosis of these lesions far simpler and allows us to identify atypical lesions e.g. cyst or hematoma which may benefit from surgical intervention.[18] Necrosis and cyst formation following radiation therapy may also be amenable to surgical palliation with minimal morbidity using the operating microscope.[19] The devastating sequelae once commonly seen following surgery in the region of the brainstem are infrequent with modern techniques. A subset of benign exophytic brainstem gliomas has been identified by Hoffman et al.[20] They stressed the accessibility of these lesions and their benign course following subtotal surgical resection.

Craniopharyngioma. This tumor is closely adherent to the tuber space cinereum and can infiltrate the adjacent brain and hypothalamus. Elsewhere the tumor is covered by meninges and is distinct from brain tissue. The operating microscope has been invaluable in allowing radical resection and dissection of the filmy adhesions between the capsule and adjacent structures. The major limiting factor in total removal is adherence to the internal carotid artery and posterior communicating artery. Generally the capsule, once freed from the optic nerve and chiasm and the surrounding blood vessels, can be pulled off the hypothalamus, sacrificing the tuber cinereum and pituitary stalk.[21] Diabetes insipidus is almost invariably present in those patients in whom total removal has been obtained.

Opticochiasmatic and Hypothalamic Glioma. Biopsy of these lesions (usually via a subfrontal approach) is a relatively benign procedure with negligible postoperative morbidity. However, controversy continues over the management of the lesion in the very young child in whom radiation to this area is associated with significant long-term morbidity. Many neurosurgeons have adopted an expectant attitude in the child less than three years of age and withhold radiation unless there is documented worsening of the patient's condition either clinically or radiologically. Why, then, the need for biopsy?[22] Differentiation from a suprasellar germinoma may be very difficult and the sensitivity of these lesions to cisplatin makes differentation vitally important. Occasionally a solid craniopharyngioma or the rare meningioma in the child with von Recklinghausen's syndrome will mimic a hypothalamic glioma. The need for identification of these potentially resectable lesions is self evident. In the uncommon lesion in which there is pre-chiasmatic involvement intracranially from a unilateral optic nerve glioma, successful resection back to 5 mm anterior to the chiasm has been accomplished.[23]

Pinealoma. The high mortality and postoperative morbidity associated with the operative approach to lesions in the pineal region led to a conservative approach in which shunting was done for control of hydrocephalus followed by radiation therapy.[24] Before CT scanning became available, judgement as to the effectiveness of radiation therapy was usually based on clinical assessment and survival. It was not possible (except with invasive techniques such as ventriculography) to separate the radio-resistant benign tumor e.g. teratoma, in whom shunting produced resolution of symptoms and the exquisitely radiosensitive pinealoma. Improved anesthetic techniques and the use of the operating microscope has allowed the neurosurgeon to approach this area with minimal morbidity and negligible mortality.[25] Consequently, two lines of therapy evolved: 1) surgical exploration of all lesions, and 2) a low dose of radiation is given to the tumor, if there is prompt decrease in tumor size, indicating that the lesion is a highly sensitive pinealoma then further radiation would be done without surgery. Lack of response would indicate the need for surgical exploration.

As noted earlier, certain rare tumors may have serum and cerebrospinal fluid markers which allow definitive identification. Exploration is not indicated in these tumors.

Cerebellar Astrocytoma. As with most pediatric tumors these lesions tend to be quite large. However, the majority are totally resectable. Recurrence rates have been quite variable with some series reporting a 30% recurrence rate at 5 years.[26] Conversely, residual tumor may be followed for many years without evidence of increase on CT scan. Winston, Gilles et al.[26] looked at this vexing problem and devised a classification which they felt had prognostic significance.

Supratentorial Gliomas. Astrocytomas of the cerebral hemisphere and thalamus make up from 10% to 15% of pediatric tumors[27] and the common tumors of adulthood e.g. glioblastoma and metastases are. rarely encountered.

Cerebral astrocytomas are usually poorly defined and generally avascular. On occasion they may infiltrate the corpus callosum and involve both hemispheres in which case they are unresectable. In some cases the tumor is surrounded by a pseudocapsule of gliotic brain tissue and an attempt at total resection can be made. Unfortunately, it is usually only those tumors situated in a polar location amenable to lobectomy in which total removal can be achieved with certainty. Subtotal resection of large tumors associated with brain shifts and/or intracranial hypertension, may give symptomatic relief for prolonged periods. Debulking of tumor mass is also indicated to enhance the efficacy of radiation therapy.

Deep gliomas (most often in the thalamus) may present a technically difficult surgical problem. Posterior thalamic lesions can be satisfactorily debulked and occasionally totally removed with safety using a posterior cortical incision opening the trigone.[28] CT guided stereotactic biopsy[29] or biopsy using intraoperative ultrasonography[13] may be helpful when the diagnosis is in doubt. These methods also facilitate drainage of large cystic gliomas of the thalamus with relief of symptoms.

POSTOPERATIVE MANAGEMENT

CT scan done within 24 to 48 hours of surgery is helpful in evaluating the extent of tumor resection. After 48 hours enchancement of the area in which the blood brain barrier has been temporarily altered by surgery complicates the accurate assessment of tumor resection. Serial CT scans to detect recurrence prior to onset of clinical symptoms is widely used for most tumors. As noted previously, elevation of polyamines in lumbar cerebrospinal fluid is predictive of recurrent medulloblastoma.

The following complications are encountered with a highly variable incidence depending, in part, on the difficulty of the surgical lesions referred to and institution and/or neurosurgeon:

Seizures. Are seen most often in cerebral hemisphere tumors adjacent to the sensorimotor strip (in which case seizures are often the presenting complaint). Seizures may also be seen in tumors in which significant frontal lobe retraction has been necessary. Prophylactic anticonvulsive therapy is begun preoperatively in these cases.

Hydrocephalus. Is seen most often with posterior fossa tumors. It is estimated that 30% - 40% of medulloblastomas and less than 5% of cerebellar astrocytomas will require long-term postoperative shunting.

Increased neurological deficit. This may be related to retraction (particularly in lesions adjacent to the brainstem), compromised vascular supply, postoperative hematoma or mechanical injury to the cranial nerves in the operative field.

Craniopharyngioma resection has been associated with postoperative seizures, akinetic mutism and long-term difficulty with central processing of new information. The incidence is highly variable and has caused some surgeons to abandon attempts at total resection, substituting cyst aspiration or subtotal resection, followed by radiation therapy. The adverse effect of high dose radiation on the developing brain may not be immediately apparent[30,31] and long-term follow-up of a large number of children with appropriate neuropsychological examination will be necessary to evaluate this method of therapy.

OUTCOME

In this group of tumors, only the cerebellar astrocytoma and the craniopharyngioma are potentially curable by surgery alone. Other less common tumors which may be curable by surgical resection are the choroid plexus papilloma, glioma of the anterior temporal lobe or the occipital or frontal pole (all of which can be resected with a margin of normal tissue) and other rare tumors e.g. ganglioglioma.

Brain tumor surgery in the pediatric population demands close interaction and communication between the neurosurgeon, oncologist, radiotherapist and primary physician. This cooperation is necessary, not only to plan appropriate therapy, but to insure that the parents and, when appropriate, the child, have a clear understanding of the treatment goals and potential complications.

REFERENCES

1. Bruno, L., Schut, L. Survey of pediatric brain tumors, in Pediatric Section, A.A.N.S. (eds), Pediatric Neurosurgery, New York, Grune and Stratton, pp. 361-366, 1982.
2. Raimondi, A.J., Tomita, T. Medulloblastoma in childhood: comparative results of partial and total resection. Child's Brain, 5:310-328, 1979.
3. Allen, J.C., Nisselbaum, J., et al. Alpha feto protein and human chorionic gonadotropin determination in cerebrospinal fluid. J Neurosurg 51:368-374, 1979.
4. Kubo, O., Yamasaki, N., et al. Human chorionic gonadotropin produced by ectopic pinealoma in a girl with precocious puberty. J Neurosurg, 47:101-105, 1977.
5. Marton, L.J., Seidenfeld, J. Approaches to the study of polyamines as tumor markers, in Morris D.R, and Marton, L.J, (eds), Polyamines in Biology and Medicine, New York, Marcel Dekker, 1981.
6. Miller, J.D., Sakalas, R., et al. Methyl prednisolone treatment in patients with brain tumors. Neurosurg, 1:114-117, 1972.
7. Brock, M., Zillig, C., et al. The effects of dexamethasone on ICP in cases of posterior fossa tumors, in Bek, W.F., Bosch, D.A., Brock, M. (eds), Intracranial Pressure III, New York, Springer-Verlag, pp. 236-246, 1976.
8. Albright, L., Reigel, D.H. Management of hydrocephalus secondary to posterior fossa tumor. J Neurosurg 46:52-55, 1977.
9. Hoffman, H.J., Hendrick, E.B., et al. Metastasis via ventriculo-peritoneal shunt in patients with medulloblastoma. J Neurosurg 44:562-566, 1976.
10. Epstein, F., Murali, R. Pediatric posterior fossa tumors: hazards of the "pre-operative" shunt. Neurosurg, 3:348-350, 1978.
11. Pierce, E.C., Lambertson, C., et al. Cerebral circulation and metabolism during thiopental anesthesia and hyperventilation in man. J Clin Invest 41:1164-1171, 1962.
12. Flamm, E.S., Ransohoff, J., et al. Preliminary experience with ultrasonic aspiration in neurological surgery. Neurosurg 2:240-245, 1978.
13. Knake, J.E., Chandler, W.F., et al. Intraoperative sonography for brain tumor localization and ventricular shunt placement. AJNR 3:425-430, 1982.
14. Hall, R.R., Beach, A.D., et al. Incision of tissue by carbon dioxide laser. Nature 232:131, 1971.
15. Nagao, S., Roccaforte, P., et al. Acute intracranial hypertension and auditory brain-stem responses. J Neurosurg 51:669-676, 1979.
16. Lewander, R., Bergstrom, M., et al. Stereotactic computer tomography for biopsy of gliomas. Acta Radiol Diag 19:867-888, 1978.
17. Bernstein, M., Gutin, P. Interstitial irradiation of brain tumors: A review. Neurosurg 9:741-750, 1981.
18. Weisberg, L.A. Computed tomography in the evaluation of brain stem glioma. Comput Tomog 3:145-153, 1979.
19. Reigel, D.H., Scarff, T.B., et al. Biopsy of pediatric brain stem tumor. Child's Brain 5:329-340, 1979.
20. Hoffman, H.J., Becker, L., et al. A clinically and pathologically distinct group of brainstem gliomas. Neurosurg 7:243-248, 1980.
21. Hoffman, H.J. Craniopharyngioma: The continuing controversy on management, in Am Soc Pediat Neurosurg (eds), Concepts of Pediatric Neurosurgery IV. New York, S. Karger, Inc., pp. 14-82, 1982.

22. Oxenhandler, D.C., Sayers, M.P. The dilemma of childhood optic glioma. J Neurosurg 48:340-341, 1978.

23. Sayers, M.P. Optic nerve glioma, in Am Soc Pediat Neurosurg (eds) Pediatric Neurosurgery, New York, Grune and Stratton, Inc., pp 513-522, 1982.

24. Obrador, S., Soto, M., et al. Surgical management of tumors of the pineal region. Acta Neurochil 34:159-171, 1976.

25. Stein, B.M, Supracerebellar infratentorial approach to pineal tumors. Surg Neurol 11:331-337, 1979.

26. Winston, K., Gilles, F.H., et al. Cerebellar gliomas in children. J Nat'l Cancer Inst 58:833-838, 1977.

27. Matson, D.D. Intracranial tumors - General considerations, in Neurosurgery of Infancy and Childhood - 2nd Edition. Springfield, Charles Thomas, pp. 403-409, 1969.

28. Eisenberg, H.M. Supratentorial astrocytoma, in Am Soc Pediat Neurosurg (eds), Pediatric Neurosurgery, New York, Grune and Stratton, pp. 429-512 1982.

29. Wald, S., Fogelson, H., et al. Cystic thalamic gliomas. Child's Brain, 9:981-993, 1982.

30. DiLorenzo, D., Nolletti, A., et al. Late cerebral radionecrosis. Surg Neurol 10:281-290, 1978.

31. Ross, H.S., Rosenberg, S., et al. Delayed radiation necrosis of the optic nerve. Am J Ophthalmol 76:683-686, 1973.

COLORECTAL CANCER - INTERACTIONS OF SURGERY, RADIATION AND CHEMOTHERAPY

LEONARD L. GUNDERSON, M.D., M.S., MICHAEL J. O'CONNELL, M.D., AND
ROBERT W. BEART, M.D.

## Definition of the Problem

For 1983, both the expected incidence (126,000) and expected number of
deaths (58,100) for adenocarcinoma of the large bowel ranks second only to
carcinoma of the lung.[1] The male/female incidence ratio is essentially
equal. Studies done during the last decade have shown a proximal shift of
lesion incidence within the large bowel (i.e., rectal cancers have become less
common and colon cancers more frequent). The cause for this is uncertain.

Survival rates for colorectal carcinoma have improved slightly over the
past 25 to 30 years. Such improvements, however, have been the
result of an increase in operability with little improvement by stage of
disease in those patients who have survived a "curative resection."

Recent developments have led to marked interest in a combined modality
approach for initial treatment of rectal and selected colonic carcinomas:
1) local failure or recurrence (LF) within the operative field has been
identified as a significant problem in various operative series in spite of
potentially curative surgery;[2-10] 2) although significant palliation of 75%
to 85% of such failures can be obtained with radiation alone or in combination
with chemotherapy, the duration of palliation is often limited, the curative
potential is 5% or less in most series, and therefore, prevention of local
recurrence is a necessity; 3) data is increasing to indicate the curative
potential of radiation for patients with residual or unresectable disease (10%
to 30%) or those who refuse abdominoperineal resection.[11-16] Radiation dose
levels required to accomplish such results (6000 to 7000+ rads) can, however,
result in significant complications in surrounding dose-limiting tissues and
organs unless many precautions are utilized.[14,17] Conventional supervoltage
irradiation, therefore, is not a competitive alternative to operation for
lesions which are resectable. A preferred method is to combine more moderate
radiation doses of 4500 to 5000 rad with potentially curative surgery when
high risk of local recurrence exists.

TABLE 1          STAGING SYSTEMS FOR COLORECTAL CARCINOMA

Comparison of Dukes' scheme with TNM and a
modification of the Astler-Coller system by Gunderson and Sosin[5]

| Dukes' | Modified Astler-Coller | TNM* | |
|--------|------------------------|------|---|
| A ⟨ | A | $T_1N_0$ | Nodes negative; lesion limited to mucosa |
|   | $B_1$ | $T_2N_0$ | Nodes negative; extension of lesion through mucosa but still within bowel wall |
| B | $B_2$** | $T_3N_0$ | Nodes negative; extension through the entire bowel wall (including serosa if present) |
| C ⟨ | $C_1$ | $T_2N_0$ | Nodes positive; lesion limited to bowel wall |
|   | $C_2$** | $T_3N_1$ | Nodes positive; extension of lesion through the entire bowel wall (including serosa) |

\*  By definition $M_0$ or no evidence of metastases.
\*\* Separate notation is made regarding degree of extension beyond the bowel
    wall:  microscopic only (m); gross extension confirmed by microscopy (m &
    g); adherence to or invasion of surrounding organs or structures ($B_3$ +
    $C_3$, TNM system - $T_5$).


ADJUVANT IRRADIATION

Staging Systems

A  comparison  of  common  staging  classifications  utilized  in  these
malignancies  is  shown  in  Table  1.  A  modification[5,6]  of  the  Astler-Coller
rectal  system,[2]  applicable  to  all  carcinomas  of  the  digestive  tract,  is
preferred in analyzing data because it reflects more accurately the influence
that  initial  extent  of  disease  has  on  later  patterns  and  incidence  of  failure
as  well  as  survival  rates.  In  the  past,  the  Dukes'  staging  system[18,19]  has
long  been  useful  because  of  its  ability  to  predict  the  outcome  of  survival
after  surgery,  but  it  is  less  useful  in  distinguishing  subpopulations  of
patients  at  greatest  risk  for  local  failure.  The  modified  system
differentiates  by  degree  of  extra-rectal  or  extra-colonic  involvement  and
indicates  that  within  each  Dukes'  stage  (B  and  C)  there  are  subgroups  of
patients  with  significantly  different  risks  for  local  failure.[7,8]  The
relatively equivalent TNM stage is listed on the same table.

## Operative Failures After "Curative Resection"

Rectal cancer. The risk of local recurrence in the tumor bed or regional nodes after "curative resection" is related to disease extension beyond the bowel wall as well as to nodal involvement.[2,3,8,10,20] Local recurrence in patients with nodal involvement but tumor confined to the bowel wall (i.e., Cl) is 20% to 25%, which is actually less than in the group with negative nodes but extension through the wall (i.e., B2 or B3) where the risk is 30% to 35%. The group that has both bad prognostic factors, nodal involvement and extension through the wall (i.e., C2 or C3), has nearly an additive risk of local recurrence varying from 50% to 65% in clinical series and 70% in re-operative series. In a series from Massachusettes General Hospital (MGH), the incidence of both total and local failure in node-negative patients increased with each degree of extension beyond the wall.[8] Separate analyses from MGH and M.D. Anderson Hospital suggest that the degree of extra-rectal extension even in node positive patients appears to be an independent factor influencing the risk of local recurrence.[8,10]

Colon. Increasing data is being accumulated in clinical,[3,22-24] autopsy,[21] and re-operative series[7,25] to indicate that local recurrence is frequently seen after resection of colonic as well as rectal lesions. Clinical series can, however, underestimate the incidence of local failures as they can often be asymptomatic, and excess emphasis may be placed on liver only failures. While data from clinical series[24] suggest that one-third of failures occur solely in the liver, autopsy[21] and re-operative data[7,25] indicate this may be less than 10%.

---

TABLE 2          EXTRAPELVIC COLON PATTERNS OF FAILURE
(University of Washington[23])

---

| Failure Any Component | Total group* #   %   (%) | Reoperation** #     % |
|---|---|---|
| Local failure | 54--29 (9.8) | 29/61 (47.5%) |
| Abdominal failure | 73--39 (13.3) | |
|    Retroperit. LN | ---- | 13/38 (34%) |
|    Peritoneal seeding | ---- | 28/64 (44%) |
| Liver metastasis | 74--40 (13.5) | 18/54 (33.5%) |

\* Open % are of 186 patients with failure and ( ) % of total group of 550.
\*\* 54 of 64 had symptomatic reoperation.

Failure by stage: A 1/58 (1.5%); B 9/106 (8.5%); $B_2$ 63/200 (31.5%); $B_3$ 14/23 (61%); $C_1$ 9/20 (45%); $C_2$ 75/126 (59.5%); $C_3$ 15/17 (88%).

In the University of Washington series,[23] 186 of 550 patients with colon cancer had later evidence of failure. Within the failure group, 64 of the 186 had a re-operation at some interval (symptomatic look in 54). As shown in Table 2, in the group with re-operation, one could accurately divide abdominal failures into a retroperitoneal nodal component of disease versus peritoneal seeding. In addition, a much higher percentage of patients were found to have a local failure.

A total of 230 patients had re-operative procedures following curative resection of colorectal cancer at the University of Minnesota,[7,25] and failures were defined in 152. Since this was a select high-risk group with a majority of patients having nodal involvement alone or in combination with extension beyond the bowel wall at the time of the initial procedure, data in this series cannot be compared directly with other series. Failures in the tumor bed and nodes were most common with rectal lesions (Table 3) but were not uncommon with primaries at other bowel sites (with colonic primaries, local- only failures are less likely than with rectal cancer). Peritoneal seeding was least common with rectal primaries (lesions are less accessible to the peritoneal cavity). The incidence of hematogenous failures was similar for all sites although the distribution differed. With rectal primaries, hematogenous failures were fairly evenly divided between liver and lung due to venous drainage via both the mesenteric and internal iliac routes, but with colon primaries, initial hematogenous failures were usually in the liver.

TABLE 3      PATTERNS OF FAILURE - COLORECTAL
(University of Minnesota Reoperation Series[25])

| Site of Primary | Failure total | Component of Failure* | | |
| | | LF-RF #  %  (%) | PS #  %  (%) | DM #  %  (%) |
|---|---|---|---|---|
| **Extrapelvic** | | | | |
| Transverse | 3/8 | 3--100 (38) | 1--33 (13) | 2--67 (25) |
| Cecum | 26/37 | 18---69 (49) | 6--23 (16) | 10--38 (27) |
| Asc., Desc. and Flexures | 29/46 | 23---79 (50) | 14--48 (30) | 17--59 (37) |
| **Pelvic** | | | | |
| Rectum | 52/74 | 48---92 (65) | 3---6 (4) | 26--50 (35) |

Open % are of failure group and (  )% of total subgroup at risk.
*LF-RF (local-regional failure); PS (peritoneal seeding); DM (hematogenous)

Rectum and Colon. Although proximal and distal tumor-free bowel margins are usually described by the surgeon and pathologist, the most limiting margin is often the circumferential margin when a lesion extends through the wall. In both males and females, if a rectal cancer extends posteriorly, the surgical disease-free margin is often millimeters rather than centimeters, and in males the same is true with anterior or lateral extension of low rectal lesions.

## Radiation of Rectal Cancer - Philosophy and Results

Differences of opinion exist regarding the preferred sequence of combining surgery and irradiation. In summary, the major advantage of preoperative irradiation (XRT) is the potential damaging effect on cells that may be spread locally or distantly at the time of operation. The major advantage of postoperative XRT is the ability to sub-select out groups of patients at high risk for local recurrence on the basis of operative and pathologic findings and delete patients with advanced but undiagnosed metastatic disease prior to exploration and/or a low risk for local recurrence. A well-designed combination of pre- and postoperative XRT (sandwich technique) could, in fact, combine the theoretical advantages of each.[5,6]

Preoperative XRT. Most preoperative studies have demonstrated proof of tumoricidal responsiveness at the time of surgery either by partial or total regression of the primary or the finding of a lower incidence of lymph node involvement than would ordinarily have been anticipated.[26-28] In two prospective randomized low-dose series (Princess Margaret Hospital 500 rads, single dose[15] or VA Hospital 2000 to 2500 rads in 2 to 2.5 weeks versus operation alone[27]), survival was statistically better in some irradiated patient subgroups (no demonstrable survival advantage when the overall randomized groups were compared). In the VAH series of 700 patients, local recurrence and distant metastases were also decreased in an autopsy subgroup, but both were still unacceptably high at 29% and 40%, respectively.[27] In the high dose, nonrandomized Oregon series[28] (using 5000 to 6000 rads in 6 to 7 weeks), only 1/45 patients (2.3%) with subsequent curative resection was proven to have later pelvic recurrence. This latter data suggests that adequate doses of preoperative XRT in combination with surgery may make a major impact on local recurrence (29% versus 2.3% in VAH versus University of Oregon data).

Postoperative XRT. Three major prospective but nonrandomized postoperative series utilized similar dose levels of 4500 to 5500 rads in 5 to 6.5 weeks and

TABLE 4           EXTENT OF DISEASE VS LATER LOCAL FAILURE (LF)
Clinical Series After Curative Resection of Colorectal Cancer

| Extent of Disease | Operation Alone U Florida, MDAH, MGH, Maine[2,4,8-10] | Operation + Postop XRT | | |
|---|---|---|---|---|
| | | MDAH[9] (rectal) | LDS-SLC[29] (colorectal) | MGH[30] (rectal) |
| Within Wall LN + ($C_1$) | 20% to 30% | 0/3 | 0/2 | 1/9 (11%) |
| Through Wall LN − ($B_2 \pm B_3$) | 25% to 35% | 1/18 (5.5%) | 0/10 | 2/36 (5.5%) |
| LN + ($C_2 + C_3$) | 45% to 65% | 3/33 (9.1%) | 2/16 (12.5%) | 5/50 (10%) |
| LN Status Unknown ($B_{2-3}$ or $C_{2-3}$) | ---- | 1/8 (12.5%) | 0/4 | ---- |
| TOTALS | 35 to 50% | 5/62 (8.1%) | 2/34 (6%) | 8/95 (8.4%) |

treated only those patients at high risk for local recurrence.[5,9,10,29,30] Table 4 compares local recurrence rates after curative resection alone or in combination with XRT. For equivalent total groups ($B_{2-3}$, $C_{2-3} \pm C_1$) local recurrence decreased from 37% to 48% with operation alone to 6% to 8% in the XRT series. Similar decreases were seen for each extent of disease. In the $B_{2-3}$ subgroup, the reduction was nearly ten-fold from 30% to 35% down to around 5% and in the $C_{2-3}$ subgroup, from 45% to 65% down to 10% to 12%.

Distant failures in the three nonrandomized series continued to be a problem in 25%-30% of patients in spite of the improvement in local control. Hematogenous failures are more common than peritoneal except for the $C_3$ group where the peritoneal failure incidence was 50% in the MGH series.[30]

Local recurrence was compared in nonrandomized but sequential series for operation alone (103 patients) versus operation and postoperative irradiation (95 patients) in the MGH analysis.[30] Since one cannot fairly compare overall local recurrence rates as one group is at risk for a longer time period, both groups were analyzed at the three-year period postoperatively. As shown in Table 5, there was a statistically significant reduction in local recurrence at nearly each stage level in the groups who received adjuvant postoperative irradiation [$B_2$(g), $B_3$, $C_1 + C_2$(m), $C_2$(g)].

| | | |
|---|---|---|
| TABLE 5 | RECTAL CANCER - PELVIC FAILURE AT 3 YEARS, MGH[30] | |

| Modified A-C Stage | Surgery Alone | Adjuvant Post-Op XRT |
|---|---|---|
| $B_2$(m) | (12)  8.3% | (6) 18.2% |
| $B_2$(m & g) | (32)  25% | (23)   0%* |
| $B_3$ | (15)  57.6% | (7)   0%* |
| $C_1$ | (11)  43.2% | (15)  7.2%* |
| $C_2$(m) | (11)  43.2% | (15)  7.2%* |
| $C_2$(m & g) | (27)  52.8% | (34)  8.9%* |
| $C_3$ | (6) 100% | (10) 30.5% |
| | (103) | (95) |

*Significant at $P \leq .05$

#'s in parentheses = total # pts at risk; Open #'s = % with pelvic failure

In a randomized trial from the Gastrointestinal Tumor Study Group, (GITSG)[31] patients were randomized to a surgical control arm versus treatment arms of postoperative irradiation, postoperative chemotherapy or a combination thereof. In the radiation alone arm, patients received either 4000 or 4800 rads and in the radiation plus chemotherapy arm, either 4000 or 4400 rads. The disease-free survival of all 3 treated arms was superior to surgery alone at the interval of 130 to 156 weeks. The difference between the combined arm of chemotherapy plus irradiation versus surgery alone is statistically significant ($P < .03$ to .05 dependending on method of analysis). The combined arm did not, however, result in a decrease in the incidence of distant metastases but rather a decrease in local recurrence when patterns of first site of failure were analyzed. This suggests that the effect of the chemotherapy was not a systemic effect but rather a local effect as a radiopotentiator. In spite of the improvement in disease-free survival in both arms with irradiation, the local recurrence rate with radiation alone was excessive with a minimum rate of 7 of 47 or 15% at latest analysis (may be higher as only first patterns of failure have been published).

The 6% to 8% incidence of local recurrence in the three nonrandomized but prospective postoperative series previously discussed was only approximately half that of the GITSG study treating similar patient subgroups. This is perhaps due to the fact that the minimum dose within the boost field of the nonrandomized series was usually 5000 rads, whereas approximately 50% of the patients in the GTSG radiation alone arm received only 4000 rads.

## RESIDUAL, RECURRENT, UNRESECTABLE (EXTERNAL + INTRAOPERATIVE XRT)

### External Beam ± Resection

While significant gains can be achieved with the addition of irradiation in an adjuvant setting, the job becomes more difficult if residual disease has been left behind after resection or if patients present with initially unresectable or recurrent disease since the radiation dose levels required are increased in magnitude.[11,13,28,32,33] In a recent Mayo Clinic series, 44 patients with locally advanced rectal cancer (unresectable - 7, resected but residual - 7, locally recurrent - 30) received 5000 rads split course pelvic irradiation with or without adjuvant immunotherapy.[34] In the patients in whom site of initial tumor progression could be evaluated, 28 of 31 experienced local progression within the radiation port, and in 17 (55%) it was their only site of disease.

In the residual disease colorectal subgroups from MGH[11] and Albert Einstein (AE),[13] the incidence of local recurrence (LF) after external beam irradiation varied by the amount of residual disease being approximately 50% (AE - 9/18; MGH - 13/24) if there was gross residual versus 15% to 26% (AE - 2/13; MGH - 8/31) if there was only microscopic residual. In the MGH analysis, a possible dose-response correlation was seen in the group with microscopic residual with a 11% LF risk (1/9) if the boost was $\geq$ 6000 rads versus 33% (7/21) if the boost was $\leq$ 5500 rads. In the patients with gross residual, a dose-response correlation could not be discerned.

In patients with rectal cancer that is unresectable for cure due to tumor fixation, a number of institutions have given preoperative radiotherapy in an attempt to shrink the lesion, allow resection, and possibly improve local control and survival.[28,32,33] The resectability rate after doses of 4500 to 5000 rads has varied from 50% to 75% by series. Even in those patients who were resected, the incidence of local recurrence has been excessive at 36% to 45%.

### IORT ± External XRT ± Resection

While combinations of external beam radiation and surgery decrease pelvic recurrence and improve survival in the subgroups with residual or initially unresectable disease, the incidence of local recurrence is too high and improvements in this may also improve survival. Since it is difficult to achieve adequate dose levels with only external beam techniques, in view of dose-limiting organs, such as small bowel, intraoperative irradiation alone or in conjunction with external beam techniques has been utilized in pilot study fashion.

Some of the most optimistic results with intraoperative irradiation (IORT) in the U.S. have been obtained in those patients who present with colorectal lesions that are unresectable for cure, have residual after resection, or have recurrent but localized disease. This group has been a major emphasis in the MGH[14,35,36] and Mayo series[37] as opposed to a minor emphasis in the Japanese trials.[38]

Results were encouraging in the combined Japanese report in that 5/14 colon patients were alive.[38] Of the eight colon patients reported by Abe et al. (included in the combined analysis), two of eight were alive and free of disease at nine years, eight months, and at ten years in spite of retro-peritoneal invasion and unresected nodal disease in both.[39]

In the MGH series, the initial 32 patients had a minimum 20 month follow-up and were analyzed in detail.[35] All received 4500 to 5000 rads with multiple field techniques and had resection when feasible, but in addition had an intraoperative electron beam boost of 1000 to 1500 rads to the remaining tumor or tumor bed. In the Mayo series,[37] all 11 patients had surgical debulking of disease combined with similar external beam doses, and IORT doses varied from 1000 to 2000 rads depending on the amount of disease. Seven of 32 patients in the MGH series and 6 of 11 in the Mayo series received some 5-fluorouracil (5FU) during the external beam component of radiation.

Local Control. For locally advanced colorectal patients, local control in both the MGH and Mayo series has been superb when all three treatment modalities could be optimally employed (4500 to 5000 rads external beam irradiation ± 5FU, surgical resection, intraoperative electron boost) independent of sequence. In the MGH series, only 1 of 28 patients (3.6%) with all 3 modalities developed either a central or local failure, and this patient had subtotal resection of a recurrent lesion after preoperative irradiation (gross residual).[35] In the Mayo series of 11 patients, only 1 (9%) developed local recurrence to date (although a 2000 rad IORT boost was given, we could deliver only 2520 rad in 14 treatments with external beam, as the patient had received 4000 rad pelvic irradiation previously). These results are a marked improvement when compared to series of patients treated initially with resection and external beam irradiation techniques in which local recurrence is 15% to 26% for microscopic residual,[11,13] 50% to 54% for gross residual,[11,13] and 36% to 45% for patients who were initially unresectable and were resected after preoperative irradiation.[28,32,33]

Survival. In the MGH group of 32 patients with locally advanced disease,[35] survival has been superior to results seen in series employing only external beam techniques ± resection. In the residual disease and recurrent subgroups, such improvements, however, may be due in part to case selection since patients who were found to have metastasis prior to, or at the time of, exploration did not receive the intraoperative boost and are not reflected in the survival curves. The marked improvement in local control that can be achieved with the aggressive approaches utilized in this series could also be responsible for the improvement in survival. Since 4 of the 10 patients who presented with recurrent disease are currently alive and 3 are without evidence of disease (39.5, 40 and 42 months), aggressive local regional approaches may be appropriate even in this disease category.

The results in the MGH initially unresectable group of 16 patients are the most intriguing, since the group was selected in similar fashion to the previous group treated with only preoperative radiation and resection.

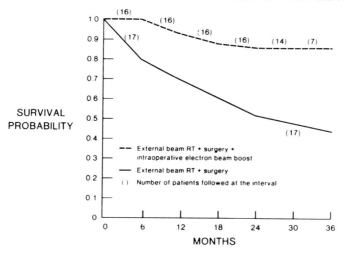

## INITIALLY UNRESECTABLE CARCINOMA OF THE RECTUM

Fig. 1. Comparison of actuarial survival in treatment of unresectable carcinoma of the rectum at MGH (p < .01 to .025 depending on method of analysis).

Survival curves comparing the two nonrandomized treatment regimens revealed a statistical advantage for the group who received the intraoperative boost that does not appear to be due to a difference in case selection (Figure 1). More patients in the intraoperative group had transection of tumor in spite of pre-operative irradiation and resection (4/16 vs. 1/14). The surgeon was usually more willing to use sharp dissection to remove all or most of the tumor since the remaining tumor or tumor bed would be within the intraoperative boost.

Morbidity. In the MGH colorectal subgroup, some problems with delayed wound healing have been encountered. Neither the magnitude nor the incidence of such problems was increased in comparison with subgroups treated with only preoperative irradiation and resection at MCH[37] or at other institutions. The healing problems are presumably related to the advanced stage of the tumor growth or regrowth (10 of the initial 32 MGH patients and 6 of the 11 at Mayo presented with recurrence), the difficulty of the surgical resection, and the aggressive radiation therapy.

Distant Failures. Distant failures are a significant problem in MGH and Mayo patients with recurrent and residual disease indicating a need for effective systemic therapy, an alteration in irradiation techniques, or both. For those patients who present with disease fixation, it may be preferable to give the external beam irradiation of 4500 - 5000 rads prior to, rather than after, surgical resection. In the MGH series, the incidence of distant failures was only 12% (2 of 16) in the primary unresectable group who received preoperative irradiation prior to resection, but in the primary residual disease subgroup is at least 50% (3/6) and is as high as 67% (6/9) if the 3 patients are included who did not have distant failure at the time of initial resection, but had such when they were reexplored for a planned IORT boost. Patient numbers are too small to prove an advantage for either treatment sequence. In the Mayo trial, 4 of 11 colorectal patients have failed. Three had only distant failure, and surgery, with transection of disease, preceded any irradiation in each patient.

THERAPEUTIC RATIO

It does little good to accomplish adequate local control if it is achieved with a high incidence of complications. A suitable therapeutic ratio between local control and complications is achieved only with close interaction between the surgeon and the radiotherapist.[14,17] Major surgical consider-ations include use of clips to mark areas at high risk as well as the use of pelvic reconstruction techniques whenever possible. There are also steps that should be taken into consideration when planning pelvic irradiation, including the use of: 1) lateral fields to avoid as much small bowel as possible while still including the area at risk, 2) shrinking or boost field techniques, and 3) treatment with bladder distension.

The incidence of small bowel obstruction requiring re-operation varies when utilizing parallel opposed versus multiple field techniques with external beam doses of 4500 to 5500 rads in an adjuvant setting. In the M.D. Anderson series which utilized parallel opposed techniques, an incidence of 17.5% occurred in irradiated patients in contrast to 5% with surgery alone.[10] When the superior extent of the radiation field was shifted from the L-2 to L-3 region down to L-5, the incidence of operative intervention decreased to 10% to 12%. This is similar to the 10% incidence in the LDS Hospital series with parallel opposed techniques.[5,29] In the MGH series[30] with multiple field and boost techniques and use of bladder distension, the incidence of small bowel obstruction requiring operative intervention is essentially equal in the group receiving irradiation (4%) as compared with operation alone (5%). The minimum follow-up in the irradiated group in the MGH series was 24 months and greater than two-thirds of patients were at risk for 3 or more years.

CONCLUSIONS AND FUTURE POSSIBILITIES

Adjuvant Irradiation

In an adjuvant setting, doses of 5000 rads in 5.5 to 6 weeks given either preoperatively or postoperatively in conjunction with resection of all known disease, produces superb local control in most patient subgroups with rectal and rectosigmoid carcinoma. Complications appear to be satisfactory provided multi-field techniques, bladder distension, etc., are utilized. In the subgroup with both node involvement and extension through the wall, the incidence of local recurrence has been reduced from 45% to 65% down to 10% to 12%, but further benefit may be anticipated if the radiation dose were increased to 5500 to 6000 rads whenever the volume of small bowel within the boost field is minimal to nonexistent.

For both colon and rectal cancer, distant failures via either the hematogenous or peritoneal route are a significant problem which occurs in 25% to 30% of resected patients receiving adjuvant radiation therapy. Whether distant failures can be reduced by combining local field radiation with systemic therapy, by utilizing a radiation technique of low-dose preoperative radiation therapy followed by postoperative when indicated[40,41] or by the use of whole abdominal[42,43] or liver treatment in conjunction with tumor bed/nodal irradiation in selected subgroups remains to be seen. For lesions at high risk for local recurrence but with extension to a peritoneal surface and positive cytology of peritoneal washings,[44,45] it would be of interest to randomize to local irradiation alone versus local XRT and whole abdominal treatment (liver and peritoneal surfaces) and for lesions below or beneath the peritoneal surface to compare local irradiation to local XRT and treatment of the liver. Careful studies will be necessary to determine whether treatment to the peritoneal surfaces should be given with intraperitoneal radiocolloids or chemotherapy, external beam irradiation, or a combination thereof, and whether the liver should be treated with infusion chemotherapy, external beam irradiation, or combined methods.

### Unresectable, Residual, Recurrent

When unresectable or residual disease is treated with conventional irradiation and resection, local control and long-term survival can be achieved in 30% to 50% of patients, but the presence of dose-limiting normal tissues prevents delivery of adequate levels of external beam irradiation in a majority of patients. In early colorectal pilot studies from MGH, the addition of intraoperative electron boosts appears to improve both local control and survival.[14,35-37] Even if such results can be duplicated in randomized trials for rectal and rectosigmoid lesions, they may not be achievable in colonic malignancies where systemic failures play a more predominant role (abdominal treatment may be necessary in addition to the aggressive local approach).

For cases found to be locally unresectable for cure prior to or at initial exploration, it would be worthwhile to obtain a baseline CT study, deliver 4500 to 5000 rads, and then restage the patient 3 to 4 weeks later. If the patient is without evidence of metastases and lesion extent is stable or reduced on a repeat CT, it would be justifiable to combine exploration and resection with an intraoperative or postoperative "boost" dose of irradiation. This sequence may be preferable to initial resection of such lesions before irradiation, since this often results in disease cut through and may produce an increased incidence of peritoneal or hematogenous failure.

For locally advanced or recurrent colorectal lesions in which the surgeon feels operative resection will never have a role, the combination of external beam irradiation and chemotherapy can achieve useful palliation in 75% to 80% of patients and an occasional cure.[5,14-16,29] If lesion size and location are such that intraoperative boosts with electrons, implantation techniques, or orthovoltage can be safely used to supplement external beam doses, further gains may be possible. Even with such boost techniques, the addition of radiation dose modifiers (radiation sensitizers, hyperthermia, etc.) may be necessary. When intraoperative boosts cannot be utilized, dose levels achievable with external beam irradiation vary depending on location of tumor and normal tissues. For rectal lesions, a boost field can occasionally be carried to 6000 to 6500 rads if small bowel can be deleted. For colonic malignancies, the dose within the boost field is often limited to 5000 to 5500 rads in view of the presence of stomach, liver, or small intestine. At these dose levels, the chance for permanent local control is minimal, and any gains in local control will be achieved with combinations of chemotherapy and irradiation, or the use of radiation dose modifiers.

In summary, it appears that radiotherapy has much to add in the therapeutic management of patients with colorectal malignancies. This can be achieved with an acceptable risk of complications only if there is close interaction between the surgeon and the radiotherapist wherein both utilize all mechanisms possible to limit dose to organs such as the small bowel.

REFERENCES
1. Silverberg, E. Cancer Statistics, 1982. Cancer 32:15-31, 1982.
2. Astler VB, Coller FA. The prognostic significance of direct extension of carcinoma of the colon and rectum. Ann Surg 139:846-851, 1954.
3. Cass AW, Million RR, Pfaff FA. Patterns of recurrence following surgery alone for adenocarcinoma of the colon-rectum. Cancer 37:2861-2865, 1976.
4. Gilbert SB. The significance of symptomatic local tumor failure following abdomino-perineal resection. Int J Rad Oncol Biol Phys 4:801-807, 1978.
5. Gunderson LL. Combined irradiation and surgery for rectal and sigmoid carcinoma. In Emerging role of Radiotherapy in Four Selected Areas. Fletcher G (ed.), Current Prob Cancer 1:40-53, 1976.
6. Gunderson LL, Sosin H. Areas of failure found at reoperation (second or symptomatic look) following "curative surgery" for adenocarcinoma of the rectum: Clinicopathologic correlation and implications for adjuvant therapy. Cancer 34:1278-1292, 1974.
7. Gunderson LL, Tepper JE, Dosoretz DE, Hopelson G, Hoskins RB, et al. Patterns of failure after treatment of gastrointestinal cancer. In Proceedings of CROS-NCI Conference on Patterns of Failure after Treatment of Cancer. Cox J (ed), Cancer Treatment Reports (in press).
8. Rich T, Gunderson LL, Galdabini J, et al. Clinical and pathologic factors influencing local failure after curative resection of carcinoma of the rectum and rectosigmoid. Cancer (in press).
9. Romsdahl M, Withers HR. Radiotherapy combined with curative surgery. Arch Surg 113:446-453, 1978.
10. Withers HR, Cuasay L, Mason KA, Romsdahl MM, Saxton JP. Elective radiation therapy in the curative treatment of cancer of the rectum and rectosigmoid colon. In: Gastrointestinal Cancer. Strocklein JR, Romsdahl MM, ed. New York, Raven Press, pp 351-362, 1981.

11. Allee PE, Gunderson LL, Munzenrider JE. Postoperative radiation therapy for residual colorectal carcinoma. ASTR Proceedings. Int J Rad Oncol 7:1208, 1981.

12. Cummings BJ, Rider WD, Harwood AR, Keane TJ, Thomas GM. External beam radiation therapy for adenocarcinoma of the rectum. Dis Colon Rectum (in press).

13. Ghossein NA, Samala EC, Alpert S, et al. Elective postoperative radiotherapy after incomplete resection of a colorectal cancer. Dis Colon Rectum 24:252-256, 1981.

14. Gunderson LL, Cohen AM, Welch CW. Residual, inoperable, or recurrent colorectal cancer: surgical-radiotherapy interaction. Am J Surg 139:518-525, 1980.

15. Rider WD. Is the Miles operation really necessary for the treatment of rectal cancer? J Can Assoc Radiol 26:167-175, 1975.

16. Wang CC, Schulz MD. The role of radiation therapy in the management of carcinoma of the sigmoid, rectosigmoid, and rectum. Radiology 79:1-5, 1962.

17. Gunderson LL, Meyer JE, Sheedy P, Munzenrider JE. Radiation Oncology. Part XVIII. In: Alimentary Tract Radiology, 3rd Edition. Margolis AR, Burhenne HJ, eds. St. Louis, CV Mosby, pp 2409-2446, 1983.

18. Dukes CE. The pathology of rectal cancer. In: Cancer of the Rectum, C. Dukes, ed. Edinburgh, E & S Livingston, pp 59-68, 1960.

19. Gabriel WB, Dukes C, Bussey HJR. Lymphatic spread in cancer of the rectum. Br J Surg 23:395-413, 1935.

20. Copeland EM, Miller LD, Jones RS. Prognostic factors in carcinoma of the colon and rectum. Am J Surg 116:875-881, 1968.

21. Welch J, Donaldson GA. The clinical correlation of an autopsy study of recurrent colorectal cancer. Ann Surg 89:496-502, 1979.

22. Malcolm AW, Perencevich NP, Olson RM, et al. Analysis of recurrence patterns following curative resection for carcinoma of the colon and rectum. Surg Gynecol Obstet 152:131-136, 1981.

23. Russell AH, Tong D, Dawson LE, Wisbeck W. Adenocarcinoma of the proximal colon: sites of initial dissemination and patterns of recurrence following surgery alone. Cancer (in press).

24. Welch JP, Donaldson GA. Detection and treatment of recurrent cancer of the colon and rectum. Am J Surg 135:505-511, 1978.

25. Gunderson LL, Sosin H. Adenocarcinoma of the colon: areas of failure in a reoperation series (second or symptomatic looks). (Submitted for)

26. Kligerman MM, Urdanetta N, Knowlton A, et al. Preoperative irradiation of rectosigmoid carcinoma including its regional lymph nodes. Am J Roentgenol 114:498-503, 1972.

27. Roswit B, Higgins GA, Keehn RJ. Preoperative irradiation for carcinoma of the rectum and rectosigmoid colon: report of a National Veteran's Administration randomized study. Cancer 35:1597-1602, 1975.

28. Stevens KR, Allen CV, Fletcher WS. Preoperative radiotherapy for adenocarcinoma of the rectosigmoid. Cancer 37:2866-2874, 1976.

29. Gunderson LL. Radiation therapy of colorectal carcinoma. In: Digestive Cancer, Vol 9. Thatcher N (ed.), XII International Cancer Congress Proceedings, New York: Permagon Press, pp. 29-38, 1979.

30. Hoskins B, Gunderson LL, Dosoretz D, Galdabini J. Adjuvant postoperative radiotherapy in carcinoma of the rectum and rectosigmoid. ASTR Proceedings. Int J Rad Oncol 6:1379, 1980 (submitted for publication).

31. Mittleman A, et al. (for GITSG group). Adjuvant chemotherapy and radiotherapy following rectal surgery: an interim report from the gastrointestinal tumor study group (GITSG). In: Salmon SE, Jones SE, eds. Adjuvant therapy of cancer III. New York, Green and Stratton, pp 547-557, 1981.

32. Dosoretz DE, Gunderson LL, Hoskins B, et al. Preoperative irradiation for localized carcinoma of the rectum and rectosigmoid: patterns of failure, survival, and future treatment strategies. Cancer (in press).

33. Emami B, Pilepich M, Wilett C, Munzenrider JE, Miller HH. Management of unresectable colorectal carcinoma (preoperative radiotherapy and surgery). Int J Rad Oncol Biol Phys 8:1295-1299, 1982.

34. O'Connell MJ, Childs DS, Moertel CG, et al. A prospective controlled evaluation of combined pelvic radiotherapy and methanol extraction residue of BCG (MER) for locally unresectable or recurrent rectal carcinoma. Int J Rad Oncol Biol Phys 8:1115-1119, 1982.

35. Gunderson LL, Cohen AM, Dosoretz DE, et al. Residual, unresectable or recurrent colorectal cancer: external beam irradiation and intra-operative electron beam boost ± resection. Int J Rad Oncol (in press).

36. Gunderson LL, Shipley WU, Suit HD, et al. Intraoperative irradiation: a pilot study combining external beam irradiation with "boost" dose intraoperative electrons. Cancer 49:2259-2266, 1982.

37. Gunderson LL, Tepper JE, et al. Intraoperative ± external beam irradiation. In: Current Problems in Cancer. RC Hickey (ed). Chicago, Yearbook Medical Publishers Inc. (in press).

38. Abe M, Takahashi M. Intraoperative radiotherapy: the Japanese experience. Int J Rad Oncol Biol Phys 7:863-868, 1981.

39. Abe M, Takahashi M, Yakumoto E, et al. Clinical experience with intra-operative radiotherapy of locally advanced tumors. Cancer 45:40-48, 1980.

40. Gunderson LL, Dosoretz DE, Hedberg SE, et al. Low-dose preoperative irradiation, surgery, and elective postoperative radiation therapy for resectable rectum and rectosigmoid carcinoma. Cancer (in press).

41. Mohuidden M, Kramer S, Marks G, Dobelbower RR. Combined pre- and post-operative radiation for carcinoma of the rectum. Int Rad Oncol Biol Phys 8:133-136, 1982.

42. Dembo AJ, Van Dyk J, Japp B, et al. Whole abdominal irradiation by a moving strip technique for patients with ovarian cancer. Int J Rad Oncol Biol Phys 5:1933-1942, 1979.

43. Turner SS, Vieira EF, Ager PJ, et al. Elective postoperative radio-therapy for locally advanced colorectal cancer. Cancer 40:105-108, 1977.

44. Creasman WT, Disaia PJ, Blessing J, et al. Prognostic significance of peritoneal cytology in patients with endometrial cancer and preliminary data concerning therapy with intraperitoneal radiopharmaceuticals. Am J Obstet Gynecol 141:921-929, 1981.

45. Nakajima T, Harashima S, Hirata M, Kajitani T. Prognostic and therapeutic value of peritoneal cytology in gastric cancer. Acta Cytol 22:225-229, 1978.

THE TREATMENT OF LIVER METASTASES

JOHN E. NIEDERHUBER, M.D.

Metastatic tumor involving the liver is a leading cause of cancer death and can result from virtually any malignancy. When the liver is the only demonstrated site of metastatic disease, there is good evidence that direct hepatic artery delivery of chemotherapy can be beneficial.[1-8] The majority of the experience leading to this conclusion has involved the hepatic artery infusion of 5-fluorouracil in the treatment of hepatic metastases from colorectal cancer.

There are a number of pharmacologic and physiologic observations to support the rationale for using intra-arterial infusions. For example, the dual blood supply to the liver, with greater than 95% of the tumor blood supply arising from the hepatic artery provides several advantages. First, the chemotherapeutic agent can be infused in high doses without excessive hepatocyte toxicity. Second, if the site of drug metabolism is the liver, providing high drug concentrations may result in higher tumor dose with minimal systemic side effects. Third, continuous infusion provides high concentrations of drug during tumor cell DNA synthesis, thus enhancing the therapeutic effect.

While the first successful delivery of drug directly to the liver via the hepatic artery was reported by Klopp et al. in 1950,[9] it was not until the 1960's that this approach gained any degree of clinical interest. During the late 1960's and 1970's a variety of methods were used for catheter placement including direct operative-positioning and percutaneous insertion via the femoral or brachial artery. The intra-arterial catheters were attached to external pumping devices and response rates were variously reported as 32% to 83% with a median response duration of 8-16 months (Table 1).[1-8]

While the responses obtained were in some instances quite impressive, the usefulness of this method of treatment was limited by technical complications and patient acceptance. The reports summarized in Table 1 indicated that more than one third of the patients did not complete an adequate trial and the duration of successful intra-arterial access ranged from two to seven months.[2,6,10-12] Improvement in catheter materials and the recent development of an implantable drug delivery system has eliminated many of the

Published 1983 by Elsevier Science Publishing Co., Inc.
Recent Trends in Radiation Oncology and Related Fields, Amendola and Amendola, Editors

TABLE 1.    RESULTS OF INTRAARTERIAL THERAPY OF HEPATIC METASTASES
            USING AN EXTERNAL PUMP IN PATIENTS WITH COLORECTAL CANCER

| Reference | Drug & Schedule | No. of Evaluable Patients | Objective Response (%) | Median Duration of Survival (Months) |
|---|---|---|---|---|
| Sullivan[1] | Multiple regimens | 39 | 62 | 9.4 |
| Watkins[2] | FUDR 20 mg/kg/day | 82 | 73 | 10.2 |
| Cady[3] | FUDR 20/mg/kg/day | 51 | 57 | 14.0 |
| Buroker et al.[4] | FUDR 0.3 mg/kg/day | 21 | 35 | 8.0 |
| Grage et al.[5] | 5-FU 20 mg/kg/day x 14 then 10/mg/kg/day x 7 | 30 | 34 | 10.0 |
| Reed et al.[8] | FUDR 0.3 mg/kg/day | 77 | 76 | 13.0 |
| Patt et al.[7] | Mitomycin 15 mg/m$^2$ day 1, FUDR 100 mg/m$^2$/day x 5 repeated every 30 days | 12 | 83 | 16.0* |
| Oberfield et al.[6] | 5-FU 20 mg/kg/day x 10 then FUDR 20 mg/kg/day | 48 | 75 | ---- |

*From time of diagnosis of metastases

previous technical problems[13-16] and provided the stimulus for a Phase I-II trial of hepatic artery therapy using a totally implanted system.

This study began at the University of Michigan in February 1979 and the experience with hepatic artery chemotherapy for colorectal cancer metastatic to the liver was recently reviewed.[17] One hundred and ten consecutive patients representing the spectrum of metastatic colorectal cancer were entered into a Phase I-II trial in a nonrandomized sequential manner between February 1979 and July 1982. All patients had biopsy proven liver involvement and measurable disease by technetium-99m sulfur colloid (TcSc) liver scan. Patients were evaluated preoperatively with selective visceral angiography to determine the blood supply to the liver.

Each patient underwent abdominal exploration and a careful search for the presence of intraabdominal extrahepatic tumor. At the time of surgery the hepatic arterial system was isolated by careful dissection and a silastic catheter[16] was placed in an appropriate artery, usually the gastroduodenal artery. Two catheters were used when necessary to insure total liver perfusion and care was taken to completely isolate the vessels between the site of the catheter placement and their entrance into the liver to preclude drug delivery to the gastrointestinal tract and pancreas. The implanted drug delivery system was a model 400 INFUSAID Pump (Infusaid Corp., Norwood, MA) and is shown in Figure 1 and 2. The pump was placed in a subcutaneous pocket

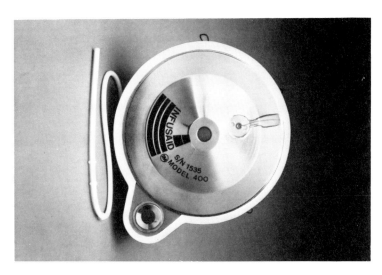

Fig. 1. Model 400 Infusaid pump weighs approximately 200 g and has overall dimensions of 3 x 9 cm. This photograph courtesy of Metal Bellows Corp.

usually in the lower abdomen and refilled approximately every 14 days by a percutaneous injection through a resealable rubber septum.

The correct position of the catheter and the ability to totally infuse the liver was demonstrated by injecting 6 MCi of Tc-99m MAA over one minute through the pump SIDEPORT$^{TM}$ and scanning the liver.[18] The first course of chemotherapy was started between the 5th and 14th postoperative day and consisted of FUDR 0.3 mg/kg/d for 14 days. The FUDR was mixed with 50 ml normal saline, 10,000 units of heparin and injected into the pump reservoir. A short infusion over 30 min of Mitomycin C, 15 mg/M$^2$ was given via the sideport every 6-8 weeks if there was extrahepatic tumor at operation or if extrahepatic metastases developed while the patient was receiving hepatic artery FUDR.

At the end of 2 weeks of continuous infusion of FUDR, the pump is emptied and refilled with 50 ml of normal saline containing 10,000 units of heparin for a two week rest cycle. Tumor response was evaluated by radionuclide scanning and physical examination. Serial serum CEA determinations were followed but were not used as a sole indication of response. The intial evaluation was performed at two months and then every four months.

A response on liver scan was defined as 50% reduction in tumor mass as measured by the product of the two largest perpendicular diameters. On

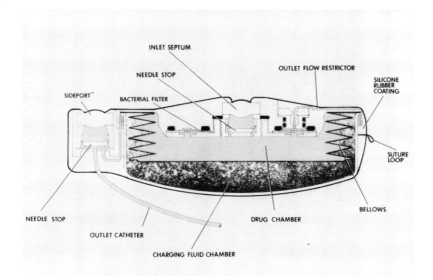

Fig. 2. Scheme of model 400 Infusaid pump produced by Metal Bellows Corp.
This pump has a driving mechanism similar to that of an earlier model
developed by Blacksear et al.[18] for continuous heparin infusions and used
without side port for a small study for hepatic arterial infusion.[19] Model
400 has a side port with an auxiliary septum which bypasses the pumping
mechanism for direct catheter injection. The disc-shaped pump is separated
into 2 chambers by a titanium bellows. The inner drug chamber contains the
solution to be infused; the outer charging chamber contains a fluorocarbon
liquid in equilibrium with its vapor phase. At 37 C, the vapor pressure
exerted by this substance is approximately 300 mm Hg greater than atmospheric
pressure. This vapor pressure provides the power source, exerting pressure on
the bellows and forcing infusate through a 0.22 bacterial filter and a
flow-regulating resistance element. The pump is placed beneath the skin, and
the inner drug chamber is refilled by percutaneous injection through a
self-sealing septum. The pressure of this injection condenses the driving
power source, thus simultaneously filling the pump and recharging the power
source. The pump has a 50 ml capacity, and flow rates of individual pumps are
factory calibrated to deliver a constant set rate, as desired, in the range of
3-6 ml/day. Diagram courtesy of Metal Bellows Corp.

physical exam a response was defined as a 30% reduction in the sum of the

liver measurements below the right costal margin in the midclavicular line

(RMCL), below the xyphoid (SX), and below the left costal margin in the left

midclavicular line (LMCL), when one of these measurements was greater than

4 cm. The CEA response was defined as a 50% reduction when the pretreatment

CEA level was increased more than 10 ng/ml.

Ninety-three of the 110 patients successfully completed two or more cycles of chemotherapy and were considered evaluable. Of the 17 patients that were not evaluable, 10 patients treated during the first phase of this study had extensive extrahepatic involvement as well as extensive hepatic tumor and did not survive long enough to complete two cycles of drug. Four patients had postoperative thrombosis of segments of their hepatic circulation or for anatomic reasons could not have total liver perfusion. An additional three patients lived considerable distances from Ann Arbor and were managed on other drug regimens by their own oncologist and were not followed at the University.

As noted, these patients represented the spectrum of metastatic colorectal cancer with 42/93 (45%) having failed previous systemic chemotherapy and 43 presenting with both extrahepatic and hepatic involvement. No patients were excluded on the basis of liver size or liver function. The mean preoperative alkaline phosphatase, serum bilirubin and serum albumin for these patients is presented in Table 2 and indicates the advanced disease status of the majority of these patients.

Table 2      HEPATIC ARTERY CHEMOTHERAPY OF METASTATIC COLORECTAL
             Cancer Preoperative Liver Function

| Test* | Met. Liver Only SE (50 Patients) | | Liver and Extrahepatic SE (43 Patients) | |
|---|---|---|---|---|
| Alk. Phos. (IU) | 282 | 32 | 269 | 26 |
| Bilirubin (mg%) | .08 | .02 | .09 | .02 |
| Albumin (mg%) | .39 | .01 | 3.5 | .01 |

*These liver function tests have been shown by multifactorial analysis to be the most significant predictors of survival (alkaline phosphatase, $p$ 0.0004; bilirubin, $p$ 0.0005; albumin, $p$ 0.0217).[19,20]

The number of complications related to operative placement of the catheter and delivery system were minimal with only 20 patients having complications which extended their hospital stay (Table 3). More important was the fact that none of the 93 treated patients had their duration of treatment limited because of technical problems with the catheter or the pump.

While there was no limit to successful hepatic artery treatment, four patients did have significant problems requiring reoperation. One patient in this group developed a hematoma in the pump pocket at seven months which

TABLE 3      SURGERY RELATED COMPLICATIONS IN 93 EVALUABLE PATIENTS

WITH METASTATIC COLORECTAL CANCER

|  | Incidence |
|---|---|
| Pulmonary (atelectasis/effusion) | 13 |
| Pump pocket seroma | 2 |
| Prolonged ileus | 1 |
| Pump pocket infection | 1 |
| Wound infection (minimal) | 1 |
| Acute pancreatitis | 1 |
| Incorrect catheter placement | 1* |

*Required reoperation to establish correct placement.

required evacuation. The bleeding point appeared to originate near the rectus muscle fascia along the catheter tract. One patient elected to stop treatment and permitted the pump to run dry only to later urge us to reoperate to place a new catheter and pump. He had experienced a good response while on therapy. One other catheter became occluded by particulate debris and required replacement and another catheter had been first established as an external line without a pump and was accidentally dislodged, requiring replacement.

The rates as determined by nuclide scan and reduction of measurable hepatomegaly by physical exam are presented in Table 4.

TABLE 4.          RESPONSE OF COLORECTAL HEPATIC METASTASES TO
INTRAARTERIAL CHEMOTHERAPY

|  | Response | Stable | Progression |
|---|---|---|---|
| Nuclide scan* | 60/79 (76%) | 16/79 (20%) | 3/79(4%) |
| Liver size** | 57/72(79%) | 10/72(14%) | 5/72(7%) |
| CEA*** | 64/70(90%) | 2/70(3%) | 4/70(6%) |

* The number of patients with measurable liver defect(s) 4 cm that demonstrated 50% reduction in the product of the perpendicular diameters.
** The number of patients presenting with one measurement of liver below costal margins by 4 cm that had 30% reduction in sum of liver extending below margin at RMCL, SX and LMCL.
***The number of patients presenting with CEA 10 ng/ml who had a 50% reduction in levels during therapy.

There were 50 patients that did not have evidence of disease outside the liver (Table 5). These patients had an 83% response rate with the median duration of response being 13 months. Initially this group of patients was treated with FUDR and mitomycin C was subsequently added to the regimen of 25 patients who demonstrated stable hepatic disease and/or extrahepatic tumor.

TABLE 5.    COMPARISON OF RESPONSE IN PATIENTS PRESENTING WITH ONLY
LIVER METASTASES vs PATIENTS WITH LIVER AND EXTRAHEPATIC TUMOR

| | Response | Stable | Progression | Median Duration of Response |
|---|---|---|---|---|
| Liver Only (50 patients) | 83% | 12% | 5% | 13 months |
| Liver & Extrahepatic (43 Patients) | 74% | 16% | 9% | 6 months |

Forty-three patients entered the study with evidence of extrahepatic tumor. This included patients with extensive abdominal involvement, lung metastases or both.  While a high percentage of these patients demonstrated a significant hepatic response, the duration of their hepatic response was much shorter.

The median survival of the patients presenting with only liver involvement was 25 months from the time of diagnosis of hepatic metastases or 18 months from the time of catheter placement.  Twenty four (48%) of the patients in this group remain alive with a median follow-up of 21 months as measured from the date of diagnosis of liver metastases or 15 months from the date of system placement (Table 6).  The median survival of the patients with extrahepatic tumor was half as long, 9 months, and only 6 of 43 patients remain alive.  The Kaplan-Meyer survival plots are presented in Figures 3 and 4.  Of the patients with tumor initially demonstrated only in the liver, 24 patients remain alive and of these, only 8 are free of extrahepatic involvement.

TABLE 6.    SURVIVAL OF METASTATIC COLORECTAL CANCER PATIENTS
TREATED WITH HEPATIC ARTERIAL FUDR MITOMYCIN C

| | From date of Diagnosis* | From date of Pump | Number Alive (3/31/83) |
|---|---|---|---|
| Liver only (50 patients) | 25 months | 18 months | 24  (48%) |
| Liver and extrahepatic (43 patients) | 14 months | 9 months | 6  (14%) |

*The median survival in months as measured from the date of confirmation of liver metastases.  The median followup of the 24 patients still alive is 24 months from the date of diagnosis of liver metastases and 15 months from pump implant date.  The median followup of the 6 patients still alive is 18 months from the diagnosis of liver metastases and 15 months from pump implant date.

134

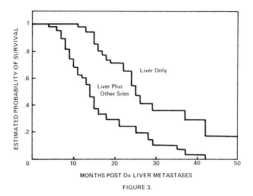

MONTHS POST Dx LIVER METASTASES

FIGURE 3.

Fig. 3. The estimated probability of survival was plotted from the first month post confirmation of recurrent colorectal cancer involving the liver by the method of Kaplan and Meyer.[22] The patient group presenting with only liver involvement at the time of hepatic artery chemotherapy was started was compared to the group of patients presenting with liver and extrahepatic tumor.

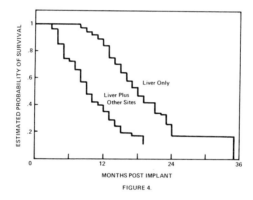

MONTHS POST IMPLANT

FIGURE 4.

Fig. 4. The estimated probability of survival was clotted from the first month of hepatic arterial therapy by the method of Kaplan and Meyer.

The two patient groups were also compared as to whether their hepatic tumor was controlled or progressing at the time of death. As can be seen in Table 7, none of the patients succumbed solely as a result of uncontrolled tumor in the liver. In fact, 78% of the patients with extrahepatic and 73% of those with only liver involvement died of progressive extrahepatic disease with their liver tumor still controlled.

TABLE 7.      THE STATUS OF TUMOR RESPONSE TO HEPATIC ARTERIAL
              CHEMOTHERAPY WITH FUDR MITOMYCIN-C AT TIME OF DEATH

|  | Presenting with Liver and Extrahepatic | Presenting with Only Liver |
|---|---|---|
| Liver tumor controlled | | |
| --unrelated death | 1  (3%)* | 3  (12%) |
| --progressive extrahepatic | 29 (78%) | 19 (73%) |
| | | |
| Progressive liver tumor | | |
| --unrelated death | 0 | 2  (8%) |
| --progressive extrahepatic | 7 (19%) | 2  (8%) |
| --no extrahepatic tumor | 0 | 0 |
| | 37 | 26 |

* Patient died of myocardial infarct.
One patient died of aspiration pneumonia with no detectable tumor at autopsy;
one patient had a long history of obstructive pulmonary disease and died of
pneumonia; one patient died of multiple liver abscesses and sepsis.

Two patients who had failed FUDR and Mitomycin C developed myelo-suppression
and sepsis on subsequent drug therapy and died at a time when there was a
progression of tumor.

The results of this study demonstrate the effective use of hepatic artery
infusion of FUDR and mitomycin C in patients with colorectal cancer involving
the liver.  The success of this treatment was due in large part to a reliable
delivery system which did not limit the duration of arterial infusion, while
providing a means for total liver perfusion without delivering drug to the
gastrointestinal tract.  With this system there was a high degree of control
of hepatic tumor and evidence of improved survival, even though almost half
the patients had failed previous systemic therapy.  The results indicated that
patients who failed did so because of progression of extrahepatic tumor, not
because of the inability to control their liver tumor.

Although this was not a randomized, controlled trial, the median survival
of 25 months from the time of diagnosis of metastatic involvement of the liver
or 18 months from the initiation of hepatic artery therapy certainly appears
to be a significant improvement.  This conclusion is supported by recent
studies at the University of Alabama (19,20).  They reviewed the records of
175 patients presenting with liver metastases from colorectal cancer.  Forty
one percent of these patients were treated with systemic 5-FU therapy and had
a median survival of 6.1 months.  They analyzed incremental risk factors and
identified 22 factors of which 7 when examined simultaneously were found to
independently influence survival.  From this data, a mathematical equation was

constructed which accurately predicted an individual patient's course. Using the two factors (alkaline phosphatase and bilirubin) with the greatest predictive value, it is possible to calculate the expected length of survival for each of the patients in our study. The predicted median survival for those patients presenting with only liver metastases was 4.6 months while the observed median survival was 18 months, an almost fourfold increase (Table 8). Patients presenting with extrahepatic and hepatic metastases had a median predicted survival of 3.1 months and a threefold increase in observed survival.

TABLE 8.        SURVIVAL WITH HEPATIC ARTERY CHEMOTHERAPY
                FOR METASTATIC COLORECTAL CANCER

|  | Predicted* | Observed | Number Alive (3/31/83) |
|---|---|---|---|
| Liver Only (50 patients) | 4.6 months | 18 months | 24    (48%) (median 15 months) |
| Liver and extrahepatic (43 patients) | 3.1 months | 9 months | 6    (14%) (median 15 months |

*Based on an integration of preoperative bilirubin and alkaline phosphatase.[19]

Side effects consisted mainly of chemical hepatitis and gastro intestinal toxicity and all resolved off treatment. Only three patients had documented gastric ulcers and all three had a prior ulcer history. All were able to be restarted on intraarterial therapy at a reduced dose (25% of original) and in no instance was treatment terminated as a result of unacceptable toxicity. The results of this initial trial have confirmed the reliability of the implanted delivery system and have provided good guidelines to select patients which can both tolerate the surgical procedure and are likely to gain a significant benefit. Clearly the response rate of liver tumor to hepatic artery therapy is superior to that obtained using systemic drug(s). These observations, while very promising, do not preclude the need for a randomized prospective trial. Furthermore, it remains unclear what role radiation therapy or hyperthermia can play in the management of metastatic liver tumor and studies which include these modalities will be necessary in the future if we are to achieve complete remission.[21]

ACKNOWLEDGEMENTS

The author would like to acknowledge the other members of the University of Michigan team involved in these studies. They include William Ensminger, M.D., Ph.D., Division of Medical Oncology; John Gyves, M.D., Division of Medical Oncology; James Thrall, M.D., Division of Nuclear Medicine; Kyung Cho, M.D., Department of Radiology; Edith Cozzi, R.N., Division of Surgical Oncology; Suzette Walker, R.N., Division of Medical Oncology.

REFERENCES

1. Sullivan RD, Zurek WZ. Chemotherapy for liver cancer by protracted ambulatory infusion. JAMA 194:481-486, 1965.
2. Watkins JR, Khazei AM, Nakea KS. Surgical basis for arterial infusion chemotherapy of disseminated carcinoma of the liver. Surg Gynecol Obstet 130:581-605, 1970.
3. Cady B, Oberfield RA. Regional infusion chemotherapy of hepatic metastases from carcinoma of the colon. Am J Surg 127:220-227, 1974.
4. Buroker T, Samson M, Correa J, Fraile R, Vaikevicius VK. Hepatic artery infusion of 5-FUDR after prior systemic 5-fluorouracil. Cancer Treat Rep 60:1277-1279, 1976.
5. Grage TB, Vassilopoulos PP, Shingleton WW, Jubert AV, Elias EG, Aust JB, Moss SE. Results of a prospective randomized study of hepatic artery infusion with 5-fluorouracil versus intravenous 5-fluorouracil in patients with hepatic metastases from colorectal cancer: a Central Oncology Group Study. Surgery 86:550-555, 1979.
6. Oberfield RA, McCaffrey JA, Polio J, Clouse ME, Hamilton T. Prolonged and continuous percutaneous intraarterial hepatic infusion chemotherapy in advanced metastatic liver adenocarcinoma from colorectal primary. Cancer 44:414-423, 1979.
7. Patt VZ, Movligit GM, Chuand VP, Wallace S, Johnston S, Benjamin R, Valdivieso M, Hersh E. Percutaneous hepatic infusion (HAI) of mitomycin C and floxuridine (FUDR): an effective treatment for metastatic colorectal carcinoma in the liver. Cancer 46:261-265, 1980.
8. Reed ML, Vaitkevicius VK, Al-Sarraf M, Vaughn CB, Singhakowinta A, Sexon-Porte M, Izbicki R, Baker L, Straatsma G. The practicality of chronic hepatic artery infusion therapy of primary and metastatic hepatic malignancies. Cancer 47:402-409, 1981.
9. Klopp CT, Alford TC, Bateman J, Berry GN, Winship T. Fractionated intra-arterial cancer chemotherapy with methyl bis amine hydrochloride; a preliminary report. Am Surg 132:811-832, 1950.
10. Clouse ME, Ahmed R, Ryan RB, Oberfield RA, McCaffrey JA. Complications of long term transbrachial arterial infusion chemotherapy. Am J. Roentgenol 129:799-803, 1977.
11. Ramming KP, Haskell CM, Tesler AS. Gastrointestinal tract neoplasms, In, Cancer Treatment (ed. by C.M. Haskell) W.B. Saunders Co., Philadelphia, PA, pp 231-357, 1980.
12. Cady B. Hepatic arterial patency and complications after catheterization for infusion chemotherapy. Ann Surg 178:156-159, 1973.
13. Ensminger WD, Rosowsky A, Raso V. A clinical-pharmacological evaluation of hepatic arterial infusions of 5-fluoro-2-deoxyuridine and 5-fluorouracil. Cancer Res 38:3784-3792,1978.

138

14. Buchwald H, Grage TB, Vassilopoulos PP, Rhod TD, Varco RL, Blackshear PL. Intraarterial infusion chemotherapy for hepatic carcinoma using a totally implantable infusion pump. Cancer 45:866-869, 1980.
15. Ensminger WD, Niederhuber JE, Dahkil S, Thrall J, Wheeler R. A totally implanted drug delivery system for hepatic arterial chemotherapy. Cancer Treat Rep 65:393-400, 1981.
16. Niederhuber JE, Ensminger WD. Surgical considerations in the management of hepatic neoplasia. In Infusion Therapy, Lokich JJ, guest ed, Seminars in Oncology, Grune and Stratton, New York, 10(2):135-146, 1983.
17. Niederhuber JE, Ensminger W, Gyves J, Thrall J, Walker S, Cozzi E. Regional chemotherapy of colorectal cancer metastatic to the liver. Cancer (In Press).
18. Yang PJ, Thrall JH, Ensminger WD, Niederhuber JE, Gyves JW, Tuscan M, Doan K, Cozzi E. Perfusion scintigraphy (Tc 99m MAA) during surgery for placement of chemotherapy catheter in hepatic artery: Concise Communication. J Nuc Med 23:1066-1069, 1982.
19. Lahr CJ, Soong SJ, Cloud G, Smith JW, Urist MM, Balch CM. A multi-factorial analysis of prognostic factors in patients with liver metastases from colorectal carcinoma. J Clin Oncol (In Press).
20. Balch CM, Urist MM, Soong SJ, McGregor M. A prospective phase II clinical trial of continuous FUDR regional chemotherapy for colorectal metastases to the liver using a totally implantable drug infusion pump. Ann Surg (In Press).
21. Barone RM, Byfield JE, Goldfarb PB, Frankel S, Ginn C, Greer S. Intra-arterial chemotherapy using an implantable infusion pump and liver irradiation for the treatment of hepatic metastases. Cancer 50:850-862, 1982.
22. Kaplan EL, Meyer P. Non-parametric estimation from incomplete observation. J Am Stat Assoc 53:457-481, 1958.

PANCREATIC CANCER - A MULTIMODALITY APPROACH

LEONARD L. GUNDERSON, M.D., M.S., J. KIRK MARTIN, M.D., AND
LAWRENCE K. KVOLS, M.D.

## INTRODUCTION

### Definition of the Problem

Cancer of the pancreas is currently the fifth leading cause of cancer deaths in the United States, and the incidence is increasing without known reason. An estimated 22,600 deaths will occur in this country during 1983.[1] Although some cures can be obtained with radical operative procedures for resectable lesions, the percentage of patients who present with such extent of disease is small. Operability with curative intent varies from 10% to 25% by series, and until the past decade operative mortality ranged from 15-20% even in the most experienced hands.[2]

The largest group of patients present with lesions in the head of the pancreas that have either spread beyond the local area via hematogenous or peritoneal routes or are technically unresectable due to the local extent of disease. For the latter group of patients, the main surgical options are palliative biliary bypass alone or in combination with elective gastroenterostomy. If gains are to be made with the unresectable group of lesions, it will have to be with radiation, chemotherapy, or a combination of both.

### Areas of Failure - Cause of Death

Little has been done to systematically analyze areas of failure with this cancer since a majority of lesions are initially inoperable. In the overall group, death results most frequently from hepatic failure due to biliary obstruction by the local tumor or hepatic replacement by metastases. Peritoneal seeding (PS) also occurs, although the exact frequency is not well documented.

Failure after "curative" resection was analyzed in a series of 31 patients from Massachusetts General Hospital (MGH).[3] Of the 26 postoperative survivors, 22 died of disease, and re-operative or autopsy information was available in 13. Local or regional recurrence (LF-RF) in the pancreatic bed (13/26 or 50%) and liver metastases were the most common areas of failure.

Approximately 50% of patients present at laparotomy with only local-regional disease. In the MGH series,[3] although only 31 patients had radical resection, an additional 35 patients had tumors which were unresectable only because of the extent of the local disease (total 66 of 145 or 46% with only local-regional disease). In Hermreck's series of 348 patients (1974), 169 or 49% had only local-regional disease at presentation, and the majority were not amenable to surgical resection.[4]

## EXTERNAL BEAM IRRADIATION + CHEMOTHERAPY-UNRESECTABLE LESIONS

It is clear that long-term palliation and occasional cures can be obtained using external beam irradiation techniques.[2,5-8] The combination of radiation therapy and chemotherapy with Fluorouracil (5-FU) for locally unresectable tumors increases survival when compared to radiation therapy alone in both randomized and nonrandomized series[5-10] and produces a median survival comparable to that obtained with surgical resection of resectable lesions (Table 1)[3]. The improvement in median survival appears to be related to both the use of chemo- therapy and to an increase in the radiation dose. However local failure remains a formidable problem, and both distant metastases to the liver and peritoneal seeding are also very common. In the series from Thomas Jefferson,[5,8] in spite of the use of radiation doses of 6300 to 7000 rad with precision high-dose external beam techniques, local control was achieved in only one-third of patients (not surprising in view of initial bulk of disease).

## INTRAOPERATIVE IRRADIATION (INTERSTITIAL IMPLANTATION OR ELECTRONS)

In order to increase the dose to the tumor volume and thus increase tumor control without increasing normal tissue morbidity, efforts have been made to utilize specialized radiation therapy techniques. This has included the use of intraoperative electrons as the sole treatment modality[11-13] or the use of Iodine$^{125}$ implants[8,14] or intraoperative electrons[15-17] as a boost dose in combination with external beam irradiation. The use of intraoperative electrons as the sole treatment modality was not effective in achieving local control or improving survival. The combination techniques have resulted in better local control and improved median survival (Table 1) when compared with conventional external beam irradiation, but some of the differences are probably due to case selection. While the combination methods deliver a much higher effective dose of irradiation than external beam alone, prospective randomized trials are needed to determine if a therapeutic gain will result from the aggressive combinations.

TABLE 1     COMPARISON OF RESULTS - CANCER OF PANCREAS
Varied Series and Techniques

| Series (reference number) | # Pts | Median SR (Months) | | | Local Failure (evaluable patients) | |
|---|---|---|---|---|---|---|
| | | Total Group | RT | RE + CT | # | % |
| Radical operation - MGH[3] (26 post op survivors) | 31 | 10.5 | --- | --- | 13/26 | 50% |
| **Regional, Unresectable** | | | | | | |
| 1. Mayo[9,10] | | | | | | |
| a. Untreated | 67 | 6.0 | --- | --- | --- | --- |
| b. 3500 rad/4 wk ± 5 FU | 64 | --- | 6.3 | 10.4 | --- | --- |
| 2. GITSG[6] | | | | | | |
| a. 4000 rad/6 wk ± 5 FU | 79 | --- | --- | 6.9 | --- | --- |
| b. 6000 rad/10 wk ± 5 FU | 100 | --- | 5.1 | 8.7 | --- | --- |
| 3. Duke (Curative Group)[7] | | | | | | |
| a. 6000 rad/10 wk ± chemo (RT, 9 pts; RT ± CT, 11 pts) | 20 | --- | 8 | 10 | --- | --- |
| 4. Thomas Jefferson[5,8] | | | | | | |
| a. 6300 - 6700 rad/7-9 wks ± chemo (RT, 33 pts; RT ± CT, 15 pts) | 48 | 10 | 8.0 | 13 | 28/42 | 67% |
| b. External + implant ± chemo (RT, 6 pts; RT ± CT, 8 pts) | 14 | 12 | 8.5 | 16 | --- | --- |
| 5. Mass General Hospital[15-17] | | | | | | |
| a. I125 + External beam XRT (postop) (4000 - 4500 rad/4.5 - 5 wk) | 12 | 11 | --- | --- | 4/12 | 33% |
| b. Ext. beam + Intraop. electron boost (4500 - 5000 rad split course ± chemo) | 16 | 17.5 | --- | --- | 7/16 | 44% |

Peritoneal Seeding +/- Wound Implants by Treatment Method

In the series from Thomas Jefferson[8] it was possible to compare the incidence of either peritoneal seeding (PS) or incisional implantation by treatment method. In the group treated solely with external beam techniques, only 3 of 42 evaluable patients (7%) developed such patterns of failure after irradiation (1 diffuse PS; 2 incisional failure). In patients treated with an $I^{125}$ implant plus external beam irradiation, those who received 500 rad external beam in a single fraction prior to the implant (non-randomized basis on the day preceding or day of implant) had a lower incidence of either pattern of failure, suggesting an alteration in the implantability of cells. Only 1 of 7 or 14% receiving low-dose preoperative irradiation developed such failure versus 5 of 7 or 71% who did not receive a preoperative dose.

Intraoperative Electrons (IORT) +/- External Beam XRT

Although a large number of patients with pancreatic carcinoma have been treated with intraoperative irradiation, only 16.7% of the 108 patients in the combined Japanese series[11] received an external beam component and none of the initial 19 reported by Goldson et al. from Howard.[13] Intra-arterial chemotherapy was added during the operative procedure in 44% of the Japanese group.

Results from the Japanese series[11] are unimpressive except for relief of pain which was reported in 47 of 59 patients (79.6%) who received a single dose of more than 2000 rad (no comment on duration). Fifteen of 108 patients were alive but only 5 for longer than 1 year, with the longest survival being 3 years and 7 months. In autopsied patients, marked degeneration of tumor cells and fibrotic changes were noted in patients receiving more than 2500 rad. Abe et al.[12] commented that the potential for combining external beam and intraoperative irradiation should be examined, since such large tumors can hardly be eradicated by a single dose of irradiation.

Results from the Howard series are difficult to interpret since 10 of the initial 19 patients in their pilot series had metastases on liver scan (survival ranged from 3 months to 15 months; all 10 patients died). Three of 9 without metastases were alive at 2, 5, and 12 months. The median survival for the entire group of 19 was 5 1/2 months. Since islands of viable cancer were found amid massive tumor necrosis and fibrous reaction in all five of their autopsied patients, they are now combining intraoperative radiation with external beam irradiation and chemotherapy in an attempt to achieve the best tumoricidal effect.[18]

The most optimistic results to date are in the series using a combination of external beam and intraoperative irradiation, and the longest follow-up exists in the MGH trial.[15-17] In this series, patients were judged unresectable at an initial exploration, received low dose preoperative irradiation prior to a second exploration, and only those who still had localized disease received a 1500 rad intraoperative boost and additional postoperative irradiation. The intraoperative boost dose was increased in 250 rad increments to 1750 rad and subsequently 2000 rad since evidence of local recurrence developed at the lower dose levels, and normal tissue tolerance was acceptable. Of the 20 patients treated to date, 16 were unresectable and the others were treated after a Whipple resection. Median survival in the locally unresectable group, as calculated from onset of treatment, is 17 1/2 months (Table 1). Although survival appears to be significantly better than results obtained with external beam $\pm$ chemotherapy for unresectable disease, this is a select series in that most patients had a second exploration 6-10 weeks after the initial operation. (Currently, more patients are receiving IORT at the time of the initial exploration which is preceded by CT $\pm$ needle guided biopsies.) While local failure appears to be less than with external beam techniques, it was still a significant problem in the initial 16 patients when the IORT boost was usually 1500 or 1750 rad (7/16 or 44%).

In the Mayo series,[16] less selectivity occurs. Patients either have their initial exploration in an operating room in the radiation therapy area (Curie OR) or if the initial exploration is done at one of the two hospitals affiliated with the Clinic, the patient is reexplored in the Curie OR in 1-10 days for purpose of the intraoperative boost. In the initial 17 patients, 8 have progressed. All had either a liver or peritoneal component of failure, and none has had proven local progression. The minimum survival for patients at risk for at least one year is 13 1/2+ months (median survivor alive with disease).

In an NCI trial,[19] patients have either a total or regional pancreatectomy, with portal vein resection if indicated, and are then randomized to receive IORT to a dose of 2000 rad with misonidazole or to receive only external beam irradiation. While this approach may ultimately provide better local control rates than in other series, at present the mortality from the operative procedure is approximately 40%.

Tolerance. Morbidity was judged as acceptable in the Howard series.[13,18] Only 1 of their 19 patients experienced intra-abdominal infection. A syndrome of anorexia, nausea, and vomiting was observed in 8 patients commencing 1-5 days after the intraoperative irradiation - such symptoms were most pronounced in patients receiving 3000 rad to volumes greater than 120 $cm^3$.

An early patient in the MGH series developed gastric outlet obstruction from irradiation of most of the circumference of the first portion of the duodenum and distal stomach due to the location of the tumor. This has been avoided in subsequent patients by routinely performing a gastrojejunostomy and by limiting the amount of duodenum in the intraoperative boost to the medial wall.[15-17] Three patients in the MGH series have developed evidence of gastrointestinal bleeding. One was from a gastric ulcer secondary to the inclusion of the distal portion of the stomach in the intraoperative field; one from a duodenal bleed in the area in the intraoperative field; and the third, a diffuse gastritis, probably related to chemotherapy and external beam irradiation. Gastric problems have subsequently been minimized by surgically moving the stomach so it is completely out of the boost field and by more cautious use of combination chemotherapy. None of the aforementioned problems have thus far been encountered in the Mayo trial.[16]

## CONCLUSIONS AND FUTURE POSSIBILITIES
### Wide Field Abdominal Treatment for Locally Unresectable Disease

In view of patterns of failure in the Mayo Clinic IORT pancreas pilot (8 of 8 with failure had liver metastases and/or peritoneal seeding), and the lack of effective systemic therapy, some form of upper or total abdominal prophylaxis appears to be indicated in addition to an aggressive combined external beam and intraoperative approach to the primary lesion. Whole abdominal external beam irradiation has been utilized for a portion of treatment with acceptable toxicity in ovarian,[20,21] colon,[22,23] and gallbladder cancer.[24] For ovarian cancer, combinations of external beam irradiation and intraperitoneal installation of colloidal radioisotopes[25-27] have been used to treat areas at risk which may include tumor bed or unresected tumor, nodes, and peritoneal surfaces (all areas also at risk with pancreatic cancer). A major difference in ovarian and pancreatic cancer is that the liver is at negligible risk with ovarian cancer and has been shielded for a portion of whole abdominal treatment. For pancreatic cancer the liver is at significant risk, and more aggressive treatment may be required (external beam irradiation, infusion chemotherapy, or both). In an attempt to define the relative risks of peritoneal seeding and determine who may benefit from upper abdomen vs. total abdomen prophylaxis for pancreatic cancer (treatment risks may be significantly different), it may be valuable to do cytology on peritoneal washings obtained before resection since data in both gynecological[28,29] and gastric cancer[30] have shown that patients with positive cytology have a significantly higher risk of later cancer failure.

## Adjuvant Irradiation

The potential for radiation therapy (XRT) is considerable when used in combination with surgery and perhaps systemic therapy for lesions which are resectable but at high risk for local recurrence. Operation alone yields inadequate results for most pancreatic cancers.[2,3,10] The use of operative resection, while justifiable, does not uniformly prevent either local failures or regrowth (LF) in the tumor bed and regional lymph nodes or distant failures (DF) by hematogenous (DM) or peritoneal routes (PS).

With pancreatic lesions, there is a propensity to invade posteriorly, and the margins of normal tissue between tumor and structures such as portal vein, superior mesenteric vessels, and retroperitoneal soft tissue are often narrow or nonexistant. Progressive extension of operative procedures to increase these margins may yield slight gains in cure rates, but these gains may be offset or minimized by a corresponding increase in operative morbidity and mortality. These "margins" could possibly be obtained with less morbidity by close interactions of the surgeon and radiation oncologist in the use of combined modality treatment.

Many of the local-regional failures that occur are predictable and are due to the presence of microscopic or subclinical residual disease left in spite of "curative operative attempts". Many of these failures should be preventable with the use of moderate doses of irradiation in the range of 4500 to 5000 rad in accordance with the "subclinical disease radiation dose concept."[31] With upper abdomen sites (biliary duct, pancreas, stomach, and colon), doses of 4500 rad in 25 fractions over 5 weeks to tumor bed and regional nodes and 5000 rad in 5 1/2 to 6 weeks within a boost field have been achieved in an adjuvant setting with acceptable tolerance in our experience. Such dose levels appear preferable to the lower dose 4000 rad continuous or split-course schemes used in the GITSG rectal and pancreas trials.

A well-designed combination of pre- and postoperative irradiation could combine the theoretical advantages of each.[32-35] An approach used in rectal cancer is to deliver 500 rad in a single fraction or 1000 rad in 5 fractions with the intent of altering implantability of cells, do the surgical resection in 1 to 3 days, and give 4500 to 5000 rad postoperatively only to those patients at high risk for local recurrence.[33,35] A similar approach would

be attractive for potentially resectable pancreatic cancers since circumferential margins are often narrow and tumor manipulation may be necessary.

Many systemic failures are probably established as microscopic deposits
prior to attempts at resection. If available chemotherapy agents do not alter
the incidence of such failures when used in combination with resection and
tumor bed $\pm$ nodal irradiation, one may have to consider liver and/or abdominal
prophylaxis in high-risk groups provided the toxicity is tolerable in pilot
trials with locally advanced disease.

## ACKNOWLEDGEMENTS

The authors are indebted to Cindy Franke and the Mayo central typing pool for
preparation of the manuscript.

## REFERENCES

1. Silverberg E. Cancer statistics, 1983. Cancer J Clin 33:9-25,1983;
2. MacDonald JS, Gunderson LL, Cohn I. Cancer of the pancreas. In: DeVita VT, Hellman S, Roseberg SA, eds. Principles and practice of oncology. Philadelphia, JB Lippincott, pp 563-589, 1982.
3. Tepper J, Nardi GL, Suit HD. Carcinoma of the pancreas review of MGH experience from 1963 to 1973: analysis of surgical failure and implications for radiation therapy. Cancer 37:1519-1524, 1976.
4. Hermreck AS, Thomas CY, Friesen SR. Importance of pathologic staging and the surgical management of adenocarcinoma of the exocrine pancreas. Am J Surg, 127:653-657, 1974.
5. Dobelbower RR. The radiotherapy of pancreatic cancer. Seminars in Oncology, 6:378-389, 1979.
6. GITSG. Comparative therapeutic trial of radiation with or without chemotherapy in pancreatic carcinoma. Int J Rad Oncol Biol Phys, 5:1643-1647, 1979.
7. Haslam JB, Cavanaugh PJ, Stroup SL. Radiation therapy in the treatment of irresectable adenocarcinoma of the pancreas. Cancer, 32:1341-1345, 1973.
8. Whittington R, Dobelbower RR, Mohiuddin M, Rosato FF, Weiss SM. Radiotherapy of unresectable pancreatic carcinoma: a six-year experience with 104 patients. Int J Rad Oncol Biol Phys, 7:1639-1644, 1981.
9. Moertel CG, Childs DS, Jr., Reitemeier RJ, Colby MY, Jr., Holbrook MA. Combined 5-fluorouracil and supervoltage radiation therapy of locally resectable gastrointestinal cancer. Lancet, 2:865-867, 1969.
10. Moertel CG. Alimentary tract cancer. In: Holland J, Frei E, eds. Cancer medicine. Philadelphia, Lea and Febiger, pp 753-1866, 1982.
11. Abe M, Takahashi M. Intraoperative radiotherapy: the Japanese experience. Int J Rad Oncol Biol Phys, 5:863-868, 1981.
12. Abe M, Takahashi M, Yabumoto E, et al. Clinical experiences with intraoperative radiotherapy of locally advanced cancers. Cancer, 45:40-48, 1980.
13. Goldson AL, Ashaveri E, Espinoza MC, et al. Single-dose intraoperative electrons for advanced stage pancreatic cancer: phase I pilot study. Int J Rad Oncol Biol Phys, 7:869-874, 1981.
14. Shipley WU, Nardi GL, Cohen AM, et al. Iodine-25 implant and external beam irradiation in patients with localized pancreatic carcinoma: a comparative study to surgical resection. Cancer, 45:709-714, 1980.

15. Gunderson LL, Shipley WU, Suit HD, et al. Intraoperative irradiation: a pilot study combining external beam irradiation with "boost" dose intraoperative electrons. Cancer, 49:2259-2266, 1982.

16. Gunderson LL, Tepper JE, Biggs PJ, Goldson A, Martin JR, et al. Intraoperative ± external beam irradiation. In: Hickey RC, ed., Current problems in cancer. Chicago, Yearbook Medical Publishers Inc. (in press).

17. Wood W, Shipley WU, Gunderson LL, Cohen AM, Nardi GL. Intraoperative irradiation for unresectable pancreatic carcinoma. Cancer, 49:1272-1275, 1982.

18. Goldson AL. Update on 5 years of pioneering experience with intraoperative electron irradiation. In: Session II, Intraoperative electron therapy. Varian Users Proceedings, 21-27, 1982.

19. Sinclair WF, Kinsella T, Tepper JE, et al. Experimental and clinical studies with intraoperative radiotherapy. Surg Gyn Obstet (in press).

20. Dembo AJ, Van Dyk J, Japp B, et al. Whole abdominal irradiation by a moving strip technique for patients with ovarian cancer. Int J Rad Oncol Biol Phys, 5:1933-1942, 1979.

21. Martinez A, Coleman CN. The role of radiation therapy in the treatment of epithelial ovarian cancer. In: Whitehouse JM, Williams CJ, eds. Recent advances in clinical oncology. London, Churchill Livingstone, pp 155-164, 1982.

22. Ghossein NA, Samala EC, Alpert S, et al. Results of postoperative radiotherapy in patients who had incomplete resection of a colorectal cancer. Dis Colon Rectum, 24:252-256, 1981.

23. Turner SS, Vieira EF, Ager PJ, et al. Elective postoperative radiotherapy for locally advanced colorectal cancer. Cancer, 40:105-108, 1977.

24. Hanna SS, Rider WD. Carcinoma of the gallbladder or extrahepatic bile ducts: the role of radiotherapy. Canad Med Assoc J, 118:59-61, 1978.

25. Rosenscheim NB, Leichner PK, Vogelsang G. Radiocolloids in the treatment of gynecologic malignant disease. Am J Obstet Gynecol, 110:773-781, 1971.

26. Pezner RD, Stevens KR, Tong D, Allen L. Limited epithelial carcinoma of the ovary treated with curative intent by the intraperitoneal installation of radiocolloids. Cancer, 42:2563-2571, 1978.

27. Torres JL, Bross DS, Hernandez E, et al. Multimodality treatment of patients with advanced ovarian carcinoma. Int J Rad Oncol Biol Phys, 8:1671-1677, 1982.

28. Creasman WT, Rutledge F. The prognostic value of peritoneal cytology in gynecologic malignant disease. Am J Obstet Gynecol, 110:773-781, 1971.

29. Creasman WT, Disaia PJ, Blessing J, et al. Prognostic significance of peritoneal cytology in patients with endometrial cancer and preliminary data concerning therapy with intraperitoneal radiopharmaceuticals. Am J Obstet Gynecol, 141:921-929, 1981.

30. Nakajima T, Harashima S, Hirata M, Kajitani T. Prognostic and therapeutic values of peritoneal cytology in gastric cancer. Acta Cytol, 22:225-229, 1978.

31. Fletcher GH. Clinical dose-response curves of human malignant epithelial tumors. Br J Radiol, 46:1-12, 1973.

32. Gunderson LL. Combined irradiation and surgery for rectal and sigmoid carcinoma. In: Fletcher G, ed. Emerging roles of radiotherapy in four selected areas. Current Prob Cancer, 1:40-53, 1976.

33. Gunderson LL, Dosoretz DE, Hedberg SE, et al. Low-dose preoperative irradiation, surgery, and elective postoperative radiation therapy for resectable rectum and rectosigmoid carcinoma. Cancer 1982 (in press).

148

34. Gunderson LL, Sosin H. Areas of failure found at reoperation (second or symptomatic look) following "curative surgery" for adenocarcinoma of the rectum: Clinicopathologic correlation and implications for adjuvant therapy. Cancer, 34:1278-1292, 1974.
35. Mohiuddin M, Dobelbower RR, Kramer S. A new approach to adjuvant radio-therapy in rectal cancer. Int J Rad Oncol Biol Phys, 6:205-207, 1980.

EXTERNAL BEAM IRRADIATION IN ADENOCARCINOMA OF THE PROSTATE

BEATRIZ E. AMENDOLA, M.D. AND IHN H. HAN, M.D., PH.D.

INTRODUCTION

Prostatic carcinoma comprises 18% of the malignant tumors in men and is also the third most common cause of death in men aged 55 years and older.[1] The incidence of prostate cancer rises sharply with age. Cancer rates are higher for blacks than for whites and also the incidence in blacks is rising more rapidly. There is a world wide variation regarding its incidence, with the Western hemisphere having a higher number than the Asian population. Latent adenocarcinoma of the prostate found at autopsy increases with age; from 5% to 14% for patients 50 to 60 years old and from 20%-40% for patients 70 to 80 years old.[2]

There are two categories of carcinoma: 1) found by the pathologist a) in a TURP specimen from benign hypertrophy or b) in an autopsy from a patient who died from other disease, this category is designated as incidental carcinoma; and 2) a carcinoma clinically detected either by rectal examination or a metastatic manifestation.[3]

STAGING

Several staging systems of prostatic carcinoma have been used, however, none have received widespread acceptance. A staging system which will combine the clinical and pathological information should be used. The American Urological staging System is used at the University of Michigan Medical Center (Table 1).[4] Clinical staging is not an accurate method of determining the local extent of cancer; the combination of clinical evaluation, radiographic and laboratory findings makes the staging of prostatic cancer precise. Pathologic diagnosis will require either perineal needle biopsy or trans urethral resection of the prostate (TURP). A simple grading system based on structural differentiation and cellular anaplasia has prognostic significance.[5]

All patients should undergo a complete pretreatment evaluation since any evidence of dissemination during this period precludes any aggressive form of treatment. The pretreatment workup at the UMMC includes: complete history

Recent Trends in Radiation Oncology and Related Fields, Amendola and Amendola, Editors

| TABLE 1 | STAGING: ADENOCARCINOMA OF THE PROSTATE<br>American Urological System |
|---|---|

STAGE A.  Incidental finding (clinically undetectable).
$A_1$    Focal
$A_2$    Diffuse

STAGE B.  Confined to the prostate.
$B_1$    Single small discrete nodule
$B_2$    Large or multiple nodules

STAGE C.  Localized to the periprostatic area.
$C_1$    No involvement of seminal vesicles  > 70 gr.
$C_2$    Involvement of the seminal vesicles  < 70 gr.

STAGE D.  Metastatic disease
$D_1$    Pelvic lymph node metastasis or ureteral
         obstrucion (hydronephrosis)
$D_2$    Bone or distant lymph node
         or soft tissue metastases.

and physical examination, chest x-ray, intravenous pyelography (IVP), cystoscopy, serum acid phosphatase, urinalysis, radioisotopic bone scans, bipedal lymphangiogram and computerized body tomography. The incidence of lymph node involvement depends on the stage and degree of differentiation. Patients with disease localized to the prostate, Stage B, have between 5% and 20% of positive nodes in the pelvis. In patients with Stage C an incidence of pelvic node metastases as high as 64% has been reported.[6]

TREATMENT

   Occasional reports describing external irradiation techniques for prostatic cancer were published in the 1930's. In spite of good response to this treatment, success was obscured due to the detrimental effect to bowel. Radiation therapy was only used for palliative cases.[7] It was not until the 1950's that this modality of treatment was used as an alternative to surgery for curative purposes.[8] In 1962 and 1967 del Regato indicated that external beam irradiation with megavoltage equipment permitted adequate local control of moderately advanced carcinoma of the prostate.[8,9] At the same time Bagshaw reported 25 of 59 patients alive after 5 years treated by external irradiation (rotation).[10] Since then many series have confirmed these findings. In general, medium energy linear accelerators are recommended for treatment of prostatic carcinoma.

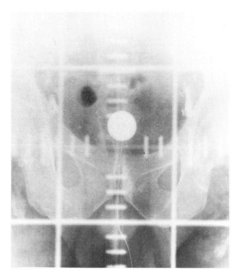

Fig. 1A. (Above) and Fig. 1B. (Below) Typical Target Volume. Mercury in the catheter and contrast material in the balloon (AP) and barium in the rectum (Lateral) delineate the urethra and the rectum.

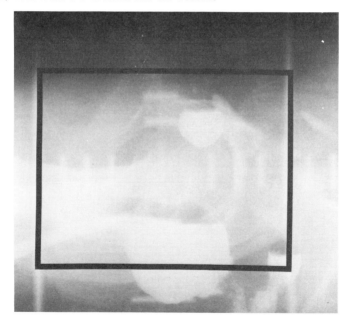

152

Patients with disease limited to the prostate as well as low grade tumor will have less than 5% chance of lymph node involvement so the treatment target should be the prostate gland and adjacent tissues (Figure 1A and 1B). Tumor localization is extremely important in these patients. Once the volume is defined, different treatment techniques can be chosen: 360° rotation, arc therapy (Figure 2), or a box technique. Simulation is essential in planning treatment for prostate cancer. Different steps are followed (Table 2).

---

TABLE 2                         RADIATION THERAPY TECHNIQUE

1) Precise localization (use of CT, etc.).

2) Foley catheter with a mercury filled balloon to outline the urethra.

3) 30 ml of 30% water soluble contrast (i.e. renographin) and 10 ml air are injected via Foley catheter into the bladder to help delineate the superior border of the prostate gland.

4) Posterior margin of the prostate is outlined by 100 ml of barium placed in the rectum.

5) CT volume verification.

---

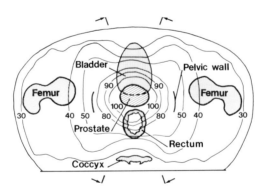

Fig. 2. Two lateral arcs used give a uniform dose in the prostate gland and less dose to bladder and rectum.

In patients with localized disease, exact knowledge of target volume is required. Regarding dose, patients should receive between 180 cGy (rad) and 200 cGy, all fields treated daily, 5 days a week, to a total dose of 6500 to 7000 cGy.

Clinical stage and histologic grade are key factors in considering treatment strategies. Patients with low grade Stage A may not require any treatment. Treatment depends on the degree of involvement, as well as the degree of differentiation. For example, patients presenting with Stage A2 (diffuse) require local irradiation when they are in the older age group and have poorly differentiated tumors (high risk group).

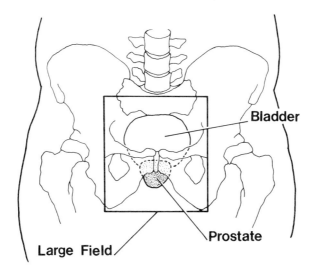

Fig. 3A. Diagram of the Treatment Volume (Whole pelvis).

Patients with Stage C or high grade tumors will require radiation to the pelvic nodes. Patients with extra capsular involvement have an incidence of 59% of pelvic nodes.[11] In one recent series, Pistenma et al. reported that 82% of patients (14 out of 17) with Stage C, poorly differentiated tumor, had pelvic lymph node involvement.[11] For these patients, a four-field box technique is recommended (Figure 3A,B,C, and D). The upper margin is at the $L_5-S_1$ level and the lower margin is at the ischial tuberosities; lateral margins are 1 to 1.5 cm lateral to the bony pelvis. The posterior border is

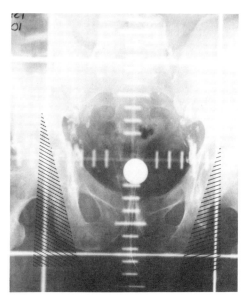

Fig. 3B. (Above) and Fig. 3C (Below). Typical Target Volume Field (AP and Lateral).

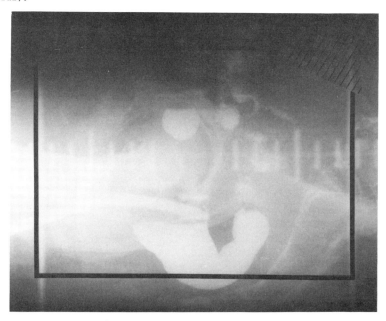

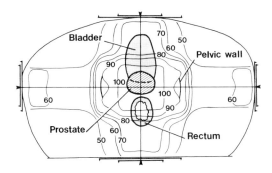

Fig. 3D. Isodose distribution from a four-field technique.

at the level of the rectum with the anterior margin at the anterior aspect of
the pubic bone.  Total dose to the large field is 4500 to 5000 cGy, then the
patient is resimulated to reduce the field to the prostate gland.  This cone
down field will receive a total dose of 7000 cGy including the previous dose
(Figure 4).  Shrinking field technique and shielding of normal tissues reduce
the side effects of treatment.

When the paraortic nodes are involved, some authors recommend treatment to
5000 cGy in 7 weeks to the paraortic nodes.[12,13]

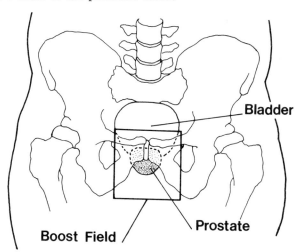

Fig. 4. Diagram of Treatment Portal, localized to the prostate gland (cone
down field).

The use of CT has been recommended to optimize treatment planning. Schlager et al., have recently reported a large number of patients in whom the prostate volume was too small when CT was used compared with conventional mode of planning. This occurred mainly when the seminal vesicles were involved.[14] These findings have been confirmed in a large series reported by Pilepich et al. in 1982.[15]

## RESULTS OF TREATMENT

Megavoltage radiation therapy is an effective and definitive mode of treatment for patients with early carcinoma of the prostate. It is also very valuable as a palliative tool for advanced disease.

Ray et al. reported 5 and 10 year uncorrected survival rates for patients with disease limited to the prostate of 72% and 48% respectively compared with 48% and 30% in patients with palpable extracapsular extension. They also demonstrated that in patients where the interval between diagnosis and initiation of treatment was less than 1 year survival was significantly higher.[15] Local recurrence based on physical examination was noted in 13% of the patients (40/310).[16]

Perez et al. reported an 80%, 5 year tumor-free actuarial survival for 42 patients with adenocarcinoma of the prostate Stage B; 56% for 141 patients with Stage C and 0% for Stage D. His reported pelvic failure rates were 7% for Stage B, 17% Stage C and 25% in Stage D. All patients were treated with curative external beam megavoltage irradiation.[13]

In general in Stage B tumor doses of 6500 cGy will produce 90%-100% local control and in patients with Stage C a tumor dose of 7000 cGy has been reported to control tumor in 80% of the patients. Relapse free actuarial survival at five years for 91 Stage C patients treated to the prostate and pelvic lymph nodes was 55.3%.[12] When the paraortic lymph nodes were involved by neoplasm, proven either by biopsy or by unequivocal lymphangio-grams, only 2 of 21 patients treated by 5000 cGy in 7 weeks (technique described by Bagshaw[12]), were reported alive, without evidence of disease at 18 months.

The Stanford experience, representing a review of 1281 cases, revealed an overall 5 year survival of 60% to 75%, and an overall 10 year survival of 40% for adenocarcinoma of the prostate.[12]

Radical radiation therapy can be used for carcinoma of the prostate with minimum morbidity when administered by an experienced radiotherapist. Regarding paraortic irradiation, controversy exists; in some individually selected patients, the results can be rewarding. It should also be noted that palliative radiation therapy in patients with prostatic carcinoma is extremely useful and beneficial.

REFERENCES

1. Silverberg, G.E., Lubera, J.A. Cancer Statistics. CA 33:2-25, 1983.
2. Hutchinson, G.B. Epidemiology of Prostatic Cancer. Seminars in Oncology, 3:151-159, 1976.
3. Mostofi, F.K. Grading of Prostatic Carcinoma. Cancer Chemotherapy Reports, Part I. 59:111-117, 1975.
4. Catalona, W.J., Scott, W.W. Carcinoma of the Prostate: A Review. Journal of Urology, 119:1-8, 1978.
5. Mostofi, F.K., Davis, C.J., Jr. Principals and Management of Urologic Cancer. NCI, Williams and Wilkins, 1979 pp: 85-94.
6. Spellman, M.C., Castellino, R.A., Ray, G.R., Pistenma, D.A. and Bagshaw, M.D. An Evaluation of Lymphography in Localized Carcinoma of the Prostate. Radiology 125:637-644, 1977.
7. Widmann, B.P. Cancer of the Prostate: The results of Radium and Roentgen Ray Treatment. Radiology 22:153-159, 1934.
8. del Regato, J.A. In, Cancer Diagnosis, Treatment and Prognosis. Ackerman, L.V. and del Regato, J.A., eds. Mosby, St. Louis, p.859 3rd edition, 1962.
9. del Regato, J.A. Radiation Therapy in the Conservative Treatment of Operable and Locally Inoperable Carcinoma of the Prostate. Radiology 88: 761-766, 1967.
10. Bagshaw, M.A., Kaplan, H.S., Sagerman, R.H. Linear Accelerator Supervoltage Radiotherapy in Carcinoma of the Prostate. Radiology 85:121-129, Jul 1965.
11. Pistenma, D.A., Bagshaw, M.D., Freiha, F.S. Extended Field Radiation Therapy for Prostatic Adenocarcinoma. Status report of a limited prospective trial. In Cancer of the Genitourinary Tract, ed. D.E.Johnson and M.L. Samuels, N. York, Raven Press, 1979, pp 229-249.
12. Bagshaw, M.D. External Radiation Therapy of Carcinoma of the Prostate. Cancer 45:1912-1921, 1980.
13. Perez, C.A., Walz, B.J., Zivnuska, F.R., Pilepich, M., et al. Irradiation of Carcinoma of the Prostate Localized to the Pelvis: Analysis of tumor response and progress. Int J. of Rad Onc Biol and Physics. 6:555-563, 1980.
14. Schlager, B., Asbell, S.O. Baker, A.S., et. al. Use of CT Scanning in Treatment Planning for Bladder Carcinoma. Int. J. Rad Onc Biol and Physics 5:99-103, 1979.
15. Pilepich, M.V., Prasad, S.C. and Perez, C.A. Computed Tomography in Definite Radiotherapy of Prostatic Carcinoma, Part 2: Definition of Target Volume. Int J Rad Onc Biol Phys, 8:235-240, 1982.
16. Ray, R.G., Cassady, R.J. and Bagshaw, M.D. Definitive Radiation Therapy of Carcinoma of the Prostate. A Report on 15 years of Experience. Rad 106:407-418, Feb, 1973.

PROSTATE CANCER:  STAGING AND ITS EFFECTS ON THERAPY


H. BARTON GROSSMAN, M.D.



Carcinoma of the prostate is the third leading cause of cancer deaths in males and has the second highest incidence, excluding skin cancer. The estimated incidence for 1982 is 73,000 new cases. In this same period, it is estimated that 23,300 men will die of prostatic cancer. Survival is related to stage, with improved life expectancy in patients with disease confined to the prostate. At the time of diagnosis, 61% of patients will have localized disease. The five year survival for localized and metastatic disease is 77% and 30% respectively.[1] Because of this significant difference, accurate staging of prostate cancer is important in determining prognosis.

DIAGNOSIS AND STAGING TECHNIQUES

The detection of prostatic cancer is so often made by rectal examination that this important finding is the cornerstone of the staging system used for the classification of this disease. It is only by careful digital examination of the prostate that early stages of carcinoma will be detected. Confirmation of the clinical impression of prostatic cancer obtained by rectal examination is usually performed by biopsy. Both needle biopsy and transurethral resection of the prostate can be expected to confirm the diagnosis with greater than 80% accuracy.[2] The method of choice varies with the presentation of disease. Needle biopsy is usually performed in patients with low stage, non-obstructing tumors while transurethral resection tends to be performed on larger neoplasms that are causing urinary outlet obstruction. Whether this method of pre-selection accounts for the reported poor prognosis of patients undergoing definitive radiation therapy for carcinoma of the prostate diagnosed by transurethral resection is unknown.[3]

Serum acid phosphatase has long been used in the staging of prostatic cancer. The enzymatic methods are readily available and are useful because they are frequently elevated in the face of untreated metastatic disease. The newer immunoassays of acid phosphatase are more sensitive and may have a tendency to more readily detect localized disease.[4] However, at this time, the immunoassays offer little clinical advantage for the routine determination

Published 1983 by Elsevier Science Publishing Co., Inc.
Recent Trends in Radiation Oncology and Related Fields, Amendola and Amendola, Editors

of serum acid phosphatase.  Because of its specificity, acid phosphatase by radio-immunoassay is superior to enzymatic analysis for the determination of bone marrow levels.[5]  However, despite this high specificity, occasional false positive results occur and the clinical usefulness of this staging method remains to be defined.

One of the two prime metastatic sites of prostatic cancer is the skeleton. For the evaluation of bone metastases, radionuclide bone imaging is markedly more sensitive than conventional radiographs.  However, because of the lack of specificity, the evaluation of these scans may occasionally be difficult.  The clinical setting in which this commonly occurs is with an individual who has one or two focal areas of increased uptake on the bone scan and normal skeletal radiographs and serum acid phosphatase.  If metastases are present, it may take up to 18 months for the lesions to be detected by conventional radiographs.  Certainly the use of a primary treatment modality with its attendant morbidity is not indicated in the face of disseminated carcinoma. On the other hand, withholding therapy when metastases may not be present is not necessarily in the patient's best interest.[6]

The second common area of metastatic spread of prostatic carcinoma is to the pelvic lymph nodes.  Lymphangiography has been used in an effort to non-operatively determine their status.  The lymphatic drainage of the prostate (as determined by contrast injection into the gland) is to the internal iliac and presacral lymph nodes.[7]  Although it is often stated that the lymph nodes surrounding the obturator nerve are not visualized on lymphangiography, Merrin and associates have demonstrated good visualization of this area.[8]  While the specificity (a reflection of the number of false positive studies) is over 90%, the sensitivity (a measure of false negative studies) is low (approximately 60%, with a range of 33% to 75%).[9]  In comparison, the reported specificity and sensitivity for computerized tomography is 100% and 18%-33% respectively.[10,11]

The only absolute way to diagnose pelvic lymphatic metastases is with bilateral pelvic lymphadenectomy.  However, the accuracy of this operative procedure is dependent both on the completeness of the dissection by the surgeon and the thoroughness of the pathologic examination of the excised tissue.  Despite these limitations, this is the standard against which other methods of diagnosis of regional lymphatic spread must be compared.

CLINICAL AND PATHOLOGIC STAGING EVALUATION

The most common staging system in current use in the United States divides prostatic cancer into four stages with several sub-groups. Stage A carcinoma is composed of those tumors that are not suspicious for neoplasm by digital rectal examination. By definition, the diagnosis is made by the pathologist, most often on tissue resected from men clinically presenting with obstructive symptoms. The pathologic extent and clinical spectrum of this stage is broad. Because of this, Stage A prostatic carcinoma has been recently sub-divided into focal (A1) and diffuse (A2) disease. The rationale to support this division is the excellent survival (equal to that of the general population) of patients with Stage A1 and the relatively poor survival associated with A2.[12] To evaluate the accuracy of individuals staged as having focal disease, a group of 34 individuals with focal carcinoma of the prostate were further staged with repeat transurethral resection. Of these, 67.6% had no neoplasm in the second specimen. Focal neoplasm was again found in 23.5% and A2 (diffuse) disease was found in 8.8%. This data highlights two points, first the lack of residual tumor in the majority of patients with focal carcinoma accounts for the excellent prognosis seen with stage A1 disease. Second, a small but important group of individuals will be understaged by a transurethral resection and these individuals are at increased risk from their neoplasm.

Stage B tumors are composed of those palpable neoplasm that are confined to the prostate. In a similar fashion as that seen in Stage A, this group has been divided into B1 (nodule of 2 cm or less) and B2 (neoplasms greater than 2 cm in size). The rationale for the subdivision is the same as discussed earlier with Stage A, i.e., improved survival associated with B1 lesions. Stage C tumors have local extension outside the prostatic capsule and may involve the seminal vesicle. Stage D tumors are metastatic.

NATURAL HISTORY

The morbidity and mortality of any neoplasm is related to the rate of growth of the tumor, its response to therapeutic intervention, and the time at risk. Obviously with an agressive neoplasm in a young individual the prognosis is poor unless a specific highly effective therapy is available. An excellent example of this is illustrated by the survival results with non-seminomatous testicular tumors prior to and after effective chemotherapy was available. Many men present with prostatic cancer in their seventh decade of life and have other simultaneous medical problems that may shorten their life expectancy. In addition, the low stage, well differentiated tumors are particularly slow growing and may take years to become symptomatic if first diagnosed at an early stage. Because of the great variability of these two factors and the resultant interplay which determines the clinical manifestations of this disease, accurate staging becomes particularly important in comparing treatment protocols. This will not avoid problems associated with individual variability but at least will minimize those associated with the neoplasm. In addition, an adequate followup time is required to evaluate the results of therapy. For low stage tumors, a ten to fifteen year study is required during which time significant changes in general medical care are often made, further confusing treatment results.

STAGING ERROR

   Staging error therefore becomes an important part of the analysis of any therapeutic study. There are multiple points at which staging error can occur, thus confounding accurate interpretation of data. Local staging is affected by the experience of the physician performing the digital examination, by the selection of tissue for histologic examination by the pathologist, and by the completeness of the transurethral resection, e.g., understaging of stage A2 disease. All of these factors exist, but fortunately they do not appear to be significant problems. The difficulty in identifying early skeletal metastases has already been mentioned and awaits further technological advances for its resolution.

| TABLE 1 | INCIDENCE OF LYMPHATIC METASTASES BY STAGE | | | | |
|---|---|---|---|---|---|
| | $A_1$ | $A_2$ | $B_1$ | $B_2$ | C |
| Golimbu (1978)[16] | 0/4 | 6/16 | 3/17 | 10/16 | |
| Freiha (1979)[13] | | 0/2 | 2/13 | 10/44 | 24/41 |
| Golimbu (1979)[17] | 0/1 | 3/9 | 2/6 | 5/9 | 5/5 |
| Lieskovsky (1980)[18] | 0/2 | 1/8 | 3/16 | 12/39 | 11/17 |
| Donohue (1981)[19] | 0/9 | 10/44 | 20/104 | 29/58 | |
| Fowler (1981)[20] | | | 5/75 | 56/129 | 58/96 |
| Prout (1981)[21] | | 2/13 | 0/7 | 9/51 | 34/67 |
| TOTAL | 0/16 (0%) | 22/92 (24%) | 35/238 (15%) | 131/346 (38%) | 132/226 (58%) |

   The major error of understaging occurs when pelvic lymphatic spread is misdiagnosed. It is easy to make this diagnosis unequivocally by pelvic lymphadenectomy, but because of the associated morbidity of an operative

| TABLE 2 | INCIDENCE OF LYMPHATIC METASTASES BY GRADE | | |
|---|---|---|---|
| | Well Differentiated | Moderately Differentiated | Poorly Differentiated |
| Golimbu (1978)[16] | 6/23 | 8/19 | 5/11 |
| Freiha (1979)[13] | 2/10 | 17/65 | 17/25 |
| Donohue (1981)[19] | 11/93 | 27/65 | 18/37 |
| Fowler (1981)[20] | 23/86 | 67/149 | 7/10 |
| Prout (1981)[21] | 0/22 | 24/77 | 21/39 |
| TOTAL | 42/234 (18%) | 143/375 (38%) | 68/122 (56%) |

procedure, various alternatives are being investigated. Lymphangiography is not sufficiently accurate to be solely relied upon. As an alternative, the grade and stage of tumor and serum acid phosphatase have been evaluated as indicators of pelvic metastases with clinically localized prostatic cancer.

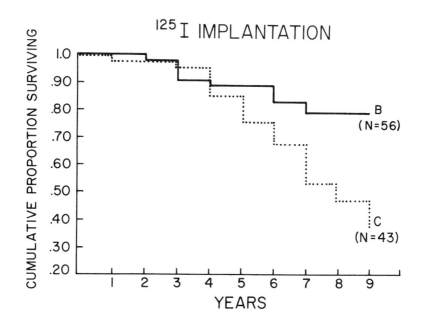

Fig. 1. Cumulative survival of clinical Stage B and Stage C patients after [125]I implantation (Reprinted with permission, Grossman et al.[14]).

The incidence of pelvic lymphatic metastases has been demonstrated to correlate with both stage and grade (Tables 1 and 2). Using stage, grade, and acid phosphatase, Freiha and associates could separate patients into three groups according to their chances of having pelvic metastases.[13] The low risk group (Stage A2, B1, and B2 with normal acid phosphatase) had only a 7% (2/28) incidence of pelvic metastases. The high risk group (Stage C, high grade, elevated acid phosphatase) had a 93% (13/14) chance of having lymphatic disease. The intermediate group had a 36% (21/58) incidence of lymphatic metastases. Stratification by stage, grade, and serum acid phosphatase helps to select out high and low risk groups but does not completely eliminate error. The real question is: What is the significance of staging error caused by the incomplete evaluation of pelvic lymph nodes?

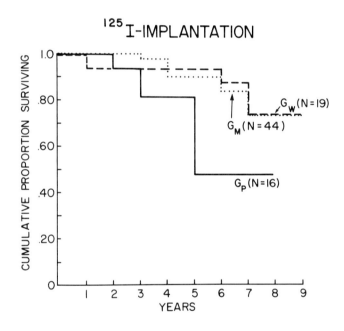

Fig. 2. Cumulative survival of patients with well differentiated (Gw), moderately well differentiated (Gm) and poorly differentiated (Gp) tumors after [125]I implantation (Reprinted with permission, Grossman et al.[14]).

$^{125}$I IMPLANTATION

To examine some of the possible ramifications of staging error on prognosis, a review of the $^{125}$I implantation data from Memorial Sloan-Kettering Cancer Center is instructive. At Memorial Hospital, $^{125}$I implantation and bilateral pelvic lymphadenectomy have been performed in selected patients with carcinoma of the prostate since 1970. An analysis of the initial experience encompassing a group of 100 patients with clinical stage B and C disease provides information both on the usefulness of this technique and on the impact of various tumor related variables on survival.[14]

The mean age of the group was 60 years. Five and nine year survival for all patients was 83% and 52% respectively with stage B patients having a significantly better prognosis than that of Stage C (Figure 1). Similarly, patients with well and moderately well differentiated tumors had a significantly better survival than patients with poorly differentiated tumors (Figure 2). If survival is examined in relationship to the presence or absence of pelvic lymph node metastases, two striking findings become apparent (Figure 3).

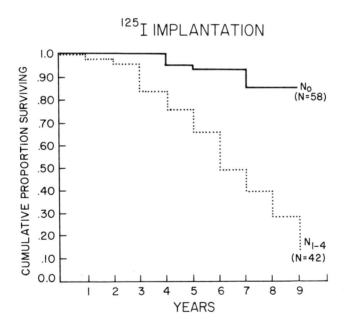

Fig. 3A. Cumulative survival of patients stratified into lymph node negative (No) and positive ($N_{1-4}$). (Reprinted with permission, Grossman et al.[14])

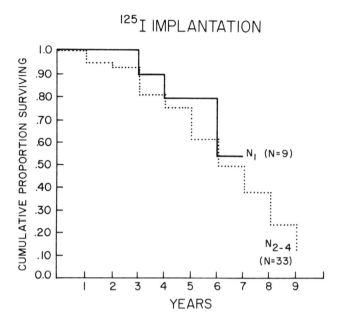

Fig. 3B Cumulative survival of patients with a single positive node (N1) versus more extensive noded disease ($N_{2-4}$). (Reprinted with permission, Grossman et al.[14])

First, survival was dramatically decreased in the presence of pelvic lymphatic metastases at the time of implantation. Second, the adverse effect of nodal metastases on prognosis persisted even if only one lymph node harbored neoplasia.

This strong adverse affect of nodal disease obscures survival differences seen between local extent of tumor. In other words, patients with Stage B and C tumors who had nodal metastases had no statistically significant differences between their survival curves. However, individuals without nodal metastases had improved survival with Stage B disease. Similarly, patients with poorly differentiated tumors had poor survival regardless of clinical stage while patients with more differentiated neoplasms had improved survival with smaller local disease.

This data demonstrates the importance of accurate staging in the evaluation of this relatively new therapeutic method. Although the overall survival data is comparable to other treatment modalities, the analysis afforded by the performance of lymphadenectomy clearly demonstrates the excellent survival afforded to individuals who are treated with [125]I implantation and whose lymph nodes are tumor free at the time of therapy. The role of patient and tumor selection in this group and their respective impacts on survival are uncertain.

CONCLUSION

The final clinical outcome of carcinoma of the prostate depends on a number of factors related to the agressiveness of an individual tumor, its response to therapy, and the relationship of the host to the neoplasm. Although many of these factors cannot be controlled for, accurate staging and grading of neoplasms helps in the categorization of some of the tumor related variables. In prostatic cancer, the status of the pelvic lymph nodes is probably the most important factor that can be, but is not always, adequately evaluated. Although lymphangiography with needle biopsy is often diagnostic,[15] the most accurate way of assessing metastatic disease in the regional lymphatics is by operative excision. This, of course, has associated morbidity which is particularly significant in the patients who would not otherwise be operated upon.

Pelvic lymphadenectomy cannot be recommended as a routine staging procedure because it is simply that. It has little, if any, therapeutic value as evidenced by the poor survival in patients with only one involved lymph node. It does, however, have applicability in several clinical settings. One is in the evaluation of new therapeutic methods for which staging is particularly important. A second is in treatment methods that have their own morbidity and which would not usually be performed in the presence of metastatic disease, e.g., radical prostatectomy. An additional application is in the performance of [125]I implantation, where pelvic lymphadenectomy can be performed at the same time as the therapeutic procedure with little increase in morbidity and considerable gain in prognostic information.

REFERENCES
1. Silverberg, E. Cancer Statistics, CA 32:15, 1982.
2. Bissada, N.K. Accuracy of Transurethral Resection of the Prostate Versus Transrectal Needle Biopsy in the Diagnosis of Prostatic Carcinoma. J Urol 118:61, 1977.
3. McGowan, D.G. The Adverse Influence of Prior Transurethral Resection on Prognosis in Carcinoma of Prostate Treated by Radiation Therapy. Int J Rad Onc Biol Phys 6:121, 1980.
4. Quinones, G.R., Rohner, T.J., Jr., Drago, J.R., and Demers, L.M. Will Prostatic Acid Phosphatase Determination by Radioimmunoassay Increase the Diagnosis of Early Prostatic Cancer? J Urol 125:361, 1981.

5.  Belville, W.D., Mahan, D.E., Sepulveda, R.A., Bruce, A.W., and Miller, C.F. Bone Marrow Acid Phosphatase by Radioimmunoassay: 3 Years of Experience. J Urol 125:809, 1980.

6.  Ball, J.D. and Maynard, C.D. Nuclear Imaging in Urology. Urol Clin N.A. 6:321, 1979.

7.  Raghavaiah, N.V. and Jordon, W.P., Jr. Prostatic Lymphography. J Urol 121:178, 1979.

8.  Merrin, C., Wajsman, Z., Baumgaurtner, G., and Jennings, E. The Clinical Value of Lymphangiography: Are the Nodes Surrounding the Obturator Nerve Visualized? J Urol 117:762, 1977.

9.  Liebner, E.J., Stefanis, S., and Uro-Oncology Research Group. An Evaluation of Lymphography with Nodal Biopsy in Localized Carcinoma of the Prostate. Cancer 45:728, 1980.

10. Golimbu, M., Morales, P., Al-Askari, S. and Shulman, Y. CAT Scanning in Staging of Prostatic Cancer. Urology 18:305, 1981.

11. Morgan, C.L., Calkins, R.F., and Cavalcanti, E.J. Computed Tomography in the Evaluation, Staging, and Therapy of Carcinoma of the Bladder and Prostate. Radiology 140:751, 1981.

12. Cantrell, B.B., DeKlerk, D.P., Eggleston, J.C., Boitnott, J.K., and Walsh, P.C. Pathological Factors that Influence Prognosis in Stage A Prostatic Cancer: The Influence of Extent Versus Grade. J Urol 125:516, 1981.

13. Freiha, F.S., Pistenma, D.A., and Bagshaw, M.A. Pelvic Lymphadenectomy for Staging Prostatic Carcinoma: Is it Always Necessary? J Urol 122:176, 1979.

14. Grossman, H.B., Batata, M., Hilaris, B., and Whitmore, W.F., Jr. $^{125}$I Implantation for Carcinoma of Prostate: Further Follow-up of First 100 Cases. Urology 20:591, 1982.

15. Correa, R.J., Jr., Kipp, C.R., Burnett, L., Brannen, G.E., Gibbons, R.P., and Cummings, K.B. Percutaneous Pelvic Lymph Node Aspiration in Carcinoma of the Prostate. J Urol 126:190, 1981.

16. Golimbu, M., Schinella, R., Morales, P., and Kurusu, S. Differences in Pathological Characteristics and Prognosis of Clinical A2 Prostatic Cancer from A1 and B Disease. J Urol 119:618-622, 1978.

17. Golimbu, M., Morales, P., Al-Askari, S., and Brown, J. Extended Pelvic Lymphadenectomy for Prostatic Cancer. J Urol 121:617-620, 1979.

18. Lieskovsky, G., Skinner, D.G., and Weisenburger, T. Pelvic Lymphadenectomy in the Management of Carcinoma of the Prostate. J Urol 124:635-638, 1980.

19. Donohue, R.E., Fauver, H.E., Whitesel, J.A., Augspurger, R.R., and Pfister, R.R. Prostatic Carcinoma: Influence of Tumor Grade on Results of Pelvic Lymphadenectomy. Urology 17:435-440, 1981.

20. Fowler, J.E., Jr. and Whitmore, W.F., Jr. The Incidence and Extent of Pelvic Lymph Node Metastases in Apparently Localized Prostatic Cancer. Cancer 47:2941-2945, 1981.

21. Prout, G.R., Jr., Griffin, P.P., Daly, J.J., and Shipley, W.U. Nodal Involvement as Prognostic Indicator in Prostatic Carcinoma. Urology (March Supplement) 17:72-79, 1981.

COMPUTED TOMOGRAPHY OF PROSTATIC MALIGNANCY

MARCO A. AMENDOLA, M.D., BEATRIZ E. AMENDOLA, M.D., AND
H. BARTON GROSSMAN, M.D.

INTRODUCTION

Prostatic carcinoma is the third most common cause of cancer in American males. It is estimated that in 1983, 75,000 new cases of prostatic carcinoma will be diagnosed in the United States and that approximately 24,000 men will die of this disease.[1] The incidence of latent carcinoma, as judged by pathological examination of prostate glands at autopsy in men not suspected of having prostatic cancer, increases dramatically after age 40, rising to 20%-40% for men 70 to 79 years of age.[2,3] Proliferative changes of the prostate also develop in many men so that by the age of 80 years, more than 80% will have benign prostatic hyperplasia (BPH) of some degree. Although the prostate is accessible to transrectal palpation, the accuracy of this method in determining the presence of prostatic cancer may be as low as 50%.[4] Knowledge of periprostatic spread, distant metastases and tumor size are of paramount importance in the treatment of prostatic cancer. Digital rectal examination, excretory urography, bone scan, serum acid phosphatase, and cystoscopy are common clinical studies utilized for the diagnosis, staging, and followup of prostatic cancer. Despite these studies, periprostatic spread and lymphatic metastases continue to be difficult to accurately diagnose and quantify unless invasive procedures are performed. Computed tomography (CT) is a noninvasive test which is applicable for the evaluation of disease extent and for radiation therapy treatment planning. In selected patients, CT may be an alternative to more invasive procedures.

TECHNIQUE FOR COMPUTED TOMOGRAPHY OF THE PROSTATE

Diluted oral contrast material is administered to all patients prior to CT scanning in order to opacify the bowel lumen. Our standard protocol calls for the oral administration of 16 oz of 3% Hypaque, 10 to 12 hours before the CT scan, a repeat dose 2 hours prior to the exam, plus 8 oz when on the scanning table. Unless contraindicated, all patients additionally receive intravenous contrast to outline the urinary bladder and to opacify pelvic vascular structures. For the abdominal part of the examination, scans with 10 mm collimation and 1 or 2 cm spacing are obtained from the diaphragm down to the iliac crest.[5] To image the pelvis, 10 mm consecutive transverse CT scans are obtained from the level of the iliac crests to below the level of the ischial tuberosities according to scout views (computed digital radiographs) obtained for localization.

To evaluate local disease as completely as possible, optional techniques[6] to be used include:

1. Contiguous 5 mm sections throughout the prostate region.
2. High-resolution, small-field-of-view scans.
3. Application of multiplanar reconstruction to obtain sagittal and coronal reformatted images.
4. Selected use of ultrathin 1.5 mm. sections through a region of interest.
5. Scanning in supine, prone and decubitus positions.
6. Direct coronal CT scans of the pelvis obviating the need for computer reconstructon of multiple contiguous axial images.[7-9]
7. Rapid sequence scanning during IV bolus injecton of contrast to opacify pelvic vascular structures.

In selected patients, additional bladder and rectal opacification is employed using diluted water soluble contrast instillation by catheter.

COMPUTED TOMOGRAPHY OF PROSTATE CARCINOMA

CT can directly image the prostate and outline the size, contour and density of the gland (Figure 1).[10] However, even with high quality, high resolution scans, CT currently is unable to identify the different prostatic lobes and to separate prostatic capsule from prostatic parenchyma.[11]

Normal glands and BPH cannot be differentiated by CT from those harboring carcinoma unless irregular prostate enlargement or spread of tumor beyond the capsule is present.[12] Regardless of size and intravenous contrast enhancement, prostate carcinoma has similar tissue attenuation as the normal glandular substance.[11,12] A rare exception is the mucinous adenocarcinoma of the prostate which can be seen as a localized area of decreased CT density within the gland because of the characteristic mucin secretion. In the recent case reported by Dunnick, et al.[13] a gelatinous tumor mass of well differentiated mucinous adenocarcinoma measured 12 Hounsfield units (HU) compared with 46 HU for the normal portion of the gland. Another prostate malignancy which in our experience has demonstrated areas of diminished

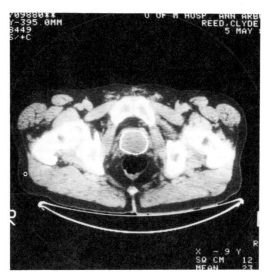

Fig. 1. CT scan through symphisis pubis: prostate outlined by a region of interest marker which indicates a surface area of 12 cm² at this level. From sequential CT scans through the gland the prostate volume can be calculated.

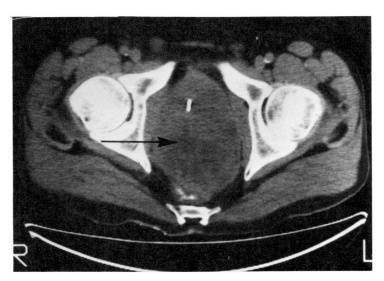

Fig. 2. Large prostatic sarcoma containing areas of lower CT density consistent with necrotic foci within lesion. Note radiopaque catheter outlining the prostatic urethra.

attenuation within the tumor is prostatic sarcoma. These areas most likely represent focal necrosis (Figure 2). Massive tumor size, younger age group and marked invasiveness are characteristics of prostatic sarcoma which will help in differentiating these tumors from the more common adenocarcinoma. In summary, CT is used primarily to assess periprostatic and distant spread of tumor after needle biopsy or histology from prostatic resection has confirmed the presence of cancer.[14] The classification used for the clinical staging of prostatic carcinoma is listed in Table 1.[15]

---

TABLE 1          STAGING:   ADENOCARCINOMA OF THE PROSTATE

STAGE A.  Incidental finding (clinically undetectable).
              $A_1$  Focal
              $A_2$  Diffuse

STAGE B.  Confined to the prostate.
              $B_1$  Single small discrete nodule
              $B_2$  Large or multiple nodules

STAGE C.  Localized to the periprostatic area.
              $C_1$  No involvement of seminal vesicles $>70$ gr.
              $C_2$  Involvement of the seminal vesicles $<70$ gr.

STAGE D.  Metastatic disease.
              $D_1$  Pelvic Lymph node metastasis or ureteral
                    obstruction (hydronephrosis)
              $D_2$  Bone or distant lymph node or soft tissue
                    metastases

---

As previously discussed, CT cannot accurately diagnose patients with Stage A or most Stage B tumors. However, it can separate neoplasms confined to the prostate from Stage C or D prostatic carcinomas.

CT signs of periprostatic extension include obscuration and asymmetry of normal fat planes with invasion of the pelvic side wall, and/or adjacent viscera, i.e., bladder, urethra and especially the seminal vesicles. The rectum is usually free of local tumor extension. Gross invasion of the seminal vesicles, is of particular impact since it may influence therapeutic management. The incidence of pelvic lymph node metastasis in patients with Stage C disease is approximately 60% (see the chapter, "Prostate Cancer: Staging and Its Effects on Therapy"). A subtle, but definite sign of Stage C disease is the positive "seminal vesicle angle sign" described by Seidelmann et al.[16,17] With the patient in the supine position, the normal seminal vesicles are separated from the postero-inferior aspect of the bladder by an intervening fat plane (Figure 3).  Its obliteration indicates tumor extension (Figure 4).   False positive signs may be produced by a distended rectum or scanning in the prone position so care must be exercised in its evaluation.[18]

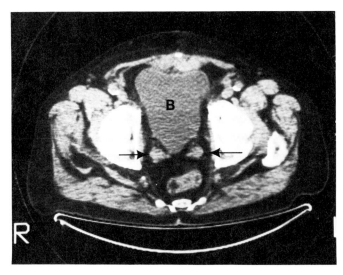

Fig. 3. Normal seminal vesicles (arrows) separated from bladder (B) by an intervening fat plane.

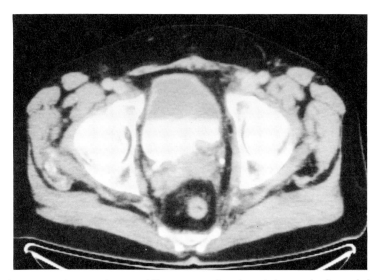

Fig. 4. Prostatic carcinoma with gross extension into seminal vesicles and bladder. Note the bilateral obliteration of both seminal vesical angles.

CT may understage patients by missing microscopic tumor extension into the periprostatic fat or minimal seminal vesicle invasion. Even though the sensitivity of CT in detecting extracapsular extension is low, in a series with surgically proven correlation there were no false positives indicating high specificity.[19] It has therefore been advocated that CT should be reserved for those patients in which there is high clinical suspicion of Stage C or D disease.[20] CT may also be used to screen candidates for definitive therapy of clinically localized neoplasms based on the ability of CT to demonstrate more advanced disease than was suspected clinically.[21]

At the University of Michigan Hospitals, selected patients with localized carcinoma of the prostate (Stage $A_2$ or B) have a bilateral staging pelvic lymphadenectomy followed by implantation of radioactive $^{125}I$ seeds into the prostate or radical prostatectomy. CT is routinely obtained as a preoperative study to spare patients with locally invasive tumor or gross adenopathy (Figure 5) an inappropriate surgical procedure. CT is also used to: 1) evaluate the size of the prostate gland; 2) assess periprostatic extension of tumor; and 3) provide a baseline for monitoring response to therapy. Tumors that are large or grossly locally invasive are treated with external beam radiation therapy.

LYMPH NODE METASTASES FROM PROSTATIC CARCINOMA

From the prostatic lymphatic network, collecting trunks drain to the external iliac, hypogastric and presacral lymph nodes.[22,23] Since tumor tends to spread along this drainage pattern, metastases from prostatic cancer rarely, if ever, occur in the para-aortic lymph nodes unless the primary pelvic nodes have first become involved.[24] The incidence of histologically proven lymph node metastases depends on several factors: 1) clinical stage of the disease; 2) histologic differentiation of the primary tumor; 3) extent of involvement of the prostate by carcinoma; and 4) size of the malignant prostate. When there are no distant metastases, the incidence of lymph node metastases increases with advancing clinical stage: 23% for Stage B disease and 56% for Stage C.[24]

The accuracy of bipedal lymphangiography (LAG) in detecting pelvic node metastases from prostatic carcinoma varies widely according to different researchers, but it is generally accepted that it fails to agree with the microscopic findings in at least 30% of the patients. The sensitivity of LAG in detecting metastases (i.e., the fraction of patients whose nodal metastases are detected) ranges from 35% to 75%, and the specificity (the fraction of

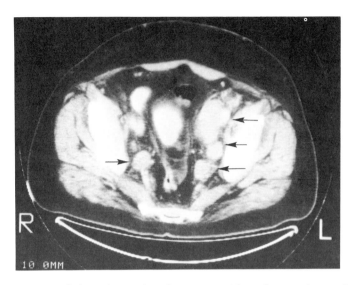

Fig. 5A. Gross pelvic adenopathy from prostatic adenocarcinoma involving external and internal iliac nodes.

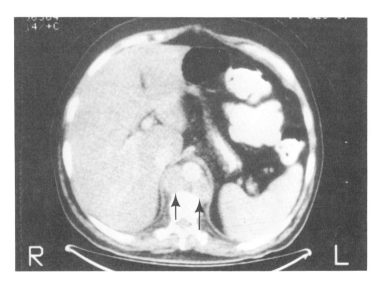

Fig. 5B. Another patient with retroperitoneal adenopathy involving retrocrural nodes (arrows).

patients correctly identified as having no nodal metastases) ranges from 21%
to 95%.[25-30] In the Uro-Oncology Research Group series of 114 patients with
negative lymphangiograms, biopsy at staging surgery proved that 21 patients
had nodal metastases.[25] Recently, the performance of percutaneous fine
needle biopsy of suspected abnormal nodes,[23,31] and even of radiographically normal nodes[32] opacified by lymphangiography has been advocated to
overcome the diagnostic limitations of lymphangiography. However, LAG remains
a tedious, time consuming, and invasive procedure which limits its general
acceptability and widespread use. Also LAG may not be feasible in patients
with impaired pulmonary function or with history of sensitivity to the
lymphangiographic contrast. Some have argued that the obturator and
hypogastric lymph nodes, those most frequently involved with prostatic
metastases, fail to be visualized on lymphangiography. Although it is true
that the internal iliac (hypogastric) nodes can be seen in only about one half
of the cases studies by LAG, the lymph nodes surrounding the obturator nerve
are consistently opacified.[26,33]

The presence of lymphatic metastases from prostatic carcinoma adversely
affects prognosis and often changes therapy. For this reason, once the
diagnosis of prostatic cancer has been confirmed histologically, and after
physical, laboratory, radiographic and radionuclide examinations have failed
to demonstrate distant metastases, additional studies to assess regional lymph
node status are usually recommended. The most accurate method currently
available for determining extension of prostatic carcinoma to the regional
lymph nodes is histologic examination of the nodes after lymphadenectomy.
Therefore, a staging bilateral pelvic lymphadenectomy is often done although
this may be associated with a 7% to 10% morbidity rate.[34-36]

The lack of a readily available, noninvasive, reliable method for detecting
lymph node metastases has forced clinicians to recommend treatment without
proper knowledge of the regional lymph node status or to perform a staging
pelvic lymphadenectomy (of questionable therapeutic value) with its attendant
risks.

Several reports have documented the ability of CT to detect metastatic
lymphadenopathy from primary pelvic neoplasms.[6,37-40] CT criteria for
abnormal pelvic lymph nodes include: 1) asymmetry around the external iliac,
internal iliac and femoral vessels, 2) discrete round masses along the pelvic
side walls, and 3) separation of these masses from the primary tumor by
pelvic fat.[38]

In our experience, pelvic lymph nodes measuring 2 cm or more on a CT scan are abnormal and are important indicators of metastatic disease in patients with prostatic carcinoma. Recently, the use of 1.5 cm as the upper limit of normal for paraaortic, common iliac and external iliac lymph nodes and 1.2 cm for deep internal iliac and obturator lymph nodes has been advocated.[39,40] However, it must be kept in mind that CT cannot differentiate benign from malignant lymph node enlargement and chronic lymphadenitis, fibrosis or fatty replacement can cause false positive results especially in minimally enlarged nodes measuring 1.5 to 2 cm. For this reason, percutaneous needle biopsy which may be performed under CT guidance is recommended to further evaluate abnormal or questionably abnormal nodes (Figure 6).

False positive CT diagnosis due to misinterpretation of atypical common iliac and external iliac vessels for abnormal pelvic lymph nodes can be obviated by using rapid sequence scanning of the questionable areas during IV injection of contrast. According to Weinerman et al.[40] vessels usually enhance to greater than 75 Hounsfield units. In addition, complete filling of the alimentary tract with oral and/or rectal contrast is essential to avoid confusion of unopacified bowel with pelvic masses. External iliac node

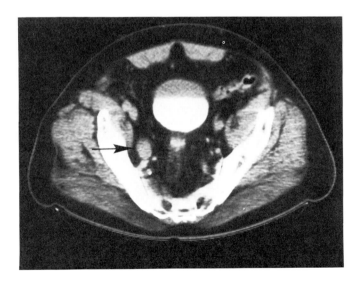

Fig. 6A. Mildly enlarged right pelvic node (arrow). This CT finding was the only suggestion of metastatic disease in this patient.

178

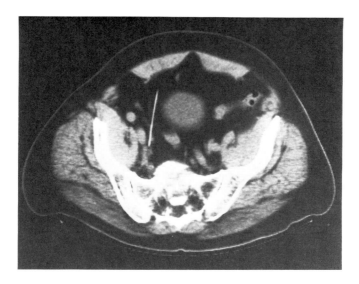

Fig. 6B. Percutaneous fine needle aspiration biopsy performed under CT guidance.

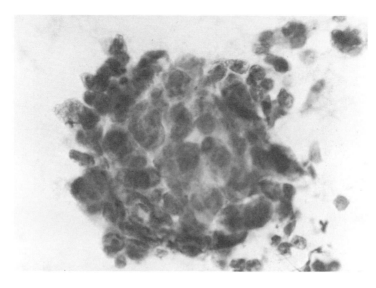

Fig. 6C. Cytologic specimen positive for malignancy. Surgery was cancelled and the patient referred to radiation therapy.

metastases are best detected on CT scans obtained through the inferior sacroiliac joint where the external iliac vessels are separated anteriorly from the internal iliac vessels which are in a more posterior location.

Lymph nodes surrounding the obturator nerve may represent the first point of lymphatic metastases in carcinoma of the prostate.[33] Metastases to the obturator nodes are best seen on sections obtained 1 to 3 cm above the acetabula, showing the characteristic teardrop shape of the supraacetabular iliac bone.[38] Our data indicate that the "surgical" obturator node is part of the medial chain of the external iliac node group and is located below and medial to the external iliac vein and above the obturator nerve[22,41] and that it does opacify on lymphangiography.[23,26,33,43]

CT has also been able to detect adenopathy in hypogastric nodes (which rarely opacify at lymphangiography) in patients without significant involvement of the common or external iliac nodes.[39] Published reports regarding the CT evaluation of pelvic adenopathy in prostatic cancer have accuracy figures ranging from 70% to 93% (Table 2). A negative CT scan cannot exclude the presence of small tumor deposits in normal size nodes. Lymphangiography may then be obtained in an effort to detect discrete tumor filling defects in these patients prior to surgery (lymphadenectomy). However, microscopic foci of tumor, are undetectable both with CT and LAG.[6,37,38]

TABLE 2      CT EVALUATION OF PELVIC ADENOPATHY IN PROSTATIC CARCINOMA

| | TP | FN | TN | FP | Sensitivity (%) | Specificity (%) | Accuracy (%) |
|---|---|---|---|---|---|---|---|
| Morgan, et al.[6] | 2 | 4 | 10 | 0 | 33 | 100 | 75 |
| Walsh, et al.[38] | 3 | 1 | 2 | 1 | 75 | 66 | 71 |
| Levine, et al.[39] | 7 | 0 | 7 | 1 | 100 | 87 | 93 |
| Weinerman, et al.[40] | 7 | 3 | 7 | 2 | 70 | 78 | 74 |
| Golimbu, et al.[19] | 5 | 12 | 27 | 2 | 30 | 93 | 70 |

$$\text{Sensitivity} = \frac{TP}{TP+FN} \qquad \text{Specificity} = \frac{TN}{TN+FP} \qquad \text{Accuracy} = \frac{TP+TN}{TP+TN+FN+FP}$$

If it is recognized that CT requires significant lymph node enlargement before metastases can be detected and that patients may present with macroscopic metastatic disease in nodes of normal size or disease recognizable only on microscopy, studies that report sensitivity rates approaching 100% must be viewed cautiously since it is likely that a highly selected group of patients has been evaluated.[44]

SKELETAL METASTASES FROM PROSTATIC CARCINOMA:  ROLE OF CT

Skeletal scintigraphy is the most accurate method currently available for the early detection of bone metastases.[44]  In carcinoma of the prostate, where osseus involvement is so common, no patient should have a radical prostatectomy or high dose radiation therapy for curative intent until bone metastases have been excluded by a radionuclide bone scan.  The bone scan is a more sensitive indicator of occult bone metastases than plain radiographs and either serum acid or alkaline phosphatase.[45,46]  Bone scans, however, are nonspecific and increased uptake may be produced by Paget's disease, arthritis, trauma, and other nonmalignant conditions.  Correlation with radiographs of areas of increased uptake or symptomatic sites is recommended to avoid false results.[47,48]  Despite careful examination of bone scans and radiographs, diagnostic uncertainty may remain in some patients.  This is particularly true of elderly male patients with cancer of the prostate, when differentiation between sclerotic metastases and Paget's disease may be difficult to ascertain.[49]  Although CT of the pelvis for the primary evaluation of metastic bone lesions is not recommended, the value of the CT in equivocal circumstances has been recognized.[50]

CT IN TREATMENT PLANNING OF PROSTATIC CARCINOMA

CT can be used to estimate prostate size which may be an important factor in selecting between therapeutic alternatives.  Serial measurements of prostatic size are also important in monitoring the response of prostatic carcinoma to therapy.[51]  When interstitial implantation of radioactive seeds is used for therapy of prostatic carcinoma, an accurate estimate of the volume or average dimension of the gland is needed for correct dosimetry.[52]  Presurgical evaluation of prostatic size permits a better estimation of the number of [125]I seeds that are required (Figure 7).  Intravenous urography and digital rectal examinations are not sensitive indicators of prostate size.  Even with radio-opaque contrast in the bladder and rectum for x-ray simulation, the size and location of the prostate are not accurately estimated from conventional radiographic studies.[53] In certain patients, such as those who have undergone abdomino-perineal resections, determination of prostatic size by manual palpation is impossible.

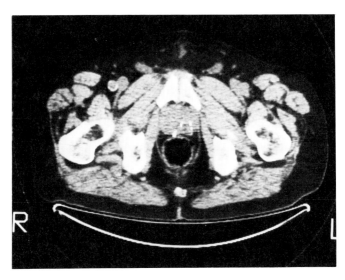

Fig. 7. CT scan demonstrating implanted [125]I seeds within the prostate. Accurate information is provided regarding distribution of seeds for dosimetry and position in the gland.

CT tends to overestimate gland weight and size.[6,10,52] Possible explanations include: 1) inclusion of the thickness of the urogenital diaphragm laterally and Denonvilliers fascia posteriorly, leading to overestimation of the transverse and anteroposterior dimensions; 2) the longitudinal axis of the prostate is actually obliquely oriented to the vertical axis (i.e., to the transverse plane of section); thus, the gland might be longer than estimated directly from transverse scans. Due to this shortcoming of conventional CT scanning in the transverse plane, sagittal and coronal reconstruction in CT of the prostate has been advocated for more accurate determination of the length and depth of the gland.[6,54-56]

Despite this limitation of axial CT images, the technique has been helpful for determination of prostatic volume, [125]I seed distribution and dosimetry and in following tumor response.[52] As previously discussed, CT also has a significant role in the selection of candidates for radioactive implantation by evaluating periprostatic tumor spread.

CT has been used to great advantage in the delineation of radiation portals for external beam radiation therapy by transferring the enlarged CT images to the treatment planning device. Therapy planning programs incorporated into the CT software providing for the use of computerized dosimetry have recently become commercially available.[6] In the extensive experience of Pilepich et al.,[57,58] treatment plan changes using CT scans were most dramatic in Stage C patients with seminal vesicle involvement. Fifty-three percent (17/32) of these patients required an enlargement of conventional treatment fields to adequately encompass the target volume.

In summary, CT is a highly useful noninvasive diagnostic modality with an important role in the evaluation of tumor extent, helpful in surgery and radiation therapy treatment planning. It also shows great promise in the evaluation of response to treatment.

REFERENCES

1. Silverberg, E., Lubera, J.A. Cancer statistics: 1983. CA 33:2-25, 1983.
2. Hutchinson, G.B. Epidemiology of prostatic cancer. Semin Oncol 3:151-155, 1976.
3. Robbins, S.L. Pathologic Basis of Disease. Saunders, Philadelphia 1190-1198, 1974.
4. Resnick, M.I., Williard, J.W., Boyce, W.H. Ultrasonic evaluation of the prostate nodule. J Urol 120:86-89, 1978.
5. Glazer, G.M., Goldberg, H.I., Moss, A.A., Axel, L. Computed tomographic detection of retroperitoneal adenopathy. Radiology 143:1476-149, 1982.
6. Morgan, C.L., Calkins, R.F., Cavalcanti, E.J., Computed tomography in the evaluation, staging and therapy of carcinoma of the bladder and prostate. Radiology 140:751-761, 1981.
7. Lee, J.K.T., Barbier, J.Y., McClenan, B.L., Stanley, R.J. Technical note: A support device for obtaining direct coronal CT images of the pelvis and lower abdomen. Radiology, 145:209,1982.
8. Osborn, A.G., Koehler, P.R., Gibbs, F.A., et al. Direct sagittal computed tomographic scans in the radiologic evaluation of the pelvis. Radiology 134:255-257, 1980.
9. Van Waes, P.F.G.M., Zonneveld, F.W. Direct coronal body computed tomography. J. Comput Assist Tomogr 6:58-66, 1982.
10. Sukov, P.J., Scardino, P.T., Sample, N.F., Winter, J., Coner, D.J. Computed tomography and transabdominal ultrasound in the evaluation of the prostate. J Comput Assist Tomog 1:281-289, 1977.
11. Van Engelshoven, M.A., Kreel, L. Computed tomography of the prostate. J Comput Assist Tomog 3:45-51, 1979.
12. Price, J.M., Davidson, A.J., Computed tomography in the evaluation of the suspected carcinomatous prostate. Urol Radiol 1:39-42, 1979.
13. Dunnick, N.R., Walther, P.J., Ford, K.R., Korobkin, M., Paulson, D.F. Mucinous adenocarcinoma of the prostate. J. Comput Assist Tomogr 6:1198-1199, 1982.
14. Weinerman, P.M., Arger, P.H., Pollack, H.M. CT Evaluation of bladder and prostate neoplasms. Urol Radiol 4:105-114, 1982.

15. Murphy, G.P., Gaeta, J.F., Pickren, J., Wajsman, Z. Current status of classification and staging of prostatic cancer. Cancer 45:1889-1895, 1980.

16. Seidelmann, F.E., Reider, N.E., Cohen, W.N., et al. Computed tomography of the seminal vesicles and seminal vesicle angle. Computed Axial Tomogr 1:281-285, 1977.

17. Seidelmann, F.E., Cohen, W.N. Pelvis in Computed Tomography of Abdominal Abnormalities, ed Haaga, J., Reich, W.E. C.V. Mosby Co, St. Louis 7:221-276, 1978.

18. Seidelmann, F.E., Cohen, W.N., Bryan, P.J. Computed tomographic staging of bladder neoplasms. Radiol Clin North Am 15:419-440, 1977.

19. Golimbu, M., Morales, P., Al-Askari, S., Shulman, Y. CT scanning in staging prostatic cancer. Urology 18:305-308, 1981.

20. Lee, J.K..T, Balfe, D.M. Pelvis in Computed Body Tomography, eds Lee, J.K.T., Sagel, S.S., Stanley, R.J. Raven Press, New York, pp 393-413, 1983.

21. Giri, P.G.S., Walsh, J.W., Hazra, T.A., Texter, J.H., Koontz, W.W. Role of computed tomography in the evaluation and management of carcinoma of the prostate. Int J Radiat Oncol Biol Phys 8:283-287, 1982.

22. Rouviere, H. Anatomy of the human lymphatic system. Edwards Brothers, Ann Arbor, MI pp. 224-226, 1938.

23. Prando, A., Wallace, S., VonEschenbach, A.E., Jing, B.S., Rosengren, J.E., Hussey, D.H. Lymphangiography in staging of carcinoma of the prostate Radiology 131:641-645, 1979.

24. Johnson, D.E., VonEschenbach, A.E. Roles of lymphangiography and pelvic lymphadenectomy in staging prostatic cancer. Urology (Suppl) 18:66-71, 1982.

25. Liebner, E.J., Stefanie, S. Uro-Oncology Research Group: An evaluation of lymphangiography with nodal biopsy in localized carcinoma of the prostate. Cancer 45:728-734, 1980.

26. Spellman, M.C., Castellino, R.A., Ray, G.R., Pistenma, D.A., Bagshaw, M.D. An evaluation of lymphography in localized carcinoma of the prostate. Radiology 125:637-644, 1977.

27. Cerny, J.E., Fara, R., Rian, R., Weckstein, M.L. An evaluation of lymphangiography in staging carcinoma of the prostate. J Urology 113:367-370.1975.

28. O'Donohue, E.P.N., Shridar, P., Sherwood, T., Williams, J.P., Chisholm, G.D. Lymphography and pelvic lymphadenectomy in carcinoma of the prostate. Br J Urol 48:689-696, 1976.

29. Hilaris, B.S., Whitmore, W.F., Batata, M., Barzell, W. Behavorial patterns of prostate adenocarcinoma following an [125]I implant and pelvic node dissection. Int J Radiat Oncol Biol Phys 2:631-637, 1977.

30. Leoning, S.A., Schmidt, J.D., Brown, R.C., Hawtrey, C.E., Fallon, B., Culp, D.A. Comparison between lymphangiography and pelvic node dissection in the staging of prostatic cancer. J Urol 117:752-756, 1977.

31. Efremidis, S.C., Dan, S.J., Nieburgs, H., Mitty, H.A. Carcinoma of the prostate: Lymph node aspiration for staging, AJR 136:489-492, 1981.

32. Gothlin, J.H., Holm, L. Percutaneous fine-needle biopsy of radiographically normal lymph nodes in the staging of prostatic carcinoma. Radiology 141:351-354, 1981.

33. Merrin, C., Wajsman, A., Baumgartner, G., Jennings, E. The clinical value of lymphangiography: Are the nodes surrounding the obturator nerve visualized? J Urol 117:762-764,1977.

34. Dretler, S.P., Ragsdale, B.D., Leadbetter, W.F. The value of pelvic lymphadenectomy in the surgical treatment of bladder carcinoma. J Urol 109:414-416, 1978.

35. Grossman, I.C., Carpiniello, C., Greenber, S.H., Malloy, T.R., Wein, A.J. Staging pelvic lymphadenectomy for carcinoma of the prostate: Review of 91 cases. J Urol 124:637-634, 1980.
36. Lieskovsky, G., Skinner, D.G., Weisenburger, T. Pelvic lymphadenectomy in the management of carcinoma of the prostate. J Urol 124:635-638, 1980.
37. Lee, J.K.T., Stanley, R.J., Sagel, S.S., McClennan, B.L. Accuracy of CT in detecting intra-abdominal and pelvic lymph node metastases from pelvic cancers. AJR 131:675-679, 1978.
38. Walsh J.W., Amendola, M.A., Konerding, K.F., Tisnado, J., Hazra, T.A. Computed tomographic detection of pelvic and inguinal node metastases from primary and recurrent pelvic malignant disease. Radiology 137:157-166, 1980.
39. Levine, M.S., Arger, P.H., Coleman, B.G., Mulhern, C.B., Pollack, H.M., Wein, A.J. Detecting lymphatic metastases from prostatic carcinoma: Superiority of CT. AJR 137:207-211, 1981.
40. Weinerman, P.M., Arger, P.H., Coleman, B.G., et al. Pelvic adenopathy from bladder and prostate carcinoma: detection by rapid sequence computed tomography. AJR 140:95-99, 1983.
41. Amendola, M.A., Tisnado, J., Walsh, J.W., et al. Computed tomography of the pelvic lymph nodes: Anatomic radiologic correlation. Scientific Exhibit presented at the 80th Annual Meeting of the American Roentgen Ray Society, Las Vegas, Nevada, 1980.
42. Cuneo, B., Marsille, M. Topographie des ganglions ilio-pelviens. Bull Mem Soc Anat Paris 653-663, 1901.
43. Herman, P.G., Benninghoff, D.L., Nelson, J.H., Jr., et al. Roentgen anatomy of the ilio-pelvic-aortic-lymphatic system. Radiology 80:182-193, 1963.
44. Castellino, R.A., Margolin, S.I. Imaging of abdominal and pelvic nodes: Lymphography or computed tomography? Invest Radiol, 17:433-443, 1982.
44. O'Mara, R.E. Skeletal scanning in neoplastic disease. Cancer 37:480-486, 1976.
45. Bisso, J., Vickers, M., Fagan, W.T. Bone scan: Clinical perspective. J Urol 111:665-669, 1974.
46. Schaffer, D.L., Pendergrass, H.P. Comparison of enzyme, clinical radiographic, and radionuclide methods of detecting bone metastases from carcinoma of the prostate. Radiology 121:431-434, 1976.
47. Mall, J.C., Berkerman, C., Hoffer, P.B., Gottschalk, A. A unified radiological approach to the detection of skeletal metastases. Radiology 118:323-328, 1976.
48. Galasko, C.M. Problems associated with the detection of skeletal metastases. J R Soc Med 71:38-41, 1978.
49. Citrin, D.L., Fogleman, I. A review of bone scan evaluation of the cancer patient. Appl Radiol May-June 102-109, 1980.
50. Amendola, M.A., Shirazi, K., Amendola, B.E., Kuhns, L.K., Tisnado, J., Yaghmai, I. Computed tomography of malignant tumors of the osseous pelvis. Comput Radiol 7:107-117,1983.
51. Grossman, H.B., Batata, M., Hilaris, V., Whitmore, W.F., Jr. $^{125}I$ implantation for carcinoma of the prostate: Further follow up of the first 100 cases. Urology 20:591-598, 1982.
52. Gore, R.M., Moss, A.A. Value of computed tomography in interstitial $^{125}I$ brachytherapy of prostatic carcinoma. Radiology 146:453-458, 1983.
53. Asbell, S.P., Schlager, B.A., Baker, A.S. Revision of treatment planning for carcinoma of the prostate. Int J Radiol Oncol Biol Phys 6:861-865, 1980.
54. Paquette, FR., Ahuja, A.S., Carson, P.L., Ibbot, B.S., Johnson, M.L. A comparative study of CT and ultrasound imaging for treatment planning of prostatic carcinoma. Int J Radiat Oncol Biol Phys 5:289-294, 1979.

55. Tisnado, J., Amendola, M., Walsh, J.W., et al. Computed tomography of the perineum. AJR 136:475-481, 1981.
56. Hamlin, D.J., Cockett, A.T.K., Burgener, F.A. Computed tomography of the pelvis: Sagittal and coronal image reconstruction in the evaluation of infiltrative bladder carcinoma. J. Comput Assist Tomogr 5:27-33, 1981.
57. Pilepich, M.V., Perez, C.A., Prasad, S. Computed tomography in definitive radiotherapy of prostate carcinoma. Int J Radiat Oncol Biol Phys 6:923-926, 1980.
58. Pilepich, M.V., Prasad, S.C., Perez, C.A. Computed tomography in definitive radiotherapy of prostatic carcinoma, Part 2: Defintion of target volume. Int J Radiat Oncol Biol Phys 8:235-240, 1982.

BLADDER CANCER:   EPIDEMIOLOGY AND RECENT RADIOTHERAPEUTIC DIRECTIONS

M. ROTMAN, M.D., H. AZIZ, M.D. AND R. YAES, M.D.

## INTRODUCTION

Cancer of the urinary bladder remains a major cause of death in the United States, and despite advances in diagnosis and treatment, the age-adjusted death rate for bladder cancer remains virtually constant.[1]   The incidence of bladder cancer for white males is twice as high as for black and hispanic males, but for females, racial differences do not affect the rate.   Overall the male:female ratio of new bladder cancers in the U.S. is 2.7:1.

In 1983 in the U.S. bladder cancer accounted for 2.4% of all cancer deaths.[1-3]   While the incidence of bladder cancer is higher among whites, the five year survival rate is almost twice as high for whites than for blacks.   This may be due to differences in the treatment, higher stage at presentation, differences in the natural history of the disease, or a possible combination of these factors.

## ETIOLOGY

Investigations over the years have shown a relationship with the dyes used in paint, rubber and cable industries,[2] abnormal tryptophan metabolism,[3] smoking,[4-7] nitrates in smoked meats,[8,9] coffee,[10,11] artificial sweeteners[12-15] and analgesics.[16]   Chronic irritation due to calculi, stasis in diverticuli[17,18] schistosomiasis[19-21] or other causes can give rise to squamous metaplasia and hence to squamous cell carcinoma.[20]   In Egypt, where schistosomiasis is endemic, bladder cancer accounts for 38.5% of all cancer in men;[20] the vast majority of these being squamous cell carcinoma.   In addition, a genetic predisposition to bladder carcinoma has been noted by Herring et al.[22]

## DIAGNOSIS AND INITIAL WORK-UP

Seventy-five percent of bladder cancer patients present with hematuria; urinary frequency, urgency and dysuria are also common complaints.   Before treatment is initiated, a complete work-up including history and physical, complete blood count, blood and urine chemistries, chest x-ray, intravenous urography, cystoscopy with multiple biopsies, bimanual examination under anesthesia and computed tomography is performed.

STAGING AND HISTOLOGY

Bladder tumors are staged according to the Marshall modification[23] of the Jewett and Strong[24] staging system or the TNM system of the International Union Against Cancer.[25] Both systems are essentially equivalent with minor variations. In Jewett and Strong's original review, a positive correlation between high grade and high stage at presentation was found, confirming the supposition that high grade tumors tend to be more agressive.[24]

Baker meticulously studied multiple sections of surgical specimens and found that 50% of tumors labeled Stage B1 (superficial muscle) actually had lymphatic dissemination of tumor deep in the muscularis and should have been staged B2. All lesions staged B2 had lymphatic permeation.[26]

Bladder cancer tends to metastasize first to regional lymph nodes and then to bone, lungs, and liver.[24] However, lymph node metastases are most common in the ipsilateral pelvic nodes.

Ninety-seven percent of bladder tumors arise in the transitional epithelium. In the U.S the most common histology by far is transitional cell carcinoma followed by squamous cell carcinoma and adenocarcinoma,[28] and the latter two histologies carry a poor prognosis.

Ninety percent of transitional cell carcinomas are papillary and that they are often multifocal and have a high recurrence rate may be related to the fact that they are often preceeded by proliferative changes in the bladder mucosa.[29] Epithelial hyperplasia can progress to carcinoma in situ and changes in papillary cystitis and papilloma could lead to papillary carcinoma. On the other hand, in a recent study by Brown[30] of 104 consecutive cases of bladder cancer at the University of Kansas only 20 had a history of benign papillary lesions.

Transitional cell carcinoma is usually graded from I to IV according to Broder's system,[31] in order of increasing anaplasia. Higher grade tumors carry a poorer prognosis. In Mostofi's[32] collection of 2,678 cases of bladder cancer, Grade I papillary carcinomas had an 85% 5 year disease-free survival rate, and a 67% 10 year disease-free survival rate. The corresponding figures for the combined Grade II and Grade III tumors were 20% and 12%, respectively. In general, high grade anaplastic tumors tend to be more deeply infiltrating at diagnosis and also tend to metastasize early.

Invasion of the muscle is not readily identified in most transurethral resection of the bladder (TURB) specimens; invasion of the lamina propria is even more difficult to appreciate. Thus, the distinction between benign papilloma and Grade I Stage A papillary carcinoma is difficult to make, and it is indeed controversial as to whether such a distinction is meaningful.[32]

PROGNOSTIC FACTORS

Most prognostic factors have become apparent due to the studies of Batata,[33] and van der Werf-Messing.[34] In Batata's study, the main prognostic factor after stage is the grade of the tumor. Overall 5-year survival for high grade tumors was 20-32% as compared to 46-56% for low grade tumors. Two new factors affect the prognosis: 1) abnormal urogram[33,34] and 2. vascular invasion by the tumor.[34] The size of the tumor is also a prognostic factor. Batata[33] estimates that only 27% of patients whose tumor was more than 4 cm in diameter survive for 5 years as compared to more than 50% of patients whose tumor was less than 4 cm.

TREATMENT

Surgery

Transurethral resection of the bladder (TURB) is a commonly practiced method of treatment for early stage carcinoma for well differentiated papillomatous lesions. These should be single and located in an area accessible for resection.

Segmental resection is indicated for solitary tumors. The location and site of the tumor should be such as to allow full thickness excision with a 2 cm margin. Recurrences are common in high grade tumors. Preoperative irradiation, consisting of 1050 rads in three treatments, is given to the patient to reduce the wound implants from 14% to 4.2%.[35]

Cystectomy may be total or radical. Total cystectomy is done without lymph node dissection. It is indicated for multicentric, low or high grade tumors, where a lesser procedure would prove ineffective. Radical cystectomy is indicated for high stage carcinomas where lymph nodes may be involved.[36] Cystectomy is a major operative procedure which produces a significant morbidity of 30-50%, and a mortality of 3-10%.[36] The 5 year survival for cystectomy alone is limited to 30%.[36] Moreover, a large percentage of patients selected for cystectomy, prove inoperable.

## Irradiation

Interstitial implantation. Ideally, the tumor selected for implant should be localized, with muscle invasion not beyond Stage IB(T2), and the total area not more than 5 cm in diameter. The technique requires a prior cystostomy and resection of the tumor to its base. The base with a 1 cm margin establishes the target-volume. In the past, other centers have used "tantalum hair pins" and radium needles.[35] Iridium 192 has certain advantages over both tantalum and radium because its energy is only 0.3 MeV as compared to 1.1 MeV and 1.4 MeV for tantalum and radium, respectively.

Interstitial implantation seems to be the most promising method of treatment. Van der verf Messing[35] has not only shown good long-term survival for superficial tumors, but also for T3A(B2) tumors, if the size of the tumor was limited to 5 cm, and if external irradiation produced a Stage reduction. Total tumor dose given by this technique is 6,000 to 6,500 rads in 6 or 7 weeks .

## Definitive Irradiation with External Beam

The combined 5 year survival for all stages and all grades treated with definitive radiation is 30-40%.[33,37-39] Recent reports[40-43] suggest that surgical salvage of irradiation failures is entirely feasible.

Selection of optimum dose. In 1975, Morrison[37] collected data from the world literature concerning tumor control and complications at various dose levels. He observed that complications started to develop after a dose of 1,500 rets was given and that complications rose steeply to about 40% when the dose level reached 2,000 rets. Tumor control also starts at about 1,500 rets, and the probability of tumor control increases as the dose is increased. A tumor dose of 6,000 rads in 6.5 weeks or 6,500 rads in 7 weeks, which is equivalent tO 1,750 rets and 1,800 rets, respectively, is well tolerated with an acceptable complication rate.

## Complication from Irradiation

After analyzing 101 patients who received a definitive course of irradiation, Bloedorn[44] found several factors which predispose patients to severe radiation reaction. These factors are: 1) any kind of recent surgery, 2) obstructive uropathy, 3) presence of infection and 4) faulty radiation techniques. Bloedorn[44] therefore suggested that if there is any obstruction or infection, they should be relieved before the initiation of irradiation. Since 75% of the patients who developed severe radiation reaction had recent surgery, Bloedorn[44] strongly felt that such patients should wait for a least three weeks before initiation of irradiation.

Acute complications occur either during irradiation or immediately following completion of the therapy. Acute complications may be: 1) severe cystitis, 2) uremia (occurs only rarely when both ureteral orifices are involved by tumor), 3) rectal reaction in the form of diarrhea and tenesmus, 4) bladder ulcers due to faulty irradiation techniques and subsequent overdose and 5) fistula formation due to regression of the tumor.

Late complications include hemorrhagic cystitis resulting from the development of telangectasia. Contracted bladder may develop one or more years after the completion of treatment. In extreme cases, bladder capacity is reduced to only 50-60 mls. Ureteral or bladder neck obstruction occurs as a result of chronic fibrosis or invasion by recurrent tumor. Late fistula formation is usually due to overdosage. Small bowel obstruction and necrosis usually occurs in postoperative cases where the small bowel gets entrapped in the pelvis due to adhesions.

COMBINED MODALITY THERAPY

Pre-operative Irradiation and Planned Cystectomy

Patients with low stage tumor O, A or Bl (Tis, Tl,T2) have shown no definite improvement with pre-operative irradiation.[36] However, in cases beyond Stage Bl(T2), there has been definite improvement with pre-operative irradiation.

A variety of pre-operative regimens have been used, ranging from 5,000 rads in 5 weeks[45] to 2,000 rads in 1 week;[46] and recently, only 1,600 rads in 4 treatments has been given.[47] These differing regimens have all produced practically the same results.[47] The beneficial effect of pre-operative irradiation on survival has been seen in patients in whom T reduction to a lower pathologic stage P has been demonstrated.[34] Overall, T reduction occurs in 89% of patients, and in about 30% of cases, the stage is reduced to PO.[34] One of the recently published series[34] demonstrates that patients who were stage T3 initially and received 4,000 rads in 4 weeks as pre-operative irradiation showed best results. In PO patients, 5 year survival was 85%. For Pl, P2 and P3 it was 75%, 50% and 45%, respectively.[34] Among all of the preoperative series, Miller's[50] was the only one which was randomized and showed definite improvement in survival; viz., 51% for B2 and C (T3A, T3B) carcinomas, as compared to 20% if the same patients were treated with irradiation only. In a retrospective study, Miller

showed that there was a higher local recurrence rate for postoperative
irradiation (33%) compared to pre-operative irradiation (16%).[48]

## Definitive Irradiation and Salvage Cystectomy

The rationale of salvage cystectomy is based on the fact that cystectomy
may still be feasible after definitive irradiation[41-43] and that the salvage
rate may not differ greatly from patients with similar tumors who have been
treated with cystectomy alone.[36] Batata also reported on a group of 109
patients who received 6,000 rads in 30 treatments with curative intent and who
underwent cystectomy after the tumor had recurred or persisted.[33] In this
group also, the 5 year survival rate was 41%. Blandy et al.[41] reported on a
large series of 704 patients who were treated with definitive irradiation with
a tumor dose of 5,000 to 5,500 rads in 20 fractions. The 5-year survival for
T3(B2,C) was 38%, which is comparable to some preoperative series. However,
what is more important is that Blandy et al.[41] found two distinct tumor
populations; viz., a radiosensitive and a radioresistant group. Nearly half
of these tumors appear to be radiosensitive, giving a crude 5-year surival
rate for T3(B2,C) tumors of 56%, compared to 17.5% for the radioresistant
group with radiation alone. Blandy[41] suggests that following completion of
definitive irradiation, the patients should undergo cystoscopy and bimanual
examinations at 3 and 6 months. If by the end of six months, the tumor is
still present, cystectomy should be performed. The result of the salvage
cystectomy in patients who were judged as partial responders and
non-responders was impressive as the 5-year survival rate in these patients
rose to 38%.[41]

Mortality rate from pre-operative irradiation and radical cystectomy is
between 5%-7%[36] versus salvage cystectomy where the mortality rate increases
to about 11%.[41,43]

## Intravesical Chemotherapy

Intravesical chemotherapy may be indicated in multifocal Stage O or A
carcinomas or for prevention of recurrence following TURB for superficial
carcinomas.

In 1948, Semple[49] first tried podophyllin to deal with this problem.
Since then, several authors[50,51] have used thiotepa or mitomycin C. They
reported that the tumor was destroyed in a third of the patients.
Intravesical instillation of thiotepa or mitomycin C in these patients has the
potential of reducing neoplastic changes in the urothelium.[50-52] For chemo-

prevention in patients at high risk for recurrence, 13-Cis retinoic acid and vitamin A (Retinoids) hold promise.[51-53]

CONCLUSION

Progress in the treatment of bladder cancer has not been rapid, however, the use of combined therapy has considerably improved survival. There is still ample room for progress in this important area of oncology.

BIBLIOGRAPHY

1.  Silverberg, E. Cancer Statistics 1983. CA - A Journal for Clinicians 33:9, 1983.
2.  Veys, C.A. Bladder Tumors and Occupations: A Coroner's Notification Scheme. Brit J Indus Med, 31:65, 1974.
3.  Boyland, E. and Williams, D.C. The Metabolism of Tryptophan II, The Metabolism of Tryptophan in Patients Suffering from Cancer of the Bladder. Biochem J 64:578, 1956.
4.  Morgan, R.W., Jain, M.G. Bladder Cancer: Smoking, Beverages and Artifical Sweeteners. CMAJ III:1067, 1974.
5.  Armstrong, B., Doll, R. Bladder Cancer Mortality in England and Wales in relation to cigarette smoking and saccharin consumption. Brit J Prev Soc Med 28:233, 1974.
6.  Hoffman, D., Masuda, Y., Wynder, D.L. Alpha-napthylamine and B naphthylamine in cigarette smoke. Nature (London) 221:254, 1969.
7.  Morrison, A.S. Public Health Value of Using Epidemiologic Information to Identify High Risk Group for Bladder Cancer Screening. Seminar on Oncology 6(2):184, 1979.
8.  Richardson, W.E. The Occurrence of Nitrates in Vegetable Foods, in Meats and Elsewhere. J Am Chem Soc 29:1757, 1907.
9.  Wolf, I.A., Wasserman, A.E. Nitrates, Nitrites and Nitrosomines. Science 177:15, 1972.
10.  Cole, P. Coffee Drinking and Cancer of the Lower Urinary Tract. Lancet 1:1335, 1971.
11.  Simon, D., Yen., S., Cole, P. Coffee Drinking and Cancer of the Lower Urinary Tract. J Nat Canc Inst 54:597, 1975.
12.  Egeberg, R.O., Seingield, J.L., Frantz, I., et al. Report to the Secretary of HEW from the Medical Advisory Group on Cyclamates. JAMA 211:1358, 1970.
13.  Bryan, G.T., Erturke, E. Production of Mouse Urinary Bladder Carcinomas by Sodium Cyclamate. Science 167:966, 1970.
14.  Richardson, H.L., Richardson, M.E., Wallace, H. Urinary Bladder Carcinoma and Other Pathologic Alterations in Rats Fed on Cyclamates. Proc Am Assoc Cancer Res 13:2, 1972.
15.  National Academy of Sciences Subcommittee on Non-nutritive Sweetners, Dec. 1974.
16.  Angervall, L., Bengtsson, U., Zetterlund, C.G. and Zsigmond, M. Renal Pelvic Carcinoma in a Swedish District with Abuse of Phenacetin Containing Drugs. Brit J Urol 41:405, 1969.

17. Mayer, R.F., Moore, T.D. Carcinoma Complicating Vesical Diverticula. J Urol 71:307, 1954.

18. Knappenberger, S.T., Uson, A.C., Milicow, M.M. Primary Neoplasms Occurring in Vesical Diverticula: A report of 18 cases. J Urol 83:153, 1960.

19. Gelfand, M., Weinberg, R.W., Castle, M.W. Relation Between Carcinoma of the Bladder and Infestation of Schistosoma Hematobium. Lancet 1:1249-1251, 1967.

20. Chevlen, E.M., Awwad, A.K., Zeigler, J.L., Elsebai, I. Cancer of the Bilharzial Bladder. Int J Rad Onc Biol and Phys 5:921-1138, 1979.

21. Dimette, R.M., Sproat, H.F., Sayegh, E.S. The Classification of Urinary Bladder Carcinoma Associated with Schistosomiasis and Metaplasia. J Urol 75:680, 1956.

22. Herring, D.N., Cartwright, R.A., Williams D.D.R. Genetic Associates of Transitional Cell Carcinoma. Brit J Urol 51:173, 1979.

23. Marshall, V.F. The Relations of Pre-Operative Estimate of the Pathologic Demonstration of the Extent of Vesical Neoplasm. J Urol 68:714, 1952.

24. Jewett, H.J., Strong, G.H. Infiltrating Carcinoma of the Bladder: Relation of Depth of Penetration of the Bladder Wall to Incidence of Local Extension and Metastasis. J Urol 55:366, 1946.

25. TNM Classification of Malignant Tumors (Second Edition). International Union Against Cancer, Geneva, Switzerland, 1974.

26. Baker, R. The Accuracy of Clinical vs. Surgical Staging. JAMA 206:1770, 1968.

27. Friedman, N., Ash, J. Tumors of the Urinary Bladder. Atlas of Tumor Pathology - Section VIII, Fasicle 31a. Armed Forces Institute of Pathology, Washington, D.C. 1959.

28. U.S. Dept. of Health Education and Welfare, Cancer Patient Survival Report #5, 1976.

29. Mostofi, F.K. The Role of Tumor Histology in Recurrence of Early Bladder Cancer in Syllabus: Genitourinary Malignancy, M. Rotman, ed., Radiological Society of North America, 1980.

30. Brown, P.N. The Origin of Invasive Carcinoma of the Bladder. Cancer 50:515, 1982.

31. Broders, A.C. Carcinoma Grading and Practical Application. Arch Path.2:376, 1926.

32. Mostofi, F.K. Pathological Aspects and Spread of Carcinoma of the Bladder. JAMA 206:1764, 1968.

33. Batata, M.A., Chu, F.C.H., Hillaris, B.S., Lee, M.Z., Chung, S. and Whitmore, W.F. Factors of Prognostic and Therapeutic Significance in Patients with Bladder Cancer. Int J Rad Onc Bio and Phys 7:575-579, 1981.

34. Van der Werf-Messing, B., Friedell, G.H., Menon, R.S., Hop, W.C.J. and Wassif, S.B. Carcinoma of the Urinary Bladder T3NxMO Treated by Preoperative Irradiation Followed by Cystectomy. 8:1849-1855, 1982.

35. Van der Werf-Messing, B. Cancer of the Urinary Bladder Treated by Interstitial Radium Implant. Int J Rad Biol Physics 4:272, 1978.

36. Whitemore, W.F., Jr. Management of Bladder Cancer. Current Problems in Cancer, 1979.

37. Morrison, R. The Results of Treatment of Cancer of the Bladder - A Clinical Contribution to Radiotherapy. Clin Radiology 26:67, 1975.

38. Cummings, K.R., Taylor, W.J., Correa, R.J., Gibbons, R.P. and Mason, J.T. Observations In Definitive Cobalt 60 Radiation for Cure in Bladder Carcinoma: 15 Year Follow-up. J Urol 48:595, 1976.

39. Rider, W.D. and Evans, D.H. Radiotherapy in the Treatment of Recurrent Bladder Cancer. Br J Urol 48:595, 1976.

40. Wallace, D.M. and Bloom, H.J.G. The Management of Deeply Infiltrating T3 Carcinoma: Controlled Trial of Radical Radiotherapy Versus Preoperative Radiotherapy and Radical Cystectomy (First Report). Br J Urol 48:587, 1976.

41. Blandy, J.P., England, H.R., Evans, S.J.W., Hopstone, H.F., Mair, G.M.M., Mantel, B.S., Oliver, R.T.D., Paris, A.I. and Risondman, R.A. T3 Bladder Cancer - The Case for Salvage Cystectomy. Brit J Urol 52:506-510, 1980.

42. Johnson, D.E., Lamy, S. and Bracken, R.B. Salvage Cystectomy After Radiation Failure in Patients with Bladder Carcinoma. South Med Journal 70:1279, 1977.

43. Goodman, G.B., Hislop, T.G., Elwood, J.M. and Balfour, J. Conservation of Bladder Function in Patients with Invasive Bladder Cancer Treated by Definitive Irradiation and Selective Cystectomy. Int J Radiation Onc Biol Physics 77:569-573, 1981.

44. Bloedorn F.G., Young, J.D., Cuccia, C.A., et al. Radiotherapy in Carcinoma of the Bladder: Possible Complications and their Prevention. Radiology.

45. Miller, L.S. and Johnson, D.E. Megavoltage Irradiation for Bladder Cancer Alone, Postoperative and Preoperative? Proc 7th Natl Cancer Conf (Philadelphia) J.B. Lippincott, p. 771, 1973.

46. Whitemore, W.F., Jr., Batata, M.A., Hillaris, B.S., Reddy, G,N., Unal, A., Ghoneim, M.A., Grabstald, H. and Chu, F. A Comparative Study of Two Preoperative Regimes with Bladder Cancer. Cancer 40:1077, 1977.

47. Skinner, D.G., Tift, J.P. and Kaufman, J.J. High Dose, Short Course Preoperative Irradiation Therapy and Immediate Single Stage Radical Cystectomy with Pelvic Node Dissection in the Management of Bladder Cancer. J Urol 127:1274, 1982.

48. Miller L.S. Bladder Cancer: Superiority of Post Operative Irradiation and Cystectomy in Clinical Stage B2 and C. Cancer 39:973, 1977.

49. Semple, J.E. Papillomata of Bladder Treated with Preliminary Report. Br Med J 1:1235, 1948.

50. Veenema, R.J., Romas, N.A. and Fuigerhurst, B. Chemotherapy for Bladder Cancer. Urology 3:135, 1974.

51. Soloway M.S. and Martino, C. Prophylaxix of Bladder Tumor Implantation. Urology 7:29, 1976.

52. Koontz, W.W., Jr. Intravesical Chemotherapy and Chemoprevention of Superficial Low Grade, Low Stage Bladder Carcinoma. Seminars in Oncology 6(2):217-219, 1979.

53. Sporn, M.D., et al Prevention of Chemical Carcinogenesis by Vitamin A and Its Synthetic Analogues. Fed Proc 32:1332, 1976.

BLADDER CANCER:  CURRENT THERAPY AND FUTURE PROSPECTS

H. BARTON GROSSMAN, M.D.

INTRODUCTION

Bladder cancer is a significant clinical problem, with approximately 37,000 new cases occurring annually.[1]  The male to female ratio of these cases is 2.7:1.  Bladder cancer is the cause of death of approximately 10,600 people annually.  Despite extensive knowledge of the etiology and natural history of this disease, the age adjusted cancer death rate for bladder cancer in males in the United States has not changed since 1930.  Perhaps one cause of this is the fact that eighty-five percent of all patients with high stage bladder cancer will initially present with muscle invasion.[2]  On the other hand, only ten to twenty percent of the patients presenting with superficial bladder cancer (Ta or Tl) will subsequently develop muscle invasion.[3,4]

Staging

Currently there are two staging systems in use in the United States.  The oldest is the clinical characterization by Jewett, Strong, and Marshall which has long been met with clinical acceptance and good correlation with the disease course.[5,6]  The most useful subdivision of this system is into superficial versus deep carcinoma of the bladder.  In this staging system, patients with superficial disease have a much better life expectancy than those with deep disease despite the most aggressive therapy currently used for patients with more invasive tumors.  A significant problem with this staging system occurs in patients who have more advanced disease.  Patients who have invasion of adjacent organs, lymph node metastases, or distant metastases are all grouped into stage D.  Although the prognosis for all of these patients is rather poor, it is helpful to subdivide them when evaluating new forms of therapy.  Because of this, the tumor, node, metastasis (TNM) system has gained favor among those physicians whose primary interest is oncology (Table 1).  The two systems are very similar, the primary difference is in their handling of higher stage disease.  The TNM system groups patients with B2 and C disease into one group called T3, although this can be subdivided respectively into T3a and T3b.  The clinical significance of this differentiation, however, is

Recent Trends in Radiation Oncology and Related Fields, Amendola and Amendola, Editors

rather insignificant because these patients are treated in a similar fashion. Patients with more advanced disease are better stratified in the TNM system with differentiation regarding tumor extent, nodal involvement, and distant metastasis.

| TABLE 1 | | | STAGING OF BLADDER CANCER | |
|---|---|---|---|---|
| **TNM** | | **Jewett Strong Marshall** | | **Tumor Extent** |
| | | | S | |
| TIS No Mo | | | U | Carcinoma in situ |
| | | | P | O |
| Ta No Mo | | | E | Papilloma |
| | | | R | |
| | | | F | |
| T1 No Mo | | A | I | Invasion not beyond lamina propria |
| | | | C | |
| T2 No Mo | | B1 | I | Invasion into superficial muscle |
| | | | A | |
| | | | L | |
| T3a No Mo | | B2 | D | Invasion into deep muscle |
| | | | E | |
| T3b No Mo | | C | E | Invasion of perivesical fat |
| | | | P | |
| | | | M | |
| T4 No Mo | | | E | Invasion of adjacent organs |
| | | D1 | T | |
| Tx N1-3 Mo | | | A | Regional lymphatic involvement |
| | | | S | |
| | | | T | |
| Tx N4 Mo | | | A | Juxtaregional lymphatic involvement |
| | | D2 | T | |
| Tx Nx M1 | | | I | Distant Metastasis |
| | | | C | |

## Superficial Bladder Cancer

The most common presenting symptom/sign of bladder cancer is hematuria, a finding that is often grossly apparent to both patient and physician. Since this is usually evaluated endoscopically, most patients have their disease initially diagnosed at the time of cystoscopy. Because the majority of patients initially present with superficial disease, definitive treatment of their tumor by transurethral resection is usually carried out at the time of diagnosis. The obvious advantages of this therapeutic approach include preservation of bladder function, little morbidity, and good survival in individuals with low grade, low stage tumors. Five-year survival rates in patients with Tl neoplasms range from 62 to 73%, and patients with grade 1 tumors have even a better prognosis. However, when superficial neoplasms become too extensive for transurethral resection, more agressive treatment is required. (Tables 2 and 3).

| TABLE 2. | FIVE-YEAR SURVIVAL BY CLINICAL STAGE | | | | | | |
|---|---|---|---|---|---|---|---|
| Investigators* | Treatment ** | O | A | B1 | B2 | C | D |
| Cummings et al.[19] | 6000 R | | -----73----- | | --36--- | | |
| Buschke & Jack[20] | 6000 R | | | --44--- | --14--- | | O |
| Rider & Evans[21] | 6000 R | | 55 | 50 | --15--- | | 25 |
| Barnes et al.[22] | TUR | | 73 | ---31--- | | | |
| O'Flynn et al.[23] | TUR | | 62 | 59 | --20--- | | O |
| Whitmore et al.[9] | Rad Cyst | | -----53----- | | --16--- | | O |
| | 4000 R + Rad Cyst | | -----59----- | | --34--- | | O |
| | 2000 R + Rad Cyst | | -----54----- | | --40--- | | O |
| van der Werf-Messing[24] | 1050 R + Radium | | | | --35--- | | |
| | 4000 R + Cyst | | | | --50--- | | |
| Miller[7] | 7000 R | | | | --22--- | | |
| | 5000 R + Cyst | | | | --46--- | | |
| Bloom et al.[8] | 6000 R | | | | --29--- | | |
| | 4000 R + Rad Cyst | | | | --38--- | | |

\* Underlined investigator denotes prospective randomized studies.
\*\* R = number of rads external radiotherapy; TUR = transurethral resection;
   Rad Cyst = Cystectomy with Pelvic Lymphadenectomy; Radium = Radium
   Implantation; Cyst = Cystectomy

## Deep Tumors

For those few patients who have bladder tumors invading more deeply into muscle in one localized area of the bladder away from the trigone and with the remainder of the bladder normal on endoscopic and biopsy evaluation, segmental resection or partial cystectomy remains a viable alternative for definitive therapy while preserving bladder function. Isolated series in which patients have been highly selected have resulted in excellent survival with this form of therapy. With higher grade tumors, the chance for tumor recurrence in the operative incision increases.

TABLE 3          FIVE-YEAR SURVIVAL BY PATHOLOGIC STAGE

| Investigators | Treatment * | 0 | A | B1 | B2 | C | D |
|---|---|---|---|---|---|---|---|
| Resnick & O'Connor[25] | Seg Res | 75 | 71 | 77 | 19 | 12 | 20 |
| Cummings et al.[26] | Seg Res | 100 | 79 | 80 | 45 | 6 | |
| Wajsman et al.[27] | Cystectomy | -----50----- | | | ---32--- | | 0 |
| Cardonnier[28] | Cystectomy | | 46 | 52 | 40 | 31 | 11 |
| Pearse et al.[29] | Rad Cyst | | --64--- | | 50 | 20 | 18 |
| Long et al.[30] | Cystectomy | 18 | 88 | ---31--- | | 10 | 0 |
| | Rad Cyst | 67 | 80 | ---45--- | | 44 | 20 |
| Whitmore et al.[9] | Rad Cyst | -----63----- | | | ---20--- | | |
| | 4000 R + Rad Cyst | -----58----- | | | ---38--- | | 11 |
| | 2000 R + Rad Cyst | -----56----- | | | ---58--- | | 14 |
| Bloom et al.[8] | 4000 R + Rad Cyst | -----68----- | | | | 32** | 18 |

* Seg Res = segmental resection
  Rad Cyst = cystectomy with pelvic lymphadenectomy
  R = number of rads of external radiotherapy
**P3 + P4 No Mo

More extensive intravesical disease has been treated with radiation therapy, surgery, or a combination thereof. Unfortunately very few prospective randomized series have been performed to adequately evaluate these therapeutic options. Radiation therapy is attractive because it avoids a major operative procedure with its attendant morbidity and mortality and preserves bladder function. Nevertheless some patients do get severe complications with radiation therapy requiring urinary and/or intestinal diversion. In addition, the local control of extensive intravesical tumor is not always complete and furthermore the remaining urothelium continues to be at risk for the subsequent development of new neoplasms. Cystectomy, of course, eliminates the possibility of neoplasm recurring in the bladder. However, the entire urothelium is at risk and the upper tracts must be continued to be monitored for the development of new tumors. Obvious disadvantages of cystectomy aside from its being a major operative procedure, include urinary diversion with its associated problems and loss of erectile function in potent males.

Two prospective randomized series have been performed comparing therapeutic radiotherapy with preoperative radiotherapy followed by cystectomy. In a report from M.D. Anderson Hospital and Tumor Institute, 68 patients with stage T3 (B2 and C) were randomly allocated to either 7,000 rads external radiation or 5,000 rads preoperative radiotherapy followed by cystectomy.[7] The five year survival for the two groups were respectively 16% and 46%, P < 0.01. The addition of two patients who were radiation failures that were salvaged by cystectomy brings the five year survival for the radiotherapy group to 22%. Included in the 46% are five patients who did not have cystectomy performed. If only patients are included who had preoperative radiotherapy and cystectomy, the five year survival was 53%.

A second study of T3 bladder cancer has been carried out by the Clinical Trials Group, Institute of Urology.[8] This multicenter study involved 189 patients. All patients were treated with 4,000 rads to the pelvis. Those randomized to radiation therapy received an additional boost of 2,000 rads to the bladder and perivesical tissue and those patients randomized to surgery underwent cystectomy. The five year survival for the two groups by randomized treatment was respectively 29% and 38%, P=0.2. Five year survival for the two groups by treatment received was respectively 31% and 44%, P > 0.05.

As in the M.D. Anderson study, a group of patients who failed treatment with radiation therapy were then treated with subsequent cystectomy. This group (18 patients) did quite well and had a five year survival rate of 60%. This good survival in patients undergoing salvage cystectomy has been documented in other series. This probably occurs because a unique population is being selected out in which distant metastases are not apparent after longer followup. These patients do have extensive localized disease but, because of their long followup some patients with occult metastases are eliminated. If the salvage cystectomy group is excluded and one compares preoperative radiation therapy and cystectomy versus radiation alone, the difference in survival is statistically significant with radiation therapy doing much worse.[7]

In the British study there were groups of patients, however, that had significantly better survival when treated with preoperative radiation and surgery versus definitive radiation with or without salvage cystectomy. The patients with improved survival included those patients less than 60 years of age. Although the combination of preoperative radiation and surgery continued to do better in patients older than 60, the difference in survival progressively became less as the patient population became older and statistically significant differences were no longer observed. When patients were stratified according to sex, men with preoperative radiation and cystectomy appear to have superior survival prospects (P=0.06). Women on the other hand, had similar survival curves regardless of therapy. From this

large study, it is apparent that preoperative radiation and cystectomy offers
somewhat better survival prospects than radiation alone.[8] The results,
however, only attain statistical significance in those patients under 60 years
of age.

The small advantage that is seen with radiation and surgery over radiation
alone in advanced bladder neoplasms can be explained on the basis of the
occasional failure of local control by radiation therapy, as well as the
subsequent development of new neoplasms in the bladder urothelium. A very
important related question which has not been adequately answered is the
contribution of preoperative radiation to cystectomy in the control of bladder
neoplasia. There are, in fact, no controlled series to adequately evaluate
this problem. A review of the reports from Memorial Sloan-Kettering Cancer
Center are, however, helpful in addressing this problem.[9] Their therapeutic
regimens which have been consecutive over time, rather than randomized, do
offer some insight into this problem. In their series of patients with
superficial tumors who underwent either radical cystectomy, 4,000 rads
preoperative irradiation followed by radical cystectomy or 2,000 rads and
radical cystectomy, over a period of 22 years no difference was seen in
overall survival. Patients with T3 disease, however, appear to have much
better survival when treated with either preoperative radiation therapy
program as compared to surgery alone. It is, however, difficult to adequately
assess the meaning of this difference because the initial series treated with
surgery alone was performed earliest and differences in overall medical care,
as well as an improved understanding of bladder neoplasia with increasing
clinical experience, may have contributed to the inferior results seen with
this group. Nevertheless, it has been demonstrated in other therapeutic
settings that preoperative radiation does have some effect. Downstaging, that
is, the decrease in pathologic stages compared to preoperative clinical stage
following radiation therapy, is well documented and is associated with
superior survival in patients being downstaged. What is unclear is whether
this effect improves survival in the overall group or is only a method for
selecting out those patients who were initially destined to do better
regardless of their treatment. This problem of adequately defining which
patients will respond to therapy and which patients will not is very important
and continues to be a fruitful area for research.

Chemotherapy

Chemotherapy has been used primarily in two settings for the treatment of bladder carcinoma. Intravesically, a variety of agents have been used for the treatment and prophylaxis of superficial bladder tumors. Systemic therapy has usually been reserved for those patients with more advanced disease. The use of soft agar clonogenic assays offers the possibility of placing chemotherapy for urothelial tumors on a more rational basis. However, this very promising tool has not yet reached the point of routine utility in the care of the average patient.

Of the drugs used in the United States for intravesical chemotherapy, thio-tepa (N, N', N"-trietinylenethiophosphoramide) has received the most attention. It is a polyfunctional alkylating agent that is absorbed from normal bladders after intravesical instillation. Its absorption is increased with bladder neoplasms and bladder injury and may result in bone marrow depression.

In a recent report from the National Bladder Cancer Collaborative Group A, thio-tepa was shown to be effective both therapeutically and for prophylaxis.[10] In this randomized prospective study, 95 patients were treated therapeutically for incompletely resected carcinoma. Successful treatment was directly related to the amount of disease present. Patients with less than four tumors had a significantly better success rate than patients with four or more bladder tumors (62% versus 36% respectively, P=0.02). In the prophylaxis study, patients were treated at monthly intervals with either 30mg or 60mg of thio-tepa versus a controlled group. Patients who underwent prophylactic therapy had a longer interval free of disease compared to the control group, but this difference failed to achieve statistical significance. One year following onset of treatment, 50% of the patients undergoing active treatment were free of disease while only 31% of the controlled group were disease free (P=0.20). A subgroup of patients who were successfully treated with therapeutic thio-tepa, demonstrated that prophylactic therapy can be significantly better than control (P=0.05). In this group who had already demonstrated a good therapeutic response to thio-tepa, 100% of the patients receiving prophylaxis remained disease free at one year as compared to 60% in the control group.[10]

A randomized study from the European Organization on Treatment of Cancer evaluated transurethral resection (TUR), TUR and prophylactic thio-tepa, and TUR and prophylactic VM26 (epipodophyllotoxin) as therapy for superficial bladder cancer.[11] There was no difference between treatment groups in the time to first recurrence. However, the group treated with prophylactic thio-tepa had significantly fewer recurrences when compared with the control

(TUR) group, P=0.008. Although the recurrence rate with thio-tepa was also less than VM26, this difference was not statistically significant, P=0.26.

Other agents which currently appear promising include doxorubicin, mitomycin C, and others. Immunotherapy with intravesical BCG also appears to be effective.[12] The exact mechanism of action of this agent remains to be defined. Similarly, the role of intravesical chemotherapy and/or immuno-therapy in the management of carcinoma in situ remains unidentified.

Patients with metastatic disease are treated with systemic chemotherapy. Active agents against urothelial carcinomas include cisplatin, methotrexate, doxorubicin, and a wide variety of single agent and drug combinations. Unfortunately, the addition of different active agents in combination chemo-therapy, while theoretically attractive, has not caused a dramatic improvement in the response rates. Smith has recently reviewed the role of chemotherapy in the treatment of bladder cancer.[13]

## FUTURE PROSPECTS

Since patients with low stage disease have a better survival than patients with high stage disease, it would seem that earlier diagnosis should result in improved survival. A recent report from Japan sheds some light on this important question.[14] The authors used urine cytology to study a group of workers exposed to the carcinogens benzidene and -napthylamine and compared them to a similar group who were diagnosed as having cancer after clinical symptoms developed.[4] Fifteen percent of the patients in the cytology group were treated with cystectomy versus 47 percent in the symptom group implying that cytologic evaluation produced diagnosis of urothelial carcinoma at an earlier stage. Despite this fact, there was not a statistically significant difference in survival between the two groups. The five year survival for the cytology group was 68% compared with 62% for the symptom group. This means either that current therapy is not adequate to alter the natural history of bladder cancer or that effective forms of therapy are not being appropriately used in a significant number of patients.

There remains little doubt that the treatment of bladder cancer in its various stages is effective in at least some instances. It is also obvious that the optimal therapy for all patients has been far from realized. A major problem at the present time is to determine for each patient what in fact is the best form of treatment. A number of new ways of resolving this problem are currently under investigation.

Perhaps the simplest way of looking at this problem involves patients undergoing chemotherapy. It is very obvious that some people will respond to various drugs while others, who have histologically similar disease will not. The development of a clonogenic assay may prove to be of significant help in separating these groups.[15] In this experimental system, a patient's tumor cells are incubated with various chemotherapeutic drugs or control medium and then plated into soft agar. After a period of time has elapsed, the numbers of colonies of tumor cells that have grown are counted. Drugs that are assumed to show activity against a given tumor cell population will inhibit their growth in this assay. Drugs which are not active will result in tumor growth similar to the control treated cells. These results can easily be counted and quantified. Although the technique is very attractive, a variety of methodological problems remain to be resolved. In addition, although there appears to be some correlation with in vivo effect of the drugs tested, it has not been adequately demonstrated that it is sufficiently reliable to use as a prospective screening method. However, another related use would be to analyze experimental agents in vitro before testing them in wide scale clinical trials.

A second method which appears promising has been the immunologic evaluation of neoplastic cells. Again, histologically similar cells may appear very different when looked at using other criteria. Urothelial cells normally express the same blood group as a given patient's erythrocytes. Urothelial cancers may or may not express these antigens. This was initially evaluated with a red cell adherence assay and subsequently by using a more sensitive immunoperoxidase method.[16,17] A number of studies have demonstrated that tumors which no longer express the appropriate blood group tend to be more invasive. The reason for this remains unclear. However, it is tempting to speculate that these more aggressive neoplasms are more undifferentiated and therefore lose the ability to perform all of the functions of the more differentiated normal cell population. Unfortunately, although this test has been shown to correlate well with the aggressive nature of various tumors, there are enough false positive and false negative results to make application to a general patient population hazardous.

Another aspect in the immunologic evaluation of urothelial tumors utilizes the technique of monoclonal antibody production. This method of producing antibodies permits the production of multiple highly purified antibodies in large quantities from a very impure antigen preparation. Using this technique, antibodies have been produced which do react with human urothelial carcinoma.[18] Similar studies with other cell types have proved to be of

206

great clinical benefit. Monoclonal antibodies can be used along with blood group antigens to define the cell surface antigens on urothelial tumors and to determine if certain immunologic phenotypes can accurately predict the biologic behavior of a given neoplasm. In addition, they also have potential usefulness in diagnostic imaging and therapy. Whether all of these possibilities will be practically realized remains unclear at this point.

Although a great deal is known about the natural history, etiology, and therapy of urothelial carcinoma, major advances need to be made if the current survival rates for patients with this neoplasm are to improve. A number of newer methods are currently available which may have potential impact on all of these areas. While it is still too early to embrace any of these technologies as a panacea, they do show considerable promise and will need to be carefully followed in the near future. The ultimate goal continues to be the cure of clinical disease. While this goal has only been partially realized in the past, it appears that we are getting closer to accomplishing this elusive task.

REFERENCES

1. Silverberg, E. Cancer Statistics, 1982 Ca 31:15-31, 1982.
2. Kaye, K.W. and Lange, P.H. Mode of Presentation of Invasive Bladder Cancer: Reassessment of the Problem. J Urol 128:31-33, 1982.
3. Heney, N.M., Nocks, B.N., Daly, J.J., Prout, G.R., Jr., et al. Ta and Tl Bladder Cancer: Location, Recurrence and Progression. Brit. J Urol, 54:152-157, 1982.
4. Lutzever, W., Rubben, H., and Dahm, H. Prognostic Parameters in Superficial Bladder Cancer: An Analysis of 315 Cases. J Urol, 127:250-252, 1982.
5. Jewett H.J. and Strong G.H. Infiltrating Carcinoma of the Bladder: Relation of Depth of Penetration of the Bladder Wall to Incidence of Local Extension and Metastases. J Urol 53:366, 1946.
6. Marshall V.F. The Relation of the Postoperative Estimate to the Pathologic Demonstration of the Extent of Vesical Neoplasms. J Urol 68:714, 1952.
7. Miller, L.S. Bladder Cancer: Superiority of Preoperative Irradiation and Cystectomy in Clinical Stages B2 and C. Cancer, 39:973-980, 1977.
8. Bloom., H.J.G., Henory, W.F., Wallace, D.M., and Skeet, R.G. Treatment of T3 Bladder Cancer: Controlled Trial of Pre-operative Radiotherapy and Radical Cystectomy Versus Radical Radiotherapy, Second Report and Review. Brit J Urol 54:136-151, 1982.
9. Whitmore, W.F., Jr., Batata, M.A., Ghonheim, M.A., Grabstald, H., and Unal, A. Radical Cystectomy With or Without Prior Irradiation in the Treatment of Bladder Cancer. J Urol, 118:184-187, 1977.
10. Koontz, W.W., Jr., Prout, G.R., Jr., Smith, W., Frable, W.J., and Minnis, J.E. The Use of Intravesical Thiotepa in the Management of Non-Invasive Carcinoma of the Bladder. J Urol 125:307-312, 1981.

11. Schulman, C.C., Robinson, M., Denis, L., Smith, P., Viggiano, G., DePauw, et al. Prophylactic Chemotherapy of Superficial Transitional Cell Bladder Carcinoma: An EORTC Randomized Trial Comparing Thiotepa, an Epipodophyllo-toxin (VM26) and TUR Alone. Eur Urol 8:207-212, 1982.

12. Lamm, D.L., Thor, D.E., Winters, W.D., Stogdill, V.D., and Radwin, H.M. BCG Immunotherapy of Bladder Cancer: Inhibition of Tumor Recurrence and Associated Immune Responses. Cancer 48:82-88, 1981.

13. Smith, P.H. Chemotherapy of Bladder Cancer: A Review. Cancer Treat Rep 65:165-173, 1981.

14. Ohkawa, T., Fujinata, T., Poi, J., Ebisuno, S., Takamatsu, M., Nakamura, J., and Kido, R. Clinical Study on Occupational Uroepithelial Cancer in Wakayama City. J Urol 128:520-523, 1982.

15. Neill, H.B., Soloway, M.S., and Nissenkorn, I. The Clonogenic Growth of Cells Derived from Bladder Barbotage in Patients with Transitional Cell Carcinoma of the Bladder: A Preliminary Report. J Urol 127:668-670, 1982.

16. Decenzo, J.M., Howard, P., and Irish, C.E. Antigenic Deletion and Prognosis of Patients with Stage A Transitional Cell Bladder Carcinoma. J Urol 114:874-878, 1975.

17. Wiley, E.L., Mendelsohn, G., Droller, M.J., and Eggleston, J.C. Immunoperoxidase Detection of Carcinoembryonic Antigen and Blood Group Substances in Papillary Transitional Cell Carcinoma of the Bladder. J Urol 128:276-280, 1982.

18. Grossman, H.B. Monoclonal Antibody to A Bladder Tumor Associated Antigen. Abstract 290, Proceedings of the 13th International Cancer Congress, Seattle, Washington, September 8-15, p 53, 1982.

19. Cummings, K.B., Taylor, W.J., Correa, R.J., Jr., Gibbons, R.P., and Mason, J.T. Observations on Definitive Cobalt 60 Radiation for Cure in Bladder Carcinoma: 15-year Followup. J Urol 115:152-154, 1976.

20. Buschke, F. and Jack, G. Twenty-Five Years' Experience with Supervoltage Therapy in the Treatment of Transitional Cell Carcinoma of the Bladder. Am J Roentgen 99:387-392, 1967.

21. Rider, W.D. and Evans, D.H. Radiotherapy in the Treatment of Recurrent Bladder Cancer. Brit J Urol 48:595-601, 1976.

22. Barnes, R.W., Dick, A.L., Hadley, H.L., and Johnston, O.L. Survival Following Transurethral Resection of Bladder Carcinoma. Cancer Res 37:2895-2897, 1977.

23. O'Flynn, J.D., Smith, J.M., and Hanson, J.S. Transurethral Resection for the Assessment and Treatment of Vesical Neoplasms. A Review of 840 Consective Cases. Eur Urol 1:38-40, 1975.

24. van der Werf-Messing, B.H.P. Carcinoma of the Bladder T3NxMo Treated by Preoperative Irradiation Followed bv Cystectomy. Third Report of the Rotterdam Radio-therapy Institute. Cancer 36:718-722, 1975.

25. Resnick, M.I. and O'Conor, V.J., Jr. Segmental Resection for Carcinoma of the Bladder: Review of 102 Patients. J Urol 109:1007-1010, 1973.

26. Cummings, K.B., Mason, J.T., Correa, R.J., Jr., Gibbons, R.P., and Mason, J.T. Observations on Definitive Cobalt 60 Radiation for Cure in Bladder Carcinoma: 15-year Followup. J Urol 115:152-154, 1976.

27. Wajsman, Z., Merrin, C., Moore, R., and Murphy, G.P. Current Results from Treatment of Bladder Tumors with Total Cystectomy at Roswell Park Memorial Institute. J Urol 113:806-810, 1975.

28. Cardonnier, J.J. Simple Cystectomy in the Management of Bladder Carcinoma. Arch Surg 108:190-191, 1974.

29. Pearse, H.D., Reed, R.R., and Hodges, C.V. Radical Cystectomy for Bladder Cancer. J Urol 119:216-218, 1978.

30. Long, R.T.C., Grummon, R.A., Spratt, J.S., Jr., and Perez-Mesa, C. Carcinoma of the Urinary Bladder (Comparison with, Radical, Simple, and Partial Cystectomy and Intravesical Formalin). Cancer 19:98-105, 1972.

RADIATION THERAPY OF STAGE IB CARCINOMA OF THE CERVIX:
FACTORS INFLUENCING PROGNOSIS

M. ROTMAN, M.D., K. CHOI, M.D., AND J. BOYCE, M.D.

INTRODUCTION

Cervical carcinoma has a propensity to confine itself initially to the cervix and then spread progressively through regional lymphatics. In the past decade, with the increased understanding of the biological behavior of the tumor and its spread in the lymphatics, investigations have shown that certain Stage I patients have morphologic and histologic characteristics that mitigate against local tumor control.[1]

Factors such as tumor size, depth of stromal invasion, vascular infiltration, uterine extension and barrel shaped presentation affect the course of the disease and survival. Failures where such factors exist may be due to selection of localized therapy.[1] While the majority of early cases are cured, the increased incidence of early invasive carcinoma of the cervix with its proportionate increase in patients having poor prognostic features, signals the need for a refinement of our current staging and treatment techniques. This chapter discusses the possible reasons for treatment failure in early invasive cervical carcinoma, offers a revision of current staging systems based on these morphohistological factors, and suggests appropriate modification of current treatment techniques. It has been abstracted from the authors' previous publications.[1-5]

BIOLOGICAL BEHAVIOR

Tumor spread through lymphatics

Lymphatic invasion of tumors and the need for external therapy were underestimated, if not missed entirely with early radiation techniques. The classical Manchester Philosophy, states that the addition of external radiation made no appreciable differences on results in Stage I & II disease.[6,7] During the 1950's, with the advent of megavoltage irradiation, external radiotherapy was successfully used to sterilize tumor in the lymphatics, thereby adding significantly to the survival rate.[8] A full knowledge of lymphatic pathways becomes essential for proper management of cervical cancer.

Published 1983 by Elsevier Science Publishing Co., Inc.
Recent Trends in Radiation Oncology and Related Fields, Amendola and Amendola, Editors

Three primary lymphatic trunks drain the cervix and the paracervical lymph glands through the base of the broad ligament into the internal iliac, external iliac and sacral group of lymph nodes. However, metastatic proclivity for any particular group or groups of pelvic lymph nodes is uncertain. Information gleaned from surgical dissection is subject to the vagaries of surgical techniques, the accessibility or ease in dissection and the proficiency of the surgical pathologists. Furthermore, the distribution of involved lymph nodes and lymphatic channels in the diseased state are at times unpredictable and do not follow normal anatomic pathways. Surgical disruption or tumor blockage of lymphatics leads to embolization of malignant cells through collateral channels. Lymph nodes previously unobserved can become identifiable in areas perfused by tumor emboli. For example, the intercalary nodes of Henricksen lying within the vesico-vaginal and rectovaginal septae are rarely described[9] and the incidence of parametrial and paracervical lymph nodes unreported in many series varies between 2% and 35%.[10] Rich lymphatic networks about the cervix are frequently contaminated by tumor, but inexplicably remain unidentified in larger surgical series. These include the major lymphatic plexuses that (1) posteriorly invest the rectum and interconnect with ureteral sheaths, (2) form a plexus that covers the posterior wall of the bladder and (3) anastomose with the lymphatics surrounding the uterine fundus and its adnexa.[10]

Tumor Infiltration

The stromal infiltration of tumor cells can be categorized into three types: 1) the expansile type with continuous budding of neoplastic process, 2) the diffuse type with spread disseminated throughout the interstitial spaces and 3) a thromboembolic type. In the latter thromboembolic type, the tumor spreads to the lymph nodes and distant organs, and also to the pelvic tissues.[11]

The traditional concept that cervical cancer is confined initially to the cervix and later involves regional lymphatics in a progressive fashion, naturally leads one to think that cancer cells lodge in either the primary site or draining lymph nodes. However, the fact that cancer cells infiltrate through tissue planes containing the same lymphatic plexuses that envelope the pelvic organs, puts the entire pelvis at risk in the early stage of disease where certain morphohistological factors exist.

Thus, the failure to control disease loco-regionally, even in early stages of the disease, may be the direct consequence of inadequate management of tumor in the surrounding lymphatics using current locally focused therapeutics.

TABLE 1.  FACTORS INFLUENCING PROGNOSIS IN STAGE I CARCINOMA OF THE CERVIX

|  | Positive Pelvic Node | Local Recurrence | 5 Year Survival |
|---|---|---|---|
| Size of Primary |  |  |  |
| 2 cm | 31% | 44% | 58% (2-12 yrs) |
| 2 cm | 9% | 9% | 94% |
| 4 cm | 80% | 40% | 47% |
| 4 cm | 16% | 4% | 92% |
| Quadrants Involved |  |  |  |
| 3-4 | 26% | 29% | 73% |
| Depth of Invasion |  |  |  |
| 11-15 mm | 33% | 31% | 72% |
| 11 mm | 5% | 4% | 96% |
| 70% thickness | 40% | 27% | 67% |
| 70% thickness | 13% | 4% | 93% |
| Vascular Invasion |  |  |  |
| positive | 34-63% | 25-34% | 69-73% |
| negative | 4-13% | 5-8% | 93-94% |
| Corpus Extension |  |  |  |
| positive |  | 56% | 50-55% |
| negative |  | 3% | 84-95% |

MORPHOHISTOLOGICAL PROGNOSTIC FACTORS  (Table 1)

Tumor Size

FIGO stage I-B lesions range from a clinically undetectable invasive cancer in a conization specimen to a lesion of several centimeters in diameter. Numerous papers have substantiated the observation that the prognosis is directly related to tumor size.[12-15]  As the primary size exceeds 2 cm the incidence of positive nodes and local recurrence increases and the survival decreases.  In Van Nagell's surgical series, 44% of patients with lesions greater than 2 cm in diameter developed local recurrences whereas only 9% of patients with lesions less than 2cm in diameter did so.  The survival rate was 58% for patients with lesions larger than 2 cms as compared to 94% for patients with lesions smaller than 2 cms.  The incidence of lymph node metastases was as high as 31% for patients with lesions larger than 2 cms, in contrast to 9% for lesions less than 2 cms.[15]  Primary tumors less than 1 cm in diameter have been reported to reoccur at the rate of 0 to 14% in various areas.[12,14,16,17]

## Quadrant Involvement

The clinical size of the lesion has been expressed as the number of quadrants invaded by tumor or the area equivalent. Boyce reported a high incidence of positive nodes and poor outcome in patients with more than 2 quadrants invaded by tumor.[4] Burghardt and Pickel estimated tumor size in areas equivalent in giant frontal sections of the cervix.[18] The area equivalent is the product of the vertical and horizontal diameters. They reported that the quadrant areas had a positive correlation with the incidence of positive nodes and a inverse relationship with survival.

Thus the clinical size of the lesion is related to the incidence of involved nodes, pelvic recurrences, and survival. The size of the lesion is an easily assessible prognostic factor. Such information is thus useful and available before initiation of any definite treatment.

## Depth of Stromal Invasion

Boyce and Chung reported the depth of stromal invasion in the pathology specimen as a valuable prognostic factor.[4,19] Chung's criteria for poor prognosis was more than 70% thickness of invasion, but Boyce used more than 10 mm of stromal invasion as a criteria. According to a study by Boyce and associates, the single most objective method of estimating tumor size was the depth of penetration of the tumor. In their study, depth of penetration was found to be more strongly associated with disease spread outside of the cervix, with local recurrence and with survival than were other measures of the size, including the size measured by clinical examination and pathological examination.[20]

## Vascular Invasion

In assessing the presence of vascular invasion it is often difficult for the pathologist to distinguish among small venules, capillary-like spaces and lymphatics of comparable size. The flat endothelium, helpful if not necessary for a diagnosis, may in the future be better identified by using special immunoperoxidase stains.

Roche's observation of invasion of spaces resembling lymphatic spaces in more than half of the cases (57%) in microinvasive carcinoma added to the complexities of determining endolymphatic invasion.[21] In his series, the presence of tumor cells in the endolymphatic space has no correlation with lymph node metastases in the lymphadenectomy specimen. Although, somewhat controversial, the vascular or capillary-like space invasion seems to be well established as a poor prognostic factor related to increased nodal metastases, increased local recurrence and poor survivals.[22] Inversen reported that the incidence of vascular invasion can be found in tumors of less than 5 mm invasion, and that 5 out of 8 patients with vascular invasion developed a pelvic recurrence.[23] Increased incidence of positive nodes where the lesions are less than 1 cm have been reported in the presence of vascular invasion.[24] In the study made by Boyce of 138 patients with Stage I cervical carcinoma, vascular invasion was found to be significantly associated with poor outcome, controlling for the other factors such as lesion size and extra cervical spread. Further statistical analysis identified depth of invasion, vascular invasion and extra cervical spread as key prognostic variables which predict recurrence accurately in 55% of patients.[25]

## Endometrial Extension or Corpus Extension

The real incidence of endometrial extension by cervical carcinoma has not been established because dilatation and curettage is not performed routinely on these patients. A D&C is difficult to perform with bulky friable lesions or endocervical tumors. Also it is difficult to exclude contamination unless clear endometrial stromal invasion is demonstrated. Nevertheless, Perez et al. and Prempree demonstrated that patients with Stage I carcinoma and positive D&C showed significantly lower 5-year survival rates and a higher incidence of distant metastases as opposed to those with negative D&C.[26,27] In both series the incidence of distant metastases was as high as 20% in patients with positive D&C as compared to only 5% in patients with negative D&C. In a retrospective surgical series, Boyce showed that extension to the corpus in the surgical specimen are associated with high rate of pelvic recurrences and lower survival rates.[4]

## ENDOCERVICAL TUMORS: THE BARREL SHAPED CERVIX

When cervical tumors arise from the endocervical canal, they tend to expand the cervix in concentric fashion creating the distinct clinical entity known as the barrel shaped cervix. Even though the central failure in Stage I & II disease is minimal, the majority occur in patients who have an endocervical bulky disease. The tumor cell burden in this type of disease is increased with the resultant hypoxic areas in the compact stroma. This may explain the reasons for both high incidence of local failure and frequent metastases compared to the lesions arising on the exocervix.

A combined approach to the treatment of such disease using radiation and surgery has been suggested because of initial reports of increased local failure with radiation alone.[28] Further analysis made at M.D. Anderson Hospital revealed that only patients with lesions greater than 6 cms benefitted by additional hysterectomies and had almost no central recurrences.[29] However, there was no increased survival as one would have anticipated. A study by Rotman refuted the use of the combined approach and showed little advantage for this procedure over radiation alone.[2] The author has suggested that radiation alone is the preferable treatment and that combined therapy, if selected at all, should be limited to a very select group of patients.

TREATMENT LIMITATIONS:  GENERAL PRINCIPLES

Local failure in invasive cervical carcinoma may be caused by either inadequate treatment of the primary cervical mass itself or faulty management of local regional lymph nodes. Whether surgery or radiotherapy is used, it is probable that these failures occur because of deficient or improper treatment planning and limitation of techniques.

Intracavitary Irradiation Alone

Mechanical factor. Numerous intracavitary applicators currently in use are loosely derived from the historical systems such as Stockholm, Paris and Manchester. Differing treatment policies resulted in the development or modification of a variety of instruments. Study of the results helped to weed out unsatisfactory ones and emphasized the more valuable points in each method.

The selection of a proper applicator must be influenced by the experience of the personnel involved. Each system has its advantages and disadvantages requiring that the radiotherapist should be well acquainted with the applicator selected. Inherent structural shortcomings of certain instruments and their particular associated complications will limit cancer curability. For example, the Ernst applicator, with its inherent structural deficiencies, such as short source surface distance and compacting qualities, lends itself to severe complications.[3]

Radiobiological factors. When intracavitary irradiation is used alone, its efficacy may be limited in local tumors larger than 2 cm in radius, and when regional lymphatics or nodes are involved subclinically or otherwise. In these cases, planned brachytherapy is not efficacious because of the inverse square law, applicable to such therapy, which imposes an abrupt decrease in dose and dose rate with small changes in distance. The classic sigmoid curve of relationship between tumor control and radiation dose illustrates a steep gradient in possibility of cell kill within a narrow range of total dose. The tumor control probabilty rises sharply between 20% and 80% so that small dose changes within this range can result in significant reductions in tumor control. In terms of dose rate, while tumor close to a radioactive source is more efficiently radiated, the cell kill in the periphery is considerably less. As the dose rate declines the tumor cell repairs sublethal damage. Cell kill per physical dose is therefore reduced, and a much higher total dose is required to achieve the same tumor control.[30] Furthermore, the area occupied by the tumor peripherally contains the greatest number of tumor cells; this geometric disadvantage means that underkill or under-dosage (and hence, failure in the outlying tumor, its lymphatics, or nodes) is more likely with either interstitial or intracavitary radiation. In addition to the radiobiologic consideration of intracavitary radiation, the uncertainties of lymphatic drainage of the cervix have serious implication in the management of early invasive cervical cancer. Anatomic and biologic features promoting the small but significant failure rate in such disease include in part (1) the narrow senile vagina or bulky exophytic cervix that is inadequately treated by intracavitary therapy alone because poor geometry causes a low dose rate to be delivered to the tumor periphery and (2) a great incidence of lymphatic and lymph node permeation by the tumor that is clinically unappreciated. This, in turn, may be ineffectively treated because external radiotherapy is withheld.

## Radical Surgery

When surgery is used alone, local regional failure can result because of the possibility of underestimating the incidence and areas of lymphatic or lymph node metastases. Disruption of lymphatics will generate collateral-ization and back flow into alternate pathways. It is reasonable to assume that pelvic tumor contamination and distal metastases will result from anything less than total lymphadenectomy. This assumption is supported by reviewing the very poor survival results for patients with early disease who have evidence of metastases to lymph nodes.[31]

## PROPOSED MODIFICATIONS IN CLASSIFICATIONS

It has become increasingly clear that there exists a significant subpopulation of patients with apparent early invasive cervical carcinoma who

TABLE 2.         CLINICAL-PATHOLOGIC CLASSIFICATION OF CARCINOMA OF THE CERVIX

Stage O:   Carcinoma in situ, intra-epithelial carcinoma.
Stage I:   Carcinoma within uterus (cervix and fundus).
   Stage IA:      Microinvasive carcinoma, stromal invasion up to 1 mm.
   Stage IB$_1$:   Microinvasive carcinoma, stromal invasion from 1.1 mm
                  to 10 mm.
   Stage IB$_2$:   Carcinoma involving the cervix with:
                  1) Stromal invasion more than 10 mm or
                  2) Corpus involvement or
                  3) More than two quadrants involved or
                  4) Vascular involvement or
                  5) Endocervical growth, barrel-shaped cervix included or
                  6) Exophytic tumor more than 2 cm
Stage II:  Carcinoma extending beyond the cervix but not to pelvic wall
            or carcinoma involving the vagina, excluding the lower third.
   Stage IIA$_1$:  No obvious parametrial involvement.
   Stage IIA$_2$:  No obvious parametrial involvement but
                  1) Endometrial involvement or
                  2) Vascular involvement or
                  3) Endocervical invasion or barrel-shaped presentation
   Stage IIB:     Obvious parametrial involvement.
Stage III: Carcinoma extending onto the pelvic wall.  On rectal exam-
            ination, no cancer free space between the tumor and the pelvic
            wall.  Carcinoma involving the lower third of the vagina.  All
            cases with hydronephrosis or non-functioning kidney.
   Stage IIIA:    Carcinoma involving the lower third of the vagina.  No
                  extension onto the pelvic wall.
   Stage IIIB:    Extension to the pelvic wall or hydronephrosis or
                  nonfunctioning kidney, or both.
Stage IV:  Carcinoma extending beyond the true pelvis or clinically
            involving the mucosa of the bladder or rectum.  Bullous edema
            as such does not permit a case to be alloted to Stage IV.
   Stage IVA:     Spread to adjacent organs.
   Stage IVB:     Spread to distant organs.

are prone to treatment failure when managed by current, standard surgical or radiotherapeutic techniques.  The problem for the oncologist, therefore, is to identify this substrate of patients and seek appropriate alterations in their management.  The following is a modification of the currently employed clinical FIGO classification, based on morphohistologic and anatomic considerations elaborated above (Table 2).[1]  No attempt is made to change Stages III and IV, since the tumor volume and disease extent in these cases already require vigorous external and intracavitary irradiation with or without additional treatment.

The new substages suggested as Stage IB2 and IIA2 contain tumors having single or multiple factors that worsen prognosis because of decreased loco-regional control and/or increased distal lymphatic spread.  A therapeutic corollary for these substages would be maximal reliance on external beam irradiation for treatment of regional and distal disease along with extrafascial hysterectomy or intracavitary radium for local control.

## MANAGEMENT

The treatment modalities must be selected based on a careful analysis of a number of tumor prognostic factors and the limitations of each modality with respect to the biological characteristics of the primary disease.

## Intracavitary Irradiation

A typical intracavitary insertion consists of central tandem in the uterine cavity carrying three sources, and two vaginal colpostats, each carrying one source. The radiation dose from such a system falls off rapidly as the distance from the radiation sources increases. This form of irradiation is suitable for controlling tumor in and around the cervix. It is limited in its capabilities to sterilize tumors extending to the lateral parametria or pelvic nodes. Intracavitary irradiation alone is effective only in early stages of the disease where there is no risk of disease spread outside of the effective volume of intracavitary irradiation, and where there are no poor prognostic morphohistological factors. In other cases the external beam irradiation must be used in addition to the intracavitary insertion. The local failure was as high as 20% in the Volterrani series of 182 patients with Stage I-B disease treated with intracavitary insertions only.[32] Hamburger also reported local failure only in 4 out of 93 patients with the lesion less than 1 cm, but 3 out of 17 patients with lesions larger than 1 cm, developed regional failure with intracavitary treatment only.[16]

## External Beam Irradiation

Early in the history of radiation therapy, impact on curability was achieved in cervical cancer by the application of radium within the tumor bearing area. Prior to the megavoltage era the external beam was of poor quality and was not the mainstay of treatment in cervical cancers. Fletcher advocated the need for external irradiation in Stage II carcinoma of the cervix, which was a departure at the time from the Manchester technique that relied heavily on intracavitary radiation.[29] In a comparison of survival rates in Stage I and II disease, Schwartz demonstrated that in 4 leading institutions the survivals were superior over the Manchester treatment by approximately 20% where external irradiation and intracavitary irradiations were combined.[33]

In the currently proposed classification there appears to be a population of patients with early disease who are likely to benefit from additional external radiotherapy, i.e., Stages I-B2 and IIA2 (Table 2).

The combination of external treatment and intracavitary insertions must be individualized for each case to achieve maximum results with minimum complications. In general, as tumor size or stage of disease increases, the dose of the external beam increases and the amount of the intracavitary radiation decreases proportionately. The external beam radiation causes shrinkage of the tumor and as the malignancy reduces in size it becomes more vulnerable to the intense radiation delivered by the intracavitary applications.

## Surgery

Surgery has superseded radiation therapy in the management of early disease. In cases where lymphatic spread in Stage I disease is absent or limited, such as in substage I-A and I-B1 the results of surgery are rarely compromised. However, when lymphatic spread occurs, as is likely in stage I-B2, the surgeon's ability to encompass all malignancy becomes severely restricted. Most surgeons recognize inherent difficulties in accomplishing an adequate pelvic node dissection and the high probability of cutting through disease with the consequent potential for local recurrence and distal spread. The role of surgery alone is thus limited to a selected group of Stage I patients, although intracavitary irradiation alone is equally effective as shown earlier.

The local failure rate with barrel shaped tumors treated by radiation alone led to the use of additional extrafascial hysterectomies. This in turn prompted a variety of techniques, combining radiation and surgery in the management of virtually all enlarged and exophytic tumors. However, this did not result in the anticipated increased survival rates. The author, refuted the use of the combined approach in a study showing little advantage of this procedure over radiation alone. His retrospective analysis which undertook to study the feasability of a combined surgical-radiation treatment for bulky exophytic and barrel shaped tumors, showed no evidence of disease in the surgical specimen in over 90% of such cases. Among patients receiving radiation and surgery, there was an increased incidence of severe gastrointestinal and genitourinary complications in constrast to a controlled group of patients treated with radiation alone.[2]

A combination of radiation and surgery has also been advocated in treating most adenocarcinomas of the cervix, as a diagnostic procedure for evaluation of nodal disease and for debulking large tumors. These methods have been promulgated in spite of the documented increase in complications by factors ranging from 2.6 to 4 without improvement in survival. The question must be raised as to whether the operation results in: 1) blood-borne spread of tumor cells during the surgical procedure, 2) the formation of collateral channels of lymphatics forcing tumor cells outside the normal pathway or 3) lymphatic reflux of tumor cells away from the treated areas.

There are controversies in the management of the early stage of cervical cancer: surgery, intracavitary irradiation or external irradiation. There has not been a large scale prospective randomized study to date. At present, a judicious selection of treatment modality on an individualized basis with respect to the morphohistologic factors and limitations of each treatment modality should give the best benefit to the patient.

REFERENCES
1. Rotman, M., John, M., Boyce, J. Prognostic factors in cervical carcinoma. Cancer, 48:560-567, 1981.
2. Rotman, M., John, M., Moon, S.H., Chi, K.N., et al. Limitations of adjunctive surgery in carcinoma of the cervix. Int J Rad Oncol Biol Phys, 5:327-332, 1979.
3. Rotman, M., John, M., Roussis, K., Moon, S.H., Choi, K.N., et al. The intracavitary applicator in relation to complications of pelvic radiation: the Ernst System. Int J Rad Oncol Biol Phys, 4:941-956, 1978.
4. Boyce, J., Fruchter, K.G., Nicastri, A., Ambiavagar, P., Reinis, M.S., Nelson, J.J. Lesion size, extent of disease and outcome in Stage I carcinoma of the cervix. J Gynecol Oncol, 12:154-165, 1981.
5. Choi, K.N., Rotman, M. Radiation therapy in the management of invasive cervical cancer. In: Contemporary issues in clinical oncology: Gynecologic cancer. Churchill Livingstone Inc. (In press).
6. Tod, M., Meredith, W.J. Treatment of cancer of cervix uteri: A revised "Manchester Method." Br J Radiol, 26:252-257, 1953.
7. Tod, M., Meredith, W.J. Dosage system for use in treatment of cancer of uterine cervix. Br J Radiol, 11:809-823, 1938.
8. Rutledge, F.N., Fletcher, G.H., MacDonald, E.J. Pelvic lymphadenectomy as an adjunct to radiation therapy in treatment for carcinoma of the cervix. Am J Roentgenol, 93:607-614, 1965.
9. Henriksen, E. The lymphatic spread of carcinoma of the cervix and the body of the uterus. Am J Obstet Gynecol, 58:925-942, 1959.
10. Plentl, A.A., Friedman, E.A. Lymphatics of the cervix uteri. In: Lymphatic System of the Female Genitalia, Philadelphia, W.B. Saunders Co., 75-93, 1971.
11. Miller, N.F., Hinerman, D.L., Riley, G.M., Ludovici, P.P., Gosling, J.R.G., Christian, R.T., Hall, D.F. The nature of cervix cancer. Obstet Gynecol, 14:703-713, 1959.
12. Brunschwig, A. Surgical treatment of Stage I cancer of the cervix. Cancer, 13:34-36, 1960.
13. Cherry, C.P., Glucksman, A., Dearing, R., Ways, R. Observations on lymph node involvement in carcinoma of the cervix. J Obstet Gyencol Br Emp, 60:368, 1953.

220

14. Piver, M.S., Chung, M.S. Prognostic significance of cervical lesions size and pelvic node metastases in cervical carcinoma. Obstet Gynecol, 46:507-510, 1975.
15. Van Nagell, J.R., Donaldson E.S., Parker, J.D., Van Dyke, A.H., Wood, E.G. The prognostic significance of cell type and lesion size in patients with cervical cancer treated by radical surgery. Gynecol Oncol, 5:142-151, 1977.
16. Hamberger A.D., Fletcher, G.H., Wharton, J.T. Results of treatment of early Stage I carcinoma of the uterine cervix with intracavitary radium alone. Cancer, 41:980-985, 1978.
17. Tak, W.K. Munzenrider, J.E., Mitchell, G.W. External irradiation and one radium application for carcinoma of the cervix. Int J Rad Oncol Biol Phys, 5:29-36, 1979.
18. Burghardt, E., Pickel, H. Local spread of lymph node involvement in cervical cancer. Obstet Gynecol, 52:139, 1978.
19. Chung, C.K., Nahas, W.A., Stryker, J.A., Curry, S.L., Abt, A.S., Mortel, R. Analysis of factors contributing to treatment failure in Stage IB and IIA carcinoma of the cervix. Am J Obstet Gynecol, 138:550-556, 1980.
20. Boyce, J. Fruchter, R.G., Nicastri, A.D., Dottino, P. Measures of lesion size in stage I cervical carcinoma. Presented at A.C.O.G. Annual clinical Meeting, Dallas, TX, May, 1982 (Ms. available on request)
21. Roche, W.D., Norris, H.J. Microinvasive carcinoma of the cervix; The significance of lymphatic invasion and confluent patterns of stromal growth. Cancer, 36:180-186, 1975.
22. Van Nagell, J.R., Donaldson, E.S., Wood, E.G., et al. The significance of vascular invasion and lymphatic infiltration in invasive cervical cancer. Cancer, 41:228-234, 1978.
23. Iverson, T., Abeler, V., Klorstad, K.E. Factors influencing the treatment of patients with Stage IA carcinoma of the cervix. Br J Obstet Gynecol, 86:593-597, 1979.
24. Sedlis, A., Sall, S.T., Seekade, Y., et al. Microinvasive carcinoma uterine cervix: A clinical pathological study. Am J Obstet Gyencol, 133:64-74, 1979.
25. Boyce, J., Fruchter, R., Nicastri, A., DeRegt, R., et al. Vascular invasion in Stage I carcinoma of the cervix. Cancer (In press).
26. Perez, C.A., Zivnuska, F., Askin, F., Camel, H.M., Ragan, D., Power, W.E. Mechanisms of failure in patients with carcinoma of the uterine cervix extending into the endometrium. Rad Oncol Biol Phys, 2:651-659, 1977.
27. Prempree, T., Patanaphan, V., Viravathana, T., Sewchand, W., Cho, Y.K., Scott, R.M. Radiation treatment of carcinoma of the cervix with extension into the endometrium: A reappraisal of its significance. Cancer 49:2015-2020, 1982.
28. Durrance, F.Y., Fletcher, G.H., Rutledge, F.N. Analysis of central recurrent disease in Stage I and II squamous cell carcinoma of the cervix in the intact uterus. Am J Roentgenol, 106:831-838, 1969.
29. Fletcher, G.H. Textbook of Radiotherapy, 3rd ed. Phlladelphia, Lea and Febiger, 720-773, 1980.
30. Hall, E.J. Radiation dose rate: A factor of importance in radiobiology and radiotherapy. Br. J Radiol, 45:81-97, 1972.
31. Disaia, P.J. Surgical aspects of cervical cancer. Cancer, 48:548-559, 1981.
32. Volterrani, F., Lombardi, F. Long terms results of radium therapy in cervical cancer. Int J Rad Oncol Biol Phys, 6:565-648, 1980.
33. Schwarz, G. An evaluation of the Manchester System of treatment of cervix. Am J Roentgenol, 105:579-585, 1969.

RADIATION THERAPY AS PRIMARY TREATMENT FOR CANCER OF THE BREAST

LUTHER W. BRADY, M.D.,   JOHN M. BEDWINEK, M.D. AND   JOHN R. LOUGHEAD, M.D.

Radical mastectomy for carcinoma of the breast, as described by Halsted[1] in 1894, is one of the most noteworthy historical achievements in the management of this relatively common malignant disease. For about 50 years, the operation was almost universally accepted as the only definitive form for treatment for cancer of the breast. However, in 1924, Keyness[2,3] challenged this procedure and further challenge was brought by the reports of McWhirter[4] in the late 1940's. McWhirter demonstrated that total mastectomy combined with postoperative radiation therapy to the chest wall and regional lymphatics gave survivals and recurrence rates that were similar to those previously attributable to the radical mastectomy.

The reports of Keynes[2,3] led toward more conservative therapy demonstrating by a study performed at St. Bartholomew's Hospital in London that primary cancer of the breast could be treated by tumor excision and radium needle implantation. In a matched series of cases comparing this treatment technique with mastectomy carried out by Lord Moniyhan, the survival results at 10 years were the same for the two treatment techniques.

Developments during the last 30 years have created a major change in opinion regarding breast cancer management. Developments in radiation oncology afforded the potential for a major impact upon the treatment of patients with advanced breast cancer and these advances have led to the development of sophisticated and innovative programs in the use of radiation therapy as the primary means of management in the patient with early breast cancer.

In 1983, the American Cancer Society anticipates that there will be 114,900 new patients with cancer of the breast diagnosed with 37,500 patients dying with the disease process in the United States. Cancer of the breast constitutes 27% of all malignancies seen in the female and accounts for 19% of all deaths due to cancer in women.[5]

Although most patients with breast cancer initially present with disease limited to the local and regional areas, more than one-half will subsequently die with disseminated disease. Prior concepts upon which the radical

Recent Trends in Radiation Oncology and Related Fields, Amendola and Amendola, Editors

222

TABLE 1.    CANCER OF THE BREAST:    FACTORS THAT INFLUENCE PROGNOSIS

    I. Histologic
      A. Histology
      B. Degree of differentiation of the tumor
      C. Vascular invasion
      D. Lymphatic invasion
      E. perineural sheath invasion
      F. Immunologic response

   II. Stage
      A.  Tumor size
      B.  Axillary nodal status
         1) number of positive nodes
         2) level of axillary involvement
         3) micro-metastases vs macro-metastases
         4) extranodal capsular extension
      C. Location of the tumor within the breast
      D. Distant metastases

  III. Age/Menopausal Status

   IV. Receptor Studies (ER/pR)

    V. Karnofsky Status

TABLE 2.   CANCER OF THE BREAST:   AXILLARY NODE STATUS AND SIZE OF TUMOR[5]

| Size (cm) | Number of cases | Incidence of positive axillary nodes |
|---|---|---|
| 0.1 to 1 | 1423 | 302 (21%) |
| 1.1 to 2 | 5064 | 1571 (31%) |
| All cases up to 2 cm | 6487 | 1873 (29%) |

TABLE 3.    CANCER OF THE BREAST TREATED BY MASTECTOMY ALONE
Influence of Invasion on Survival

| | Number of cases | 5-Year Survival NED | Recurrence |
|---|---|---|---|
| In Situ | 323 | 240 (74%) | 24 (7%) |
| Invasive 1 cm or less | | | |
| negative nodes | 1121 | 788 (70%) | 143 (13%) |
| positive nodes | 302 | 160 (53%) | 94 (32%) |
| 1.1 cm or more | | | |
| negative nodes | 8883 | 5312 (60%) | 1675 (19%) |
| positive nodes | 6265 | 2041 (33%) | 3211 (51%) |

mastectomy was based, envisioned the disease as a localized process that gradually spreads in an orderly fashion from a single focus in the breast to the regional lymph nodes and then only after overwhelming these lymph nodes does it finally spread to more distant sites. This dogma has been in vogue for more than 75 years but has now undergone major re-evaluation. The regional lymphatics are not, as previously thought, temporary barriers to hematogenous dissemination. Blood borne metastases can occur simultaneously with or even before lymph node metastases become evident. In fact, the finding of cancer cells in the regional lymphatics is an indication that microscopic distant metastases are probably already present.

This new view of the spread of breast cancer has led to questions relative to the long-cherished concept that the radical or modified radical mastectomy was of paramount importance to survival. This has allowed for an increasingly greater use of more limited surgery combined with definitive radiation therapy. It has also made it clear that improvements in survival will come primarily through the development and the use of effective systemic chemotherapy or hormonal therapy. Thus, all modalities must be integrated in the treatment of the patient with breast cancer. It is mandatory that the individual specialties give up their chauvinism and consider how best to use surgery, radiation therapy, and chemotherapy to optimize the treatment for the individual patient.

Before making a decision about the particular treatment program to be pursued for a patient, whether that be excisional biopsy and radiation therapy, radical mastectomy, modified radical mastectomy with or without systemic chemotherapy, the well established factors that influence prognosis must be carefully considered (Table 1 through Table 10).

Every patient with cancer of the breast should have a carefully identified program for workup. This workup should include a carefully taken history and physical examination with evaluation of the patient's menstrual status. The suspicious lump in the breast should be removed by excisional biopsy with a margin of normal tissue surrounding it in order to establish the diagnosis, the histologic characteristics of the tumor, and to submit the tumor for estrogen and progesterone receptor studies. There is no evidence to substantiate a deleterious effect of separating the excisional biopsy with subsequent establishment of the diagnosis from the definitive treatment program so long as that time interval does not exceed two to three weeks.

The various diagnostic techniques to determine the true extent of the disease process as well as baselines for future comparison should include

TABLE 4.     CANCER OF THE BREAST TREATED WITH SURGERY ALONE
                Influence of Location on Survival[6]

| Location | Number of Patients | 10-Year Survival |
|----------|--------------------|------------------|
| Lateral  | 690                | 40%              |
| Central  | 262                | 28%              |
| Medial   | 216                | 38%              |

TABLE 5     PROGNOSTIC VARIABLES IN OPERABLE CANCER OF THE BREAST[7]

Histologic Grading of Primary Tumor
    Low grade 10-year survival     60%
    High grade 10-year survival     25%

Vascular Invasion in Primary Tumor
    Yes   visceral metastases     43%
    No   visceral metastases     4%

TABLE 6               CANCER OF THE BREAST
               Influence of lymph node involvement
          and axillary invasion on 8-Year survivals.[8]

| Level of Axillary Invasion | Type of Lymph Node Involvement | | Total |
| | Micro-metastases | Macro-metastases | |
|---|---|---|---|
| N − | − | − | 82% |
| N + Level I | 94% | 62% | 71% |
| N + Level II | 59% | 29% | 55% |

TABLE 7.   PROGNOSTIC VARIABLES IN OPERABLE CANCER OF THE BREAST[7]

Positive Axillary Nodes
    10-year relapse-free survival   24%
    1 to 3 Nodes   34%
    Greater than 3 Nodes   15%
    10-year survival   40%

Negative Axillary Nodes
    10-year relapse-free survival   75%
    10-year survival   82%

TABLE 8.  THE RELATIONSHIP BETWEEN LYMPH NODE IMMUNO-HISTOLOGIC PATTERNS
AND SURVIVAL RATES IN CANCER OF THE BREAST[9]

| Histologic Pattern | Survival | |
|---|---|---|
| | 5-year | 10-year |
| Lymphocyte Predominant | 84% | 75% |
| Germinal Center predominance | 72% | 54% |
| Unstimulated | 63% | 39% |
| Lymphocyte Depletion | 36% | 33% |

TABLE 9   PROGNOSTIC VARIABLES IN OPERABLE CANCER OF THE BREAST[7]

| Estrogen Receptors | 3-Year Relapse-Free Survival |
|---|---|
| ER  + | 82% |
| ER  - | 35% |
| N  - /ER  + | 79% |
| N  - /ER  - | 58% |

TABLE 10        CANCER OF THE BREAST:  PROGNOSTIC FACTORS
(Radical Mastectomy and Post-Operative Radiation Therapy)[10]
Estrogen Receptors and Recurrence

| Characteristic | Recurrence at 20 months | |
|---|---|---|
| | ER - (%) | ER + (%) |
| Age (in years): | | |
| less than 50 | 32 | 0 |
| older than 50 | 36 | 16 |
| Axillary Nodes: | | |
| Negative | 19 | 6 |
| Positive | 59 | 26 |
| 1 to 3 | 36 | 25 |
| more than 4 | 72 | 27 |
| Primary Size: | | |
| less than 2 cm | 40 | 5 |
| greater than 2 cm | 37 | 16 |
| Primary Location: | | |
| Outer quadrant | 31 | 9 |
| Inner/central | 50 | 19 |

roentgenograms of the chest, bilateral mammographic examination, biochemical profile, complete blood count, and urinalysis. Once the diagnosis of breast cancer has been established, bone scan, liver/spleen scans and other indicated studies depending upon symptoms and findings must be carried out. If there are identifiable abnormalities on the bone scan, roentgenograms of those areas should be taken for precise identification of the cause for the radionuclide localization. Computerized assisted tomographic scanning with intravenous contrast enhancement of the liver should be done when the liver scan proves to be abnormal. This becomes an important study to identify the presence or absence of metastatic disease within the liver.

Once these studies have been obtained, it is only then that an appropriate decision can be made regarding treatment. All of the potential treatment alternatives can then be discussed with the patient.

In the interval from 1970 to 1980 in the United States, there has been a major shift in the distribution of stage in the patient presenting with carcinoma of the breast (Table 11).[10] In 1980, between 8% and 10% of patients presented with disease diagnosed as Stage 0 and 57-10% presented with Stage I lesions. Patients with Stage II disease have decreased to only an incidence of about 20-22%. These data identify the greater number of patients with early disease in the breast. This results from a higher level of sensitivity among the practicing physicians as to the diagnosis and also to a more active utilization of screening techniques such as mammography. Important in this shift toward earlier diagnosis is the patient's understanding of what abnormalities in the breast may represent and her desire to seek physician advice earlier. Obviously, this shift of stage presentation to earlier stages allows for more emphasis on breast conserving treatment methods and dispels a considerable proportion of the fear among the patients relative to mastectomy when a viable alternative using radiation therapy with preservation of the breast is available for treatment.

| Table 11 | CHANGE IN PRESENTING STAGE[11] | | |
|---|---|---|---|
| Stage at Initial Presentation | 1970 | 1976 | 1980 |
| 0 | 2% | 5% | 7% |
| I | 25% | 54% | 60% |
| II | 45% | 29% | 22% |
| III | 28% | 12% | 7% |

National Cancer Institute Breast Epidemiological Studies (unpublished data).

Conservative treatment for early breast cancer using excisional biopsy followed by curative radiation therapy has become a well-established alternative to mastectomy in many reputable institutions of the world.

As has been pointed out, Sir Geoffrey Keynes[2,3] at St. Bartholomew's Hospital in London began a treatment program for primary carcinoma of the breast using tumor excision and radium needle implantation in 1924. In a matched series of cases comparing this treatment technique with mastectomy carried out by his colleague, Lord Moniyhan, the survival results at 10 years were exactly the same for the two treatment techniques (Table 12).[2,3] Peters,[11,12] between the years 1939 and 1972, treated 184 patients with Tl and $T_2N_0$ breast cancer using excisional biopsy and radiation therapy. Each of these patients was matched according to age, tumor size, and year of treatment with three patients who were treated by radical mastectomy. Thus, there were 184 patients in the excision plus irradiation group and 552 patients in the radical mastectomy group. Up to 30 years after treatment, there has been no significant difference in survival between these two treatment groups.

TABLE 12    CANCER OF THE BREAST:  Three and five year survival of patients treated by implanted radium needles (interstitial irradiation), with survival rates for a comparable contemporary surgical series.[2,3]

|  | Group | Number of Patients | Net Survival (%) | Comparable Surgical Series (%) |
|---|---|---|---|---|
| At 3 years | I | 85 | 83.5 | 79.2 |
|  | II | 91 | 51.2 | 52.3 |
|  | III | 74 | 31.4 | -- |
| At 5 years | I | 75 | 71.4 | 69.1 |
|  | II | 66 | 29.3 | 30.5 |
|  | III | 60 | 23.6 | -- |

I and II  Disease apparently confined to the breast
III.  Disease advanced or inoperable

Mustakallio[13] began in 1940 to employ simple excision with curative radiation therapy in patients with clinically negative axillary lymph nodes. By present standards, the radiation therapy employed was inadequate, yet up to 20 years following the completion of the radiation therapy program, the survival with this technique was not significantly different from that of patients treated by radical mastectomy.

Many European institutions have had a longstanding tradition of treating cancer of the breast conservatively.[14-25] The Fondation Curie in Paris has been a leader in this technique. Baclesse[17] initiated the program in 1930 and it has been subsequently carried on by Calle[14,15,21] and Batianni.[24] Calle et al. have reported 10-year survival figures from definitively administered radiaton therapy with or without excisional biopsy that are similar to those obtained by the standard radical mastectomy procedures. More than 65% of the patients had breast preservation with a satisfactory cosmetic result.

In the last 20 years, many American institutions have pursued a program of conservative management for early breast cancer. Montague[26,27] reported in 1983, 345 patients treated with conservation surgery and irradiation. The 10-year survival figures were 78% for the American Joint Committee Stage I lesions and 73% for American Joint Committee Stage II lesions with a 2% failure rate within the breast for those 210 patients treated primarily by surgery at the M.D. Anderson Hospital and an 8.8% local failure rate in the breast in those patients who had biopsy prior to referral with no re-excision (Table 13 and Table 14).

TABLE 13. COMPARISON OF SURGICAL AND RADIOTHERAPEUTIC RESULTS AT 10 YEARS

| Stage | Surgery Memorial Hospital | | Radiation Therapy Fondation Curie[15] | |
|---|---|---|---|---|
| | Number of Patients | Alive Disease Free | Number of Patients | Alive Disease Free |
| $T_1$, $N_0$, $N_{1a}$ | 66 | 59 (89%) | 40 | 36 (90%) |
| $T_2$, $N_0$, $T_1$, $T_2$, $N_{1b}$ | 176 | 92 (52%) | 129 | 69 (53%) |
| $T_3$, $N_0$, $T_3$, $N_{1b}$ | 62 | 18 (29%) | 89 | 27 (30%) |

TABLE 14. SURVIVAL AT 5 YEARS AFTER SURGERY (Mayo Clinic 1965-1968)

| | All Patients | Type of Mastectomy | |
|---|---|---|---|
| | | Modified Radical | Radical |
| Number | 541 | 205 | 336 |
| Mean Age (years) | 59.0 | 62.3 | 57.0 |
| Positive Nodes (%) | 38.4 | 31.2 | 42.9 |
| 5-Year Survival | | | |
| Total Sample (%) | 77.9 (86.4) | 78.2 (88.9) | 77.6 (83.3) |
| Negative nodes (%) | 85.2 (94.3) | 84.0 (96.0) | 86.0 (94.0) |
| Positive nodes (%) | 66.1 (71.4) | 66.0 (75.0) | 66.0 (70.00 |

Prosnitz et al.[28] reported in 1980 a group of 293 patients treated with excisional biopsy followed by definitive radiation therapy with 10-year survivals of 81% for American Joint Committee Stage I lesions and 54% for American Joint Committee Stage II lesions with a local recurrence rate of 8% for both stages. Bedwinek et al.[29] reported similar data compiled from the Radiation Therapy Oncology Group Historical Data Base for breast cancer treated by excisional biopsy and radiation therapy.

All of the above retrospective studies of patients treated by excisional biopsy and radiation therapy compared with mastectomy series strongly suggest that in early lesions the two treatment techniques produce results that are essentially equivalent in character in terms of both survival and local-regional control (Tables 13 through 19).

PRIMARY RADIATION THERAPY IN BREAST CANCER*

| Number of Patients | 5-Year Relapse Free Survival | Local Failure | Distant Metastases |
|---|---|---|---|
| | TABLE 15  Stage I | | |
| 1660 | 1348 (81.2%) | 33/324 ((10.2%) | 48/323 (14.8%) |
| | TABLE 16  Stage II | | |
| 940 | 667 (71.%) | 81/595 (13.6%) | 114/595 (19.2%) |
| | TABLE 17  Stage I-II | | |
| 3156 | 2492 (79.0%) | 134/1232 (10.9%) | 193/1232 (15.6%) |

* Cumulative Series

TABLE 18.  PRIMARY RADIATION THERAPY FOR BREAST CANCER [28]

| Clinical Stage | 5-Year Survival | | 10-Year Survival | |
|---|---|---|---|---|
| | relapse-free | total | relapse-free | total |
| I | 87% | 91% | 71% | 81% |
| II | 63% | 77% | 40% | 54% |
| Total | 73% | 83% | 47% | 65% |

Veronesi et al.[25] have recently published prospectively randomized studies which substantiate the findings of these earlier retrospective comparisons (Table 20). Other prospectively randomized studies are under way including one under the auspices of the National Cancer Institute in the United States[30] where patients with T1 or T2 lesions are randomized to modified radical mastectomy or tumor excision and axillary node dissection followed by radiation therapy to the breast and the peripheral lymphatics.

TABLE 19          TUMORECTOMY AND RADIOTHERAPY: 10-Year Results

| Group | Number of Patients | Loco-Regional Failures % | Total Stage | Survival % |
|-------|--------------------|--------------------------|-------------|------------|
| Montague[26] | 211 | 6 | I<br>II | 78%<br>60% |
| Prosnitz[28] | 279 | 8 | I<br>II | 81%<br>54% |
| Calle[13] | 100 | 16 | I, II | 76% |
| Spitalier[33] | 141 | 20 | I, II | 81% |
| Pierquin[16] | 152 | 5 (Stage I)<br>7 (Stage II) | I<br>II | 80%<br>74% |

TABLE 20    CANCER OF THE BREAST:  Actuarial 5-year survival (Mean $\pm$ S.E.M.) in patients treated with Halsted mastectomy or quadrantectomy and radiation therapy.[25]

|  | Percentage 5-Year Survival | |
|--|----------------------------|-|
|  | Halsted Mastectomy | Quadrantectomy and Rad. Therapy |
| Overall Survival | 90.1 $\pm$ 2.5 | 89.6 $\pm$ 2.6 |
| Disease-Free Survival | | |
| All Patients | 83.0 $\pm$ 2.8 | 84.0 $\pm$ 2.8 |
| Axillary nodes negative | 89.1 $\pm$ 2.4 | 86.5 $\pm$ 2.98 |
| Axillary nodes positive | 62.0 $\pm$ 9.0 | 77.5 $\pm$ 6.3 |

The other prospective randomized trial in the United States is the one being carried out by the National Surgical Adjuvant Breast project that is designated as NSABP Protocol No. 6.  In this trial patients with tumors of 4 cm or less in size are randomized to one of three treatment arms:  1) total mastectomy plus axillary node dissection (modified radical mastectomy),  2) tumorectomy plus axillary node dissection, 3) tumorectomy plus axillary node dissection followed by radiation therapy to the breast.  All patients with histologically positive axillary lymph nodes also receive adjuvant chemo-therapy (L-PAM plus 5-fluorouracil).  In addition to comparing tumorectomy and mastectomy it also addresses the very important question of whether radiation therapy is a necessary adjunct for all patients treated by tumorectomy.  This is an extremely important clinical trial and the end results of treatment will be of significant importance in identifying the various aspects of treatment. The Veronesi study continues at the National Cancer Institute in Milan and the group at the Tata Memorial Hospital in Bombay has recently initiated a randomized clinical trial between definitive radiation therapy versus mastectomy under the aegis of the Radiation Therapy Oncology Group.

The role for radiation therapy as the primary management of carcinoma of the breast has increased. This shift toward greater emphasis for primary radiation therapy has resulted from the woman's demand to preserve the breast intact, from the data that substantiate equally good survival statistics when compared to radical mastectomy or modified radical mastectomy, and from the excellent cosmetic results that can be achieved by the treatment program. The definitively administered radiation therapy program allows for local and regional control rates and survival rates that are essentially equivalent to those achieved by surgical techniques compared stage by stage. Because of the excellent results from these reports and the increasing awareness of the public of the existence of an alternative to mastectomy, more women are seeking this alternative for treatment. Moreover, the trend toward earlier diagnosis has resulted in a higher proportion of women who are eligible for conservative breast surgery and radiation therapy. Four states (Massachusetts, California, Minnesota, and Wisconsin) now require informed consent as to the various alternatives for treatment prior to the final treatment decision. The passage of a similar law is imminent in Michigan.

As had been noted, there is a need to pursue randomized control studies to document without question the validity of this comparison between radical mastectomy or modified radical mastectomy and definitively administered radiation therapy.

If a patient cannot be entered into a clinical trial or refuses to participate, her management should be based on the answers to the following questions: 1) what patients are eligible for breat conservation surgery and irradiation? 2) what type of breast conserving surgical procedure should be done? 8) what is the radiation technique that provides the maximum potential for local control, the best in long-term survival and the best cosmetic result?

WHAT PATIENTS ARE ELIGIBLE?

Tumor Size

Tumor size is an extremely important selection factor. The larger the tumor, the greater the likelihood for local recurrence. Retrospective reviews of patients treated by excisional biopsy and curative radiation therapy show a local-regional recurrence rate of less than 5% for T1 lesions. This incidence is comparable to that seen for T1 lesions treated by mastectomy and this has been confirmed by Veronesi's prospectively randomized study.[25] For T2 lesions, the local-regional recurrence rate with tumor excision and definitive radiation therapy is about 10% and again this is similar to that reported in the mastectomy series. Whether this comparability holds for both large and small T2 lesions remains to be seen. Many radiation oncologists, therefore, have made an arbitrary decision to exclude patients from the definitive program of excisional biopsy and radiation therapy if the tumor size is greater than 3 cm.

### Breast Size

A breast that is small relative to the size of the tumor may show an unacceptably large surgical defect when the entire tumor is excised, even though survival probability and local control will be similar to that obtained by mastectomy. In such cases, the best option may be modified radical mastectomy with subsequent reconstructive surgery. The opposite extreme—very large, fat, or pendulous breasts—will give a greater probability for a poor cosmetic result even though the survival statistics and local control rates will again be essentially the same as with mastectomy. A very large and pendulous breast will tend to exhibit more fibrosis and retraction following the definitive program of external beam radiation therapy than a moderate sized breast. Since a moderate amount of fibrosis and retraction may be more acceptable to a woman than having no breast at all, large pendulous breasts are not an absolute contraindication to tumor excision and the radiation therapy program. However, these patients should be informed of the potential for retraction and fibrosis.

### Multiple Breast Masses

Patients with a second mass in the breast that cannot be excised along with the excision of the dominant mass should be considered for a mastectomy rather than excisional biopsy and definitive radiation therapy. It is, therefore, important to obtain mammograms prior to tumor excision, not only to rule out undetected masses within the affected breast but also to evaluate the contralateral breast. Mammography prior to tumor excision is particularly important in infiltrating lobular carcinoma because of the high incidence of multifocal disease with this histologic subtype. Since this high incidence of multifocal disease pertains to both ipsilateral and contralateral breasts, the contralateral breast must be followed as closely as the treated breast with physical examination at least every two months and with mammographic examinations at least yearly or whenever an abnormality is noted on physical examination. In some cases of infiltrating lobular carcinoma in which the breasts are difficult to examine and in which the fear of a new primary in the contralateral breast is extremely great, bilateral mastectomy with subsequent reconstruction should be considered as an alternative to tumor excision and radiation therapy of only the symptomatic breast.

## Age Of The Patient

In general, patients 35 years or younger are not considered for the radiation therapy program because of the long-term survival probability and the potential for carcinogenesis in the irradiated breast. Data to date do not substantiate this to be a major problem.

## Distant Metastases

Patients with distant metastatic disease are usually excluded from the definitive local radiation therapy program. A workup appropriate to detect distant disease is therefore mandatory on all patients prior to the institution of any definitive treatment program.

## Patient Attitude

An important selection factor is the attitude of the woman herself. Breast conserving surgery and radiation therapy should be limited to those women with a strong desire for breast preservation.

## WHAT TYPE OF BREAST CONSERVING SURGERY SHOULD BE DONE?

There are a number of names given to breast conserving surgery: wedge excision, quadrantectomy, segmental mastectomy, partial mastectomy, excisional biopsy, tylectomy, tumorectomy, and lumpectomy. Wedge excision, segmental mastectomy, quadrantectomy, and partial mastectomy are all more or less synonymous and imply resection of the tumor with a generous margin consisting of a segment or wedge of the breast. This can range from a resection of a very modest amount of breast tissue up to a hemimastectomy. Tylectomy, excisional biopsy, tumorectomy and lumpectomy are synonymous and mean removal of the tumor itself without a large segment of surrounding normal breast tissue.

Since the sole rationale for performing tumor excision and irradiation in lieu of mastectomy is to leave the patient with two cosmetically acceptable breasts, tylectomy is preferable to segmental mastectomy. Segmental mastectomy may result in a large surgical defect that can impair the cosmetic result. This has been confirmed by the Harvard Joint Center for Radiation experience which has shown that the cosmetic results are optimum when the tumor is excised with only enough surrounding tissue to obtain a clear margin. The National Surgical Adjuvant Breast program Protocol 06 recommends that attention be given to the direction of the incision. Cosmesis is best when excisions in the upper half of the breast are circumareolar and excisions in the lower half of the breast are radial.

In addition to excision of the tumor, most patients should have either an axillary node sampling or an axillary node dissection. This is essential for premenopausal women, since the axillary nodal status will significantly influence the potential for subsequent adjuvant chemotherapy. Since a recent study by Bonadonna's group[31] has suggested that adjuvant chemotherapy in full doses is also beneficial in post-menopausal women, an axillary node dissection is also recommended for these women.

The National Surgery Adjuvant Breast program protocol 06 recommends that the incision for the axillary surgery be separate from that used for the excision of the breast mass. It is tempting to include the excision of the upper quadrant mass with the same incision used to reach the axillary lymph nodes. This, however, results in a long scar that can produce severe lateral deviation of the breast.

The question as to the performance of a low axillary node sampling or a full axillary node dissection has not been settled. As a rule, there is a higher incidence of breast and arm edema with a full axillary node dissection than with an axillary node sample at level I. On the other hand, some node "sampling" procedures can be vigorous enough to cause as high a likelihood of breast and arm edema as a full axillary node dissection. Moreover, this probability is increased even further if the axillary node sampling turns up histologically positive nodes. In this situation, the definitive radiation therapy program should be added to the already surgically violated axilla by inclusion of the axilla in the irradiated fields. If a full dissection is performed, the low axillary contents need not be irradiated even if the nodes are histologically positive. Bedwinek[32] prefers a thorough dissection of the axillary lymphatics up to and just beneath the pectoralis minor muscle (level I and level II nodes), but not the apical nodes (level III). When this is done, the low axilla need not be irradiated regardless of the status of the recovered nodes. If the nodes from this procedure are positive, the supraclavicular fossa is irradiated and the undissected level III nodes will fall within the standard supraclavicular field. When level III nodes are included in the dissection, the incidence of breast edema is unacceptably high--greater than 27% through the life of the patient.

WHAT RADIATION THERAPY TECHNIQUE IS THE BEST?

The technique for treatment of the intact breast following excisional biopsy requires meticulous attention to detail if optimum cosmetic results and maximum local-regional control rates are to be achieved. Although there is no single correct technique for radiation therapy to the intact breast, there are several crucial technical considerations that apply to all situations and deserve attention.

Fields To Be Irradiated

In the past, patients treated with tumor excision and radiation therapy did not undergo an axillary node dissection or a sampling. Therefore, it was necessary to give comprehensive irradiation to the breast and all three peripheral lymphatics--axillary, supraclavicular, and internal mammary lymph nodes. With a sampling or dissection of the axillary lymph nodes, it is possible to reduce the number of lymphatic areas to be treated depending upon the location of the tumor within the breast and the histologic status of the axillary lymph nodes (Table 20). If the axillary lymph nodes are histologically negative and a woman with an outer quadrant lesion, the axilla, supraclavicular fossa and internal mammary lymph nodes need not be irradiated. In that circumstance, only the breast is treated. If the axillary lymph nodes are histologically negative in a woman with a medial quadrant lesion, treatment needs to be delivered to the breast as well as the internal mammary and supraclavicular lymph nodes. The low axilla may be excluded. If the axillary lymph nodes are histologically positive, the supraclavicular fossa, apical axillary lymph nodes, and internal mammary lymph nodes should be treated regardless of the location of the tumor within the breast. If the positive axillary nodes come from an axillary dissection of at least level I and lateral level II nodes, the low axillary nodes need not receive treatment. If the axillary surgery was only a sampling of the lower axillary lymph nodes, the low axilla must be treated whenever those nodes are histologically positive.

Dose

If all gross disease has been removed, the total tumor dose to the entire breast and the lymphatic areas should be no less than 4500 rad delivered in 4.5 to 5 weeks at the rate of 900-1000 rad per week and no greater than 5000 rad in 5 to 5.5 weeks at the rate of 900-1000 rad per week (Table 21). The daily fraction size should be no less than 180 rad and no greater than 200 rad.

TABLE 21. CONTROL OF SUBCLINICAL DISEASE AS FUNCTION OF DOSE*[34]

| Dose in Rads | Patients | Disease Control |
|---|---|---|
| 3000-3500 | 89 | 60-70% |
| 4000 | 121 | about 80% |
| 5000 | 273 | greater than 95% |

*1000 rads/week - 5 days a week.

Boost To The Site Of Tumor Excision

The site of the tumor excision should receive a boost of 1000 rads if the tumor was excised with clear margins, and 1500-2000 rads if the excision margins were not free or were in question. This boost can be accomplished with electrons of appropriate energy or with an interstitial implantation using Iridium-192 seeds in nylon tubing. The interstitial implantation technique may be done under local anesthesia eliminating the need to take the patient to the operating room. Boosting with an external photon beam is usually unacceptable, for this can cause the boost volume to be too large and/or the dose to the underlying lung to be excessively high. The boost dose should include 2 cm around all the excision scar and should extend down into the breast to approximately 2 cm depth to the deepest resected margins. If this deep margin cannot be determined by consultation with the surgeon, then the boost volume should extend down to the pectoralis muscle group.

Wedge Or Compensating Filters

Breasts come in all sizes and shapes and are never square or rectangular. For this reason, wedges or compensating filters must be used to achieve a uniform homogeneous distribution of the radiation dosage within the breast being treated. The variation in dose from the base of the breast to its apex should be no greater than 10%.

## Beam Energy

The entire breast should be treated with Cobalt-60 teletherapy units operating at 80 cm or better FSD or with x-ray energies of 4-6 MV. Photon energies greater than 6 MV should not be used, for these energies may result in an underdose to the superficial tissues just beneath the skin surface.

## Bolus

The skin of the breast is usually not at risk for recurrence following excision of a Tl or T2 tumor as is the skin of the chest wall following radical mastectomy or modified radical mastectomy. For this reason, applying bolus to the entire breast is unnecessary and may even lead to an undesirable cosmetic result since this practice can produce not only an unnecessarily brisk skin reaction but later telangiectasia and other late skin changes. Since the skin immediately adjacent to the excision scar may be at risk, the excision scar may be bolused for 50-100% of the treatments. At some institutions, even the scar may not be bolused.[35,36]

## Matching The Supraclavicular Field With the Tangential Fields

A hot spot can exist just beneath the skin surface at the junction of the inferior border of the supraclavicular field and the superior border of the tangential fields. This hot spot is caused by divergence of the tangential beams up into the supraclavicular fields and by divergence of the supraclavicular beam down into the tangential fields. The penumbral characteristics of Cobalt-60 are such that this match line hot region is probably not intense enough or large enough to cause a significant problem. Evidence for this conclusion is based upon the experiences of the M.D. Anderson Hospital with Cobalt-60 teletherapy devices. Although approximately 60% of their patients developed match line fibrosis, this fibrosis can be detected only by palpation and does not significantly impair the cosmetic result. On the other hand, the sharp beam of a linear accelerator and the "horns" at the edge of this beam will produce a marked increase in dose beneath the match line if the divergence mentioned above is not corrected. This increase in dose may result in severe match line fibrosis or rib fractures. When using a linear accelerator, it is, therefore, important to eliminate the divergence of both the supraclavicular and the tangential beams. The divergence of the tangential fields can be eliminated by angling the tangential beams inferiorly so that the superior border of these beams line up perfectly with the inferior border of the supraclavicular field. This inferior angulation of the tangential beams is essentially accomplished by angling the foot of the treatment couch away from the radiation source. The inferior divergence of the supraclavicular beam can be eliminated by blocking off the inferior half of this beam so that the central non-diverging portion of the beam becomes the inferior border of this field.

## Alignment Of The Tangential Beam With The Chest Wall Contour

The anterior chest wall of most women slopes downwardly from the mid chest to the neck. To make the posterior edge of the tangential beam follow this downward sloping contour, the collimator of the tangential beam is usually rotated. This rotation throws the superior edge of the tangential beam off the vertical so that it no longer perfectly matches the inferior edge of the supraclavicular beam which has been made perfectly vertical by the use of the beam splitter. This can be corrected by the "hanging block" technique in which a vertical block is affixed to the superior portion of the collimator to block off the non-vertical portion of the tangential beam. An alternative technique is used at the Washington University Mallinckrodt Institute of Radiology. Here, the posterior edge of the tangential beam is made to follow the chest wall contour by means of a rotating beam splitter rather than rotation of the entire collimator. In this way, the superior edge of the tangential beam remains in the true vertical and matches perfectly the vertical inferior edge of the supraclavicular field.

## Matching The Tangential Field With The Internal Mammary Field

The match between the medial tangential field and the internal mammary field can be a problem when there is a significant amount of breast tissue beneath this match line. In this situation, a cold spot or low dose area can exist. This can be avoided in small chested patients by not using a separate internal mammary field. When this is done, it is necessary to insure that the internal mammary nodes are included within the tangential field. Some have advocated the use of internal mammary node scintigraphy to identify these lymph nodes.[37,38] In large chested women, the lack of a separate internal mammary field can cause an excessive amount of lung to be irradiated. Hence, whenever the internal mammary nodes are to be included in the tangential fields, it is necessary to check the port films to insure that the minimum amount of lung is being irradiated. There is no good solution to this match line problem in large chested women who also have a significant amount of breast tissue beneath the tangential internal mammary match line. It is necessary to be careful and consider the individual situation and choose among the following alternatives: 1) accepting the cold spot or low dose area, 2) overlapping the medial tangential field with the internal mammary field which may cause a hot spot or high dose area, 3) not using an internal mammary field which can result in the irradiation of a large volume of lung.

From the treatment techniques described, the more appropriate ones involve adequate history and examination of all patients with the establishment of the diagnosis by excisional biopsy. Evaluation for the presence or absence of metastatic disease should be carried out and those patients without metastatic disease can be selected based on the criteria previously mentioned for the definitive radiation therapy technique.

Many studies have defined that there is a lower incidence of local failure in T1 and T2 lesions having a complete tumor excision prior to the radiation therapy program. This is in keeping with the report of Spitalier et al.[22,33] in which the local failure rate was 6.9% in patients treated with excisional biopsy prior to radiotherapy compared to 21.3% in patients treated by radiation therapy alone without excisional biopsy. The Radiation Therapy Oncology Group Breast Cancer Historical Data Base reported by Bedwinek et al.[39] demonstrated that control was better with complete excision and that if complete excision was carried out, there was no difference between the use of electron beam or implantation techniques to deliver the boost to the excisional site. If excision was not complete, the implantation technique gave better results than those achieved by electron beam as the boost to the incomplete excisional site. However, the numbers of cases are small and the data may not be statistically significant. The studies carried out at the Instituto Nationale Tumori, Milan, by Veronesi et al.[25] was comprised of patients randomized to a control study in the interval from 1973 to 1980 to consider the value of conservative procedures in patients with breast cancer of small size. In this study, 701 patients were randomized with breast cancers measuring less than 2 cm in diameter, with no palpable axillary lymph nodes to radical mastectomy or "quadrantectomy" with axillary node dissection followed by radiation therapy to the ipsilateral residual breast tissue. The Halsted procedure was carried out in 349 patients and the quadrantectomy plus radiation therapy in 352 patients (Table 20). The patients were comparable in age distribution, size, and site of primary tumor, menopausal status, and frequency of axillary nodal metastases found at surgery. There were three local recurrences in the Halsted group and one in the quadrantectomy group. Actuarial survival curves showed no difference between the two groups in disease-free or overall survival. Veronesi concluded from these results that mastectomy appears to involve unnecessary mutilation in patients with breast cancer of less than 2 cm in size with no clinically palpable axillary lymph nodes. The overall survival in the Halsted mastectomy group was 90.1% and 89.6% in the quadrantectomy plus radiation therapy group. The disease-free survival for all patients following mastectomy was 83.0% and from quadrantectomy plus radiation therapy 84.0%. For those patients with negative nodes, the survival free of disease was 89.1% in the Halsted group and 86.5% in the quadrantectomy group plus radiation therapy. For those patients with positive nodes, the Halsted procedure gave disease-free survivals of 62.0% and the quadrantectomy 75.5%. Veronesi pointed out that the risk of late carcinogenesis induced by radiation therapy in the breast tissue has been stressed by many investigators. At present, the extent of this particular risk cannot be defined. However, the risk may be counterbalanced by the possible sterilizing effects of radiation therapy on the occult microfoci of breast cancer that may be present in the residual breast tissue. The range for occult microfoci of breast cancer is from 20-45%. He concludes that this protective action may even exceed the potential of carcinogenic effects from the radiation therapy. In long-term studies, there has been no demonstrated increased risk in the potential for carcinogenesis in the radiation therapy program for management.

The Guy's Hospital Trial initiated in 1961[20] was the first randomized trial testing the efficacy of excision plus irradiation versus conventional radical surgery. It should be noted that the stage grouping used in this study was different from the UICC stage grouping. The 5-year survival for the excision plus irradiation group was the same as that for the radical mastectomy group for both Stages I and II. Moreover, it was similar to the survival data shown by Bedwinek et al.[39] in the Radiation Therapy Oncology Group Breast Cancer Historical Data Base. It is now recognized that the radiation therapy program for the Guy's Hospital trial was not at the optimum levels recommended in present contemporary studies nor were the dosages adequate to insure the maximum potential for long-term control with the minimum in terms of complication for the treatment. Also, it must be noted that the radiation therapy program was not directed toward all volumes at risk for local and regional disease.

Hayward[40] has recently reported a repeat of the initial Guy's Hospital Trial comparing in a randomized manner the efficacy of excision plus irradiation versus conventional radical surgery. In this study, 132 patients were randomized to radical mastectomy and 121 patients to wide excision and definitive radiation therapy. The radiation dosage was kept the same as for the first series reported by Atkins et al.[20] The local and distant recurrence rates after the wide excision with radiation therapy was greater than in the radical mastectomy series and survival was also affected in a similar fashion being poorer in the wide excision and radiation therapy programs. The data do not explain why there is a survival difference at this time in favor of the radical mastectomy nor are there adequate explanations as to why the radiation therapy program was unchanged when it was widely known that the program does not allow for the maximum potential for long-term local and regional control.

Important from these series is the preservation of the breast intact in the radiation therapy program with excellent cosmetic results. The 5-year local-regional recurrence rates in the first Guy's Hospital Trial was significantly greater for the excision plus irradiation group than for the radical mastectomy. As pointed out above, the explanation for this relates to the dosages of radiation employed in this trial, namely, 2500-3500 rad, inadequate when compared with contemporary standards. The local-regional failure rates in the recent review of patients treated with excisional biopsy plus adequate radiation therapy (5000 rad in 5 weeks at the rate of 1000 rad per week) are much lower than those in the Guy's excision-plus-radiation therapy group.

## LOCAL RECURRENCE FOLLOWING RADIATION THERAPY FOR OPERABLE BREAST CANCER

Local recurrence following radical surgery conveys a grave prognosis to the breast cancer patient. Although local failure sometimes occurs in the setting of obvious disseminated disease, women who have apparently isolated chest wall or nodal recurrence after mastectomy have only a 13-38% five-year survival and a 5% ten-year survival, implying that only rarely are such patients curable by further local treatment programs. Data accumulated from our own experience indicates that the appearance of a local or regional recurrence following radical mastectomy is almost always associated with other identifiable evidences of disseminated disease (80-92%).[41]

This conclusion does not necessarily apply, however, to patients who recur in the intact breast or axilla following conservative treatment using excisional biopsy and radiation therapy.

Kurtz et al.[42,43] looked at a group of patients initially treated with primary radiation therapy who subsequently developed a local recurrence in the breast and were treated with salvage surgery. From this study, it was clear that local recurrence following conservative radiation therapy does not have the dire prognosis associated with recurrences after radical mastectomy. In contrast to the experience of Chu et al.[44] who observed the 5-year survival of 21% (with very few patients free of disease as demonstrated by the 5% 10-year survival), Kurtz et al. demonstrated that more than 80% of patients with Stage I disease and 52% of patients with Stage II disease having salvage surgery were alive with no further recurrence ten years later (Table 22).

TABLE 22    SALVAGE SURGERY:    Survival with No Evidence of Disease at 10 years after Primary Radiation Terapy[42]

| Inital Stage | Salvage Surgery For Proven Local-Regional Failure | |
|---|---|---|
| | Number of Patients | % |
| $T_{1-2}$, $N_0$, $M_0$ | 21/26 | 80% |
| $T_{1-2}$, $N_1$, $M_0$ | 23/44 | 52% |
| $T_3$, $N_{0-1}$, $M_0$ | 10/31 | 32% |

Data from other investigators substantiate the results as consistent with those presented by Kurtz et al. (Table 23). Local recurrence after radical primary surgery presumably reflects a more virulent tumor biology and/or a wider disease dissemination than the surgical stage indicated. It appears

TABLE 23    RESULTS OF SALVAGE SURGERY FOR POST-IRRADIATION RECURRENCES

| Author | Number of Patients | Relapse-Free Survival |
|---|---|---|
| Calle[21] | 14 | 9  (64%) |
| Papillon[23] | 21 | 14  (67%) |
| Spitalier[22] | 32 | 27  (84%) |

that non-sterilization following radiation therapy is largely an indication of a subset or relatively radioresistant tumors not necessarily correlating with tumor aggressiveness.

Another interesting feature of the Kurtz study was that 10-year survival from the time of the primary therapy for those patients who had salvage surgery or local failure did not differ, stage for stage, from the survival of those patients who did not require salvage surgery. This observation has been confirmed with even longer follow-up by Mustakallio[13] who followed 418 conservatively treated Stage I cases, 102 of whom recurred in the irradiated volume. The relative survival curve for the locally recurrent cases was identical to that of the group experiencing no such recurrence and this equivalence persisted for the entire 25-year duration of the study.

Thus, although survival following surgical salvage of local recurrence depends to some degree upon the regional extent of the disease at that point in time, survival remains chiefly a function of the initial clinical stage at the time of the primary radiation therapy program. There are few ultimate failures among Stage I patients followed beyond five to ten years after salvage surgery whereas recurrence with Stage III patients has an outlook which is most consistent with the unfavorable initial extent of the disease.

These patients, treated by definitive radiation therapy techniques, should be followed carefully over long periods of time to identify quickly as possible any evidences of local or regional failure. At the time of such a failure, the patient should have the diagnosis established by excisional biopsy, a metastatic workup carried out to identify the presence or absence of disseminated disease. If the disease process is localized, the patient should be considered for radical mastectomy or modified radical mastectomy. The reluctance to pursue such programs in the past have been associated with the potential incidence of increased morbidity from radical salvage surgery. This additional morbidity was related to prolonged wound healing and an increased incidence of arm edema. However, with contemporary, innovative and appropriate radiation therapy techniques, these complications do not occur. The wound healing following radical mastectomy occurs without difficulty and the incidence of lymphedema is no greater than what would be expected following radical mastectomy alone. The experience of Kurtz et al.[42,43] indicates that the morbidity will be significantly less if a modified radical mastectomy or just a wide excision of the recurrence is performed rather than a full radical mastectomy.

Since the evolution of distant disease will proceed independently of local treatment modalities, a proportion of patients manifesting local-regional failure will prove inoperable mostly due to the recognition of overt metastases. Kurtz reported a 22% inoperability rate in his series similar to that reported by other investigators. Many opponents of conservative radiation therapy might argue that these inoperable patients would have had a more favorable outlook had primary radical surgery been employed from the outset. However, Kurtz pointed out that it is more likely that the metastatic deposits antedated the primary treatment and this was influenced minimally by the local-regional treatment program.

Kurtz also concludes that salvage mastectomy can be accomplished with acceptable morbidity and results in survival rates at ten years from the initial treatment being similar to those seen in patients who did have a local recurrence. Survival following salvage surgery remains largely a function of the initial clinical stage. Local failure following curative radiation therapy did not have the same unfavorable prognosis as local recurrence following radical surgery (Table 24 and 25).

TABLE 24   CANCER OF THE BREAST:   5 and 10 Year Disease-free
Survival Rates (1955-1980)[27]

| | Conservation Surgery and Irradiation 345 Patients | | Radical or Modified Radical Mastectomy Alone 728 Patients | |
| --- | --- | --- | --- | --- |
| | 5-Year | 10-year | 5-Year | 10-Year |
| Minimal Breast Cancer | 97% | 92% | 97% | 95% |
| Stage I ($T_1N_0$) | 85% | 78% | 88% | 80% |
| Stage II ($T_1N_1$, $T_2N_0$, $N_1$ | 78% | 73% | 77% | 65% |

No statistical significance between any group.

TABLE 25   CANCER OF THE BREAST:   Local-Regional Recurrence (1955-1980)

| | Conservation Surgery and Irradiation 345 Patients | | Radical or Modified Radical Mastectomy Alone 728 Patients | |
| --- | --- | --- | --- | --- |
| Minimal Breast Cancer | 1/54 | 1.9% | 1/134 | 0.75% |
| Stage I ($T_1N_0$) | 8/134 | 5.9% | 11/224 | 4.90% |
| Stage II ($T_1N_1$, $T_2N_0$, $N_1$) | 8/157 | 5.1% | 29/370 | 7.80% |

CONCLUSION

Current evidence strong suggests that radiation therapy in the primary local management of Stage I and Stage II breast cancer can achieve survival and local-regional control rates that are comparable to those obtained by radical mastectomy or modified radical mastectomy. Since primary radiation therapy has the benefit of leaving the patient with intact and cosmetically acceptable breasts, it should be considered as a viable and reasonable alternative to radical mastectomy, modified radical mastectomy, or even total mastectomy. Analyses of current series of primary irradiation data suggest that total excision of the tumor should be carried out. An axillary node sampling or dissection including level I and level II axillary nodes (those lying beneath and lateral to the pectoralis minor muscle) should be carried out, in addition to tumor excision since knowledge of the axillary nodal status serves as a prognostic indicator and facilitates the intelligent selection of those patients for adjuvant chemotherapy.

All patients treated by primary radiation therapy should be followed carefully for recurrences. If an isolated recurrence occurs, salvage mastectomy can be carried out with the expectation that the ultimate survival will be the same as it would have been had the local recurrence not occurred.

ACKNOWLEDGEMENTS
Supported by Grants CA-12478 and CA-12252 from the National Cancer Institute and by the Alperin Foundation.

REFERENCES
1. Halstead, W.S. The results of operations for the cure of cancer of the breast performed at the Johns Hopkins Hospital from June 1889 to January 1894. Ann Surg 20:497-555, 1894.
2. Keynes, G. Conservative treatment of breast cancer. Brit Med J 2:643-647, 1937.
3. Keynes, G. The treatment of primary carcinoma of the breast with radium. Acta Radiologica 10:393-402, 1929.
4. McWhirter, R. The value of simple mastectomy and radiotherapy in the treatment of cancer of the breast. Br J Radiol 21:599-610, 1948.
5. American Cancer Society Facts and Figures. New York, 1983.
6. Meyer, A.C., Smith, S.S., Potter, M. Carcinoma of the breast. Arch Surg 113:364-367, 1978.
7. Nime, F.A., Rosen, P.P., Thaler, H.T., Ashikari, R., Urban, J.A. Prognostic significance of tumor emboli in intramammary lymphatics in patients with mammary carcinoma. A J Surg Pathol 1(1):25-30, March, 1977.
8. Huvos, A.G., Lucas, J.C., Poote, P.W. Metaplastic breast carcinoma: rare form of mammary cancer. NY State J Med 73:1078-1082, May, 1973.
9. McGuire, W.L., Zava, D.T., Horwitz, K.B., Chamness, G.C. Steroid receptors in breast tumors - current status. Curr Top Exp Endocrinol 3:93-129, 1978.
10. Brady, L.W. The role of the radiologist in the diagnosis and treatment of carcinoma of the breast. Proc Institute of Medicine of Chicago, vol. 32, 1978.
11. Peters, M.V. Wedge resection and irradiation: an effective treatment of early breast cancer. JAMA 200:144-146, 1967.
12. Peters, M.V. Wedge resection with and without radiation in early breast cancer. Int J Radiat Oncol Biol Phys 2:1151-1156, 1977.
13. Mustakallio, S. Conservative treatment of breast cancer - review of 25 years followup. Clinical Radiology 23:110-116, 1972.
14. Calle, R., Vilcoq, J.R., Stacey, P., Ghossein, N.A. The outcome of treatment by tumorectomy and radiotherapy of patients with operable breast cancer. Int J Radiat Oncol Biol Phys 5:124-125, 1979.

15. Calle, R., Pilleron, J.P., Schlienger, P., Vilcoq, J.R. Conservative management of operable breast cancer: ten years experience at the Fondation Curie. Cancer 42:2045-2053, 1978.

16. Pierquin, B., Owen, R., Maylin, C. Ptmezguine, Y., Raynal, M., Meuller, W., Hannoun, S. Radical radiation therapy of breast cancer. Int J Radiat Oncol Biol Phys 6:17-24, 1980.

17. Baclesse, P. Five-year results in 431 breast cancers treated solely by roentgen rays. Ann Surg 159:103-104, 1965.

18. DeLouche, G., Bachelot, P. Tumorectomie et radiotherapie de cancers du sein. Journal europeen de radiotherapie: Oncology, Radiophysics and Radiobiologie 1:131-138, 1980.

19. Otmezguine, Y., Martin, M., LeBourgeosis, J.P., Maylin C., Raynal, M. Etude de recidives parmis 202 carcereuses du sein tratees conservativement par radiotherapie. Journal europeen de radiotherapie: Oncology, Radiophysics and Radiobiologie 1:115-130, 1980.

20. Atkins, H. Hayward, J.L., Klugman, D.J., Wayte, A.B.. Treatment of early breast cancer: a report after 10 years of a clinical trial. Brit Med J 2:423-429, 1972.

21. Calle, R., Vilcoq, J.R., Schlienger, P. Radiation therapy for operable breast cancer with or without lumpectomy, 10-year results. Presented at the International Conference of Breast Cancer, Monaco, April, 1980.

22. Spitalier, J.M., Brandone, H., Ayme, Y., Pollet, J.F., Abed, R., Amalr, R., Santamaria, S. Robert, S., Seigle, J., Altschuler, C. Primary limited surgery for operable breast cancer, 5 and 10 year results at the Marseille Cancer Institute. Presented at the International Conference of Breast Cancer, Monaco, 1980.

23. Papillon, J. Conservative treatment of early breast cancer by tumorectomy and irradiation, in Current concepts in breast cancer and tumor immunology: The Proceedings of the San Francisco Cancer Symposium of 1974. Medical Examination Publishing Co., Plushing, N.Y., p 117-134, 1974.

24. Batianni, J.P., Ennuyer, A., Drermain, P. Radiotherapie exclusive du cancer du sein. Bulletin Cancer (Paris) 59:135-160, 1972.

25. Veronesi, U., Saccozzi, R., Del Vecchio, M., et al. Comparison of radical mastectectomy with quadrantectomy, axillary dissection, and radiotherapy in patients with small cancers of the breast. NEJM 305:6-11, 1981.

26. Montague, E.D., Gutierrez, A.E., Barker, et al. Conservation surgery and irradiation for the treatment of favorable breast cancer. Cancer 43:1058-1061, 1979.

27. Montague, E.D. Conservation surgery and radiation therapy in the treatment of operable breast cancer. Presented at the American Cancer Society, National Conference on Breast Cancer in Boston, MA, 1983.

28. Prosnitz, L. Goldenberg, I.S., Harris, J., Levene, M., Hellman, S., Wallner, P.E., Brady, L.W. Primary radiotherapy for Stage I and II breast cancer: followup report from four east coast university hospitals. Int J Radiat Oncol Biol Phys 6:1339-1340, 1980.

29. Bedwinek, J.M., Perez, C.A., Kramer, S., Brady, L.W., Goodman, R., Grundy, G. Irradiation as the primary management of Stage I and II adenocarcinoma of the breast: analysis of the RTOG breast registry. Can Clin Trials 3:11-18, 1980.

30. Glatstein, E. Personal communication.

31. Brambilla, C., Valagussa, P., Bonadonna, G. Squential adjuvant chemotherapy in postmenopausal (65 yrs) breast cancer (abs.) Proc A.A.C.R. 21:758, 1980.

32. Bedwinek, J. Treatment of Stage I and II adenocarcinoma of the breast by tumor excision and irradiation. Int J Radiat Oncol Biol Phys 7:1553-1559, 1981.

33. Spitalier, J.M., Pollet, J.F., Seigle, J. et al. Curative cesium therapy of operable breast cancer: 5 year results. Proceedings of the XIII International Congress of Radiology. Excerpta Medica, 1975.

34. Fletcher, G.H. Critique of irradiation techniques - 8th peripheral lymphatics in breast cancer. To be published (presented at the 59th Annual Meeting of the American Radium Society), 1977.

35. Harris, J.R., Botnick, L. Bloomer, W.B., Chaffey, J.T., Hellman, S. Primary radiation therapy for early breast cancer: the experience at the Joint Center for Radiation Therapy. Int J Radiat Oncol Biol Phys 7:1549-1552, 1981.

36. Levene, M.B., Harris, J.R., Hellman, S. Treatment of carcinoma of hte breast by radiaton therapy. Cancer 39:2840-2845, 1977.

37. Kazem, I., Brady, L.W., Croll, M.D. The living anatomy of parasternal lymph nodes as seen on the Au-198 scan. Radioacktive Isotope in Klinik und Forschung. 399-404, 1969.

38. Ege, G. Internal mammary lymphoscintigraphy in breast carcinoma: a study of 1072 patients. Int J Radiat Oncol Biol Phys 2:821-822, 1977.

39. Bedwinek, J.M., Perez, C.A., Kramer, S., Brady, L.W., Goodman, R., Grundy, G. Irradiation as the primary management of Stage I and II adenocarcinoma of hte breast: analysis of the RTOG breast registry. Cancer Clin Trials 3:11-18, 1980.

40. Hayward, J. The surgeon's role in primary breast cancer. Breast Cancer Research and Treatment 1:27-32, 1981.

41. Brady, L.W., Bedwinek, J. Personal communication.

42. Kurtz, J.M. Personal Communication.

43. Kurtz, J.M., Spitalier, J.M. Amalric, R. Results of salvage surgery for local recurrence following primary radiation therapy of operable breast cancer. Int J Radiat Oncol Bil Phys 7:1221-1222, 1981.

44. Chu, F.C., Lucas, J.C., Parrow, J.H., Nickson, J.J. Does prophylactic radiation therapy given for cancer of the breast predispose to metastasis? Am J Roentgenol Radium Ther Nucl Med 99:987-991, 1967.

THE USE OF COMPUTERIZED TOMOGRAPHY (CT) IN RADIATION TREATMENT PLANNING
OF PRIMARY BREAST CANCER

ALLEN S. LICHTER, M.D., BENEDICK A. FRAASS, PH.D., HAL A. FREDRICKSON AND
JAN VAN DE GEIJN, PH.D.

INTRODUCTION

Computerized tomography (CT) has revolutionized radiotherapy treatment planning. Instead of planning radiotherapy based on simple external body contours with internal anatomy drawn in from orthogonal radiographs or standard cross-sectional anatomy books, one can outline treatment plans directly superimposed on CT scans.[1] Not only is CT useful for external contours, but contained within the contour is the most accurate anatomic information yet available regarding tumor location and location of normal structures. While CT is frequently used to aid planning in thoracic,[2] abdominal,[3] and pelvic[4] sites, this technology is still evolving for the treatment planning of breast cancer. In an earlier paper, Munzenrider[5] showed that CT provided useful data concerning the thickness of the chest wall. However, since similar information concerning chest wall thickness can be obtained more conveniently and less expensively with ultrasound,[6-8] the use of CT cannot be justified for that purpose alone.

Over the past three years we have used CT scanning in the Radiation Oncology Branch (ROB) of the National Cancer Institute (NCI) as the primary basis for breast cancer treatment planning. We have found such scans helpful in: 1) performing treatment planning on multiple levels; 2) displaying internal anatomy so that the internal mammary lymph node (IMLN) region can be located and treated; 3) choosing between different field configurations in an individual patient; 4) employing density corrections for lung inhomogeneity. This report discusses our findings in these various areas.


METHODS AND MATERIALS

Since June 1979, 65 patients with primary, untreated breast cancer have been irradiated following excisional biopsy and axillary dissection at the NCI. Most of these patients are part of a prospective randomized trial that is comparing excisional biopsy plus irradiation, to standard modified radical mastectomy. All patients are simulated (Oldelft Simulator) and the entrance

Recent Trends in Radiation Oncology and Related Fields, Amendola and Amendola, Editors

and exit lines of the tangential breast fields marked on the skin. Shortly thereafter, the patients are scanned in a whole body CT scanner (EMI 5005) located within and operated by the ROB. Scanning takes place on a flat couch top with one or both arms raised overhead to allow entry into the 40 cm aperture of the scanner while duplicating as closely as possible the treatment position. The previously marked simulator lines noting the field edges are outlined with radio-opaque angiography catheters which allow these marks to be seen on the scan but do not alter the CT image.

Since the hard copy output from the scanner can be slightly distorted due to the curved video screen from which this film is produced,[9] we transfer the CT image from magnetic tape directly into the disc pack of our treatment planning computer (Digital Equipment Co. PDP 11/70) and the scans are then available for viewing on the video monitor of our planning system, free of any anatomic distortion.[1] External and internal contours can be entered automatically or by hand, and treatment planning can take place superimposed on the CT image. The treatment planning programs used in our system have been previously described[10] as well as the method by which inhomogeneities are

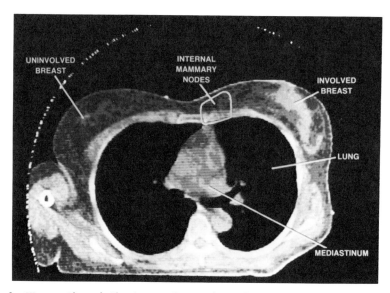

Fig. 1. CT scan through the torso of a patient about to be treated for primary breast cancer. The arm is at the patient's side next to the uninvolved breast and the arm on the treated side is raised overhead. All important anatomic structures necessary for treatment planning are easily visualized (reprinted with permission[13]).

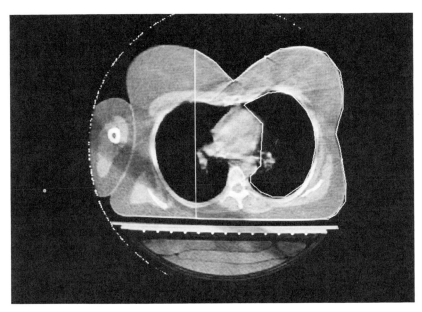

Fig. 2A. The CT scan of a large patient. The distance form skin to pleural surface in the internal mammary lymph node region is 5 cm.

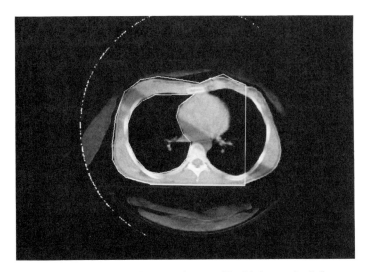

Fig. 2B. The scan of a thin patient. Chest wall thickness is 2.5 cm.

252

accounted for.[11] Lung tissue is assigned a density of 0.35, relative to the unit density of water; the variation of lung density in the range of 0.2 to 0.5 makes relatively little difference in the treatment plan.[1]

RESULTS

Figure 1 displays a CT scan of the thorax with regions of interest highlighted. The internal mammary lymph nodes, by definition, lie in close association with the internal mammary artery and vein. These vessels are superficial to the pleura and lateral to the sternal border.[12] Thus, including the point at which the sternum and pleura meet ensures coverage of the IMLN region.

In Figure 2, some extremes of anatomic configuration are shown to illustrate the variability of chest wall thickness. To assume that the IMLN lie 3 cm lateral to mid-line and 3 cm deep in every patient is to ignore these individual patient variations, previously emphasized by Munzenrider.[5]

The treatment planning in breast cancer cases can be performed superimposed on the CT scan. Figure 3 illustrates a typical isodose distribution. The sternal-pleural junction is contained within the high dose volume. Multiple

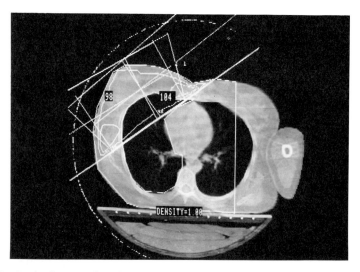

Fig. 3A. Typical central axis treatment plan performed on the CT scan. Two wedged filters are employed to compensate for the slope of the breast. The lung is assigned unit density. Dose uniformity is very satisfactory with two small "hot" spots of 104%.

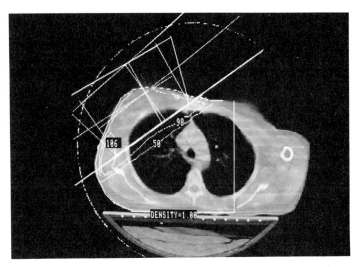

Fig. 3B. Plan in the patient illustrated in Figure 3A, 5 cm above central plane. Note that in contrast to Fig. 3A, the 50% isodose line does not follow the geometric beam edge. This is a result of collimator rotation. The beams are displayed in the unrotated position while the isodose curves are rotated to reflect the appropriate amount of collimator rotation.

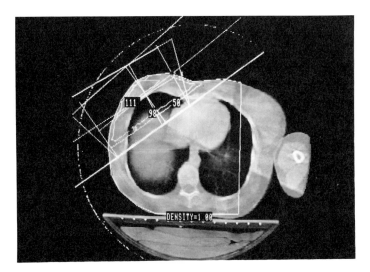

Fig. 3C. Same patient as above, 5 cm. below central ray. Again, 50% isodose line does not follow the beam edge because of collimator rotation. The thinner patient profile at this level creates additional dose non-uniformity.

The treatment planning in breast cancer cases can be performed superimposed on the CT scan. Figure 3 illustrates a typical isodose distribution. The sternal-pleural junction is contained within the high dose volume. Multiple parallel scans can illustrate the dose distribution in planes removed from the central plane where the shape of the breast can be considerably different compared to the reference plane (Figures 3B, C).

Not all patients can have the IMLN region treated within the tangential breast volume. In Figure 4, the problem is easily recognized. This large patient (from Fig. 2A) cannot be treated with tangential beams alone unless one is willing to treat excessive volumes of lung (Fig. 4A) or to encroach significantly into the contralateral breast (Fig. 4B). In order to treat the internal mammary lymph nodes, one may wish to apply a direct <u>en face</u> internal mammary lymph node field. Figure 4C illustrates such a field and with the aid of the CT one can recognize the "cold" wedge of tissue that invariably results from the junction of a vertical field with an oblique field. This cold wedge may be perfectly acceptable in patients with small amounts of chest wall

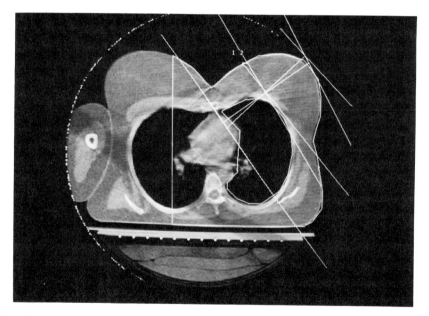

Fig. 4A. CT scan of the patient previously shown in Fig. 2A. In order to include the pleural-sternal junction without going far across midline, a majority of the underlying lung would require treatment.

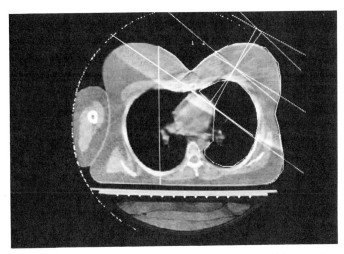

Fig. 4B. The pleural-sternal junction could be treated while sparing some lung by bringing the beams farther across midline. This would, of course, treat a substantial portion of the uninvolved breast.

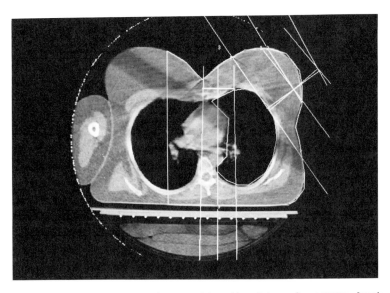

Fig. 4C. An alternate method for treating the internal mammary lymph node region employing a direct internal mammary field matched to tangential fields. Even overlapping these fields on the skin leaves a triangle of tissue that is untreated. This "cold" region would be directly in the tumor bed of this patient whose tumor was medially located in the breast.

256

tissue. However, in large patients (as in this case) this volume of under-dosage can be substantial. It is especially important to recognize this problem in patients whose tumors are located in the medial portion of the breast. In such cases, the cold wedge may lie directly within the tumor volume. In some patients, no treatment plan is "optimal" and a series of trade-offs between normal tissue tolerance, regional lymph node coverage, and tumor volume dose uniformity must be made. The CT scan is helpful in guiding these difficult decisions.

A final use of CT scanning in breast cancer therapy involves the use of tissue inhomogeneity corrections. As can be seen in CT scans and simulator or port films, a portion of lung is included in every breast cancer treatment volume. CT scans allow us to recognize the location of this lung and to quantify the amount of lung contained within the treatment plan. When an idealized dose distribution using unit density (previously illustrated in Figure 3A) is recalculated using lung density of 0.35 relative to water, the resultant plan shows a marked area of dose increase within the lung and the adjacent soft tissues (Figure 5A). One can re-plan the case using a lung

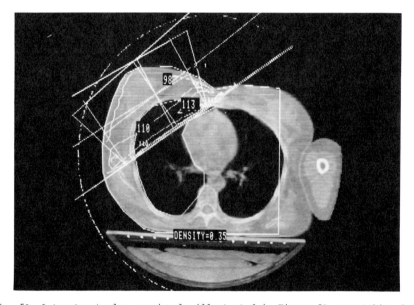

Fig. 5A. A treatment plan previously illustrated in Figure 3A, now taking into account the reduced density of lung tissue. The plan that appeared quite homogeneous is, in fact, non-uniform. A substantial volume of lung and soft tissue is treated to 110% of the prescribed dose.

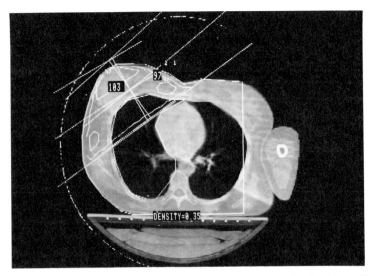

Fig. 5B. Previous case replanned and dose uniformity regained. Note that the wedges have been removed because the effective thickness of the base of the treatment volume is considerably reduced because of the lower attenuation of lung tissue.

density correction and substantially reduce the volume and intensity of the "hot spot" (Figure 5B). This often involves reducing wedge angles or in many cases (such as in this one) eliminating wedges altogether. Because of reduced lung density, the "equivalent" soft tissue thickness at the base of the breast volume that includes the lung is substantially smaller than its actual physical thickness. This means that wedged tangential fields using unit density throughout the volume have been overcompensating for this slope of the breast when lung density has not been taken into account. It should be pointed out that this area of extra dosage is contained almost entirely within normal tissue regions and not within tumor regions and thus potentially contributes far more to complications, such as rib fractures, or pneumonitis than it does to any possible improvement in tumor control.

DISCUSSION

CT scanning is useful in breast cancer for a variety of purposes. It allows one to visualize anatomy of the individual patient and to perform customized treatment planning based on both an accurate external contour and an accurate display of the patient's internal thoracic anatomy. Specifically, this is helpful in locating the sternal-pleural junction which defines the internal mammary lymph node region. The location and volume of lung contained within the plan can be accurately quantitated, allowing one to employ a tissue inhomogeneity correction to make the dose within the treatment volume as uniform as possible. It is significant that when breast treatment plans are performed using a lung density correction, little or no wedge compensation is necessary. When one takes plans that have previously been performed assuming homogeneous unit density throughout the volume and then inserts the density correction, one observes marked non-uniformity of dose (Fig. 5A). Unless the volume of lung contained within a treatment plan is quite small, it turns out that wedge compensation, in reality, decreases rather than increases, dose uniformity and treatment plans almost always are improved by removing the wedge filters.

We have used CT scanning for some additional purposes. In a previous publication the area of lung contained in breast cancer treatment plans with various field configurations was quantified[13]. From this investigation, it was shown that two tangential fields, angled deeply enough to include the internal mammary lymph node region, treat no more lung than two smaller tangential fields matched to a direct en face internal mammary photon field. The area of lung contained in the internal mammary field (directed through the thickest part of the lung) was nearly equal to the reduction in area of lung spared using shallow tangents, thus equalizing the area of lung irradiated between the two types of plans. We have also used CT scans to aid in determining the dose scattered to the opposite breast during primary breast irradiation. Using direct and extrapolated measurements we have been able to superimpose the dose scattered beyond the geometric field edge over the CT scan and show that the contralateral breast receives between 100 and 150 rads during primary breast treatment of 5000 rad total dose.[14]

An additional use of CT scanning concerns accumulating data for three-dimensional treatment volume reconstruction and three-dimensional display of dose distribution. Some of the first attempts in this area are visually dramatic[15] and will be the subject of continued research and development over the next few years.

There are, not surprisingly, some pitfalls in the use of CT scanning for primary breast cancer treatment. Our patients are treated with their arms abducted at approximately $110^\circ$ from the side. When using CT scanners with small apertures (40 cm) this arm position must be changed to an overhead position, thus potentially distorting the position of skin marks relative to their location in the treatment position. Obviously, for centers that treat their breast patients with the arm in an overhead position, this is not a problem. Similarly, scanners with 60 cm apertures allow patients to enter the scanner with the arm farther out towards the side. Those that treat with the arm supported laterally and have access to a CT scanner with a small scanner aperture must take extreme care to avoid errors in placement of the skin marks corresponding to the beam entrance and exit points.

There are other methods that can be used to obtain both external contour and internal anatomic information in breast cancer patients. Recently, we have been working with ultrasound scanning and have found that the location of lung and sternum can be accurately quantified with this technique. In our department, the advantage of ultrasound scanning is that it can be done with the patient on the simulator couch and in the exact treatment position. The disadvantage is that the image of the pleural/soft tissue interface (which indicates where the pulmonary parenchyma begins) is, at times, obscure and poorly defined. In those cases, CT scans become indispensable. We currently use input from both the CT scan and the ultrasound scan to delineate the most accurate anatomic information and plan all cases using a lung density correction. While we have used a lung density value of 0.35, recent measurements suggest this figure is closer to 0.25 for the adult lung.[16] Recognizing a change of this magnitude will alter our treatment plans by 2%-3% at best.[1] We nonetheless plan changing to this more accurate value. If the internal mammary lymph node region cannot be safely included in the tangential fields, we use CT and ultrasound information to help us choose between alternative field configurations. In this manner treatment can be optimized on an individual basis.

REFERENCES

1. Lichter, A.S., Fraass, B.A., Fredrickson, H.A., van de Geijn, J. and Glatstein, E. in Computed Tomography in Radiation Therapy, Ling, C.C., Rogers, C.C., and Morton, R.J., eds., Raven Press, New York, pp. 1-21, 1981.
2. Emami, B., Melo, A., Carter, B.L., Munzenrider, J.E. and Piro, A.J. Value of Computed Tomography in Radiotherapy of Lung Cancer. Am J Roent, 131:63-67, 1978.
3. Goitein, M., Wittenberg, J., Mendiondo, M., Doucette, J., Friedberg, C., Ferrucci, J., Gunderson, L., Linggood, R., Shipley, W.V. and Fineberg, H.V. The Value of CT Scanning in Radiation Therapy Treatment Planning: A Prospective Study. Int J Rad Onc Biol Phys, 5:1787-1793, 1979.

4.  Brizel, H.E., Livingston, P.A. and Grayson, E.V. Radiotherapeutic Applications of Pelvic Computed Tomography. J Comp Asst Tomog 4:453-466, 1979.

5.  Munzenrider, J.E., Tchakarova, I., Castro, M. and Carter, B. Computerized Body Tomography in Breast Cancer. Cancer 43:137-150, 1979.

6.  Bernardino, M.E. and Spanos, W. A Simple Technique for Determining Internal Mammary Chain Depth by Sonography. Int J Rad Onc Biol Phys 7:671-673, 1981.

7.  Brascho, D.J. Tumor Localization and Treatment Planning with Ultrasound. Cancer 39:697-705, 1977.

8.  Rhyne, T. and Birnholz, J.C. Simple Measurement of Chest Wall Thickness with Ultrasound. Radiology 108:436-438, 1973.

9.  Ibbott, G.S. Radiation Therapy Treatment Planning, Distortion of CT Imaging. Med Phys 7:261, 1980.

10. van de Geijn, J. and Fredrickson, H.A. Computation of Multi-slice Dose Distribution in Irregular Fields Modified by Irregular Blocks. Med Phys 8:560 (Poster presented at 1981 AAPM Meeting, Boston), 1981.

11. van de Geijn, J. EXTDOS 71, Revised and Expanded Version. The program for treatment planning in external beam therapy. Comp Prog Biomed 2:169-177, 1972.

12. Haagensen, C.D., Feind, C.R., Herter, F.P., Slanetz, C.A. and Weinberg, J.A. The Lymphatics In Cancer. W.B. Saunders Company, Philadelphia, pp. 322, 1972.

13. Roberson, P.L., Lichter, A.S., Bodner, A., Fredrickson, H.A., Padikal, T.N., Kelly, B.A. and van de Geijn, J. Dose to Lung in Primary Breast Irradiation. Int J Rad Onc Biol Phys 9:97-102, 1983.

14. Roberson, P.L., Lichter, A.S., Iler, V., Bodner, A. and van de Geijn, J. Proceedings of the American Society of Clinical Oncology 22:413, 1981.

15. Mansfield, C.M., Lee, K.R., Chang, C.H.J., Dwyer, S., Cook, P., Zellman, D. and Cook, L. The Role of CT SCanning in Patients With Cancer of the Breast, Cervix and Endometrium. CT 5:236-243, 1981.

16. Van Dyk, L., Keane, T.J. and Rider, W.D. Lung Density as Measured by Computerized Tomography: Implications for Radiotherapy. Int J Rad Onc Biol Phys 8:1363-1372, 1982.

INTEGRATION OF THORACIC RADIATION THERAPY AND CHEMOTHERAPY
FOR SMALL CELL CARCINOMA OF THE LUNG

JAMES D. COX, M.D., ROGER W. BYHARDT, M.D., RITSUKO KOMAKI, M.D.,
PAUL Y. HOLOYE, M.D.D AND JOHN D. NORLUND, M.D.

Concepts of the treatment of patients with small cell carcinoma of the lung (SCCL) have changed profoundly in the past decade. Radiation therapy was considered the treatment of choice for patients whose tumor seemed to be limited to the thorax and homolateral supraclavicular lymph nodes, and indeed, the only treatment that might cure such patients. This viewpoint was due to the rapid clinical and roentgenographic response of SCCL to irradiation which had been recognized for many years. In fact, the rapidity of response and the frequency with which the tumor vanished led many to conclude that total doses lower than those required with other carcinomas of the lung were sufficient. It was less widely recognized that equally rapid regrowth of the tumor ensued if total doses were not high.

A proportion of the patients who would be eligible for definitive radiation therapy actually had sufficiently limited tumors that they might have undergone surgical exploration and resection. However, the results of Britain's Medical Research Council trial which compared surgical resection with thoracic irradiation for patients with operable SCCL are well known. Of 144 evaluable patients, 73 were to receive irradiation and 71 were assigned to thoracotomy: only 48% of the latter group actually had complete resection whereas 85% of the group receiving radiation therapy received the planned treatment. Ten years after completion of this study, three patients were free of disease among those who received radiation therapy. Four percent of patients assigned to thoracotomy survived two years, and the only long-term survivor had refused thoracotomy and had been treated successfully with irradiation.[1] The irradiated patients received total doses ranging from 20 Gray (Gy) in 10 days to 66 Gy in 42 days,[20] which indicates the lack of general agreement and, more precisely, the lack of firm data about the dose-time relationships required for local control of SCCL. Another example of the lack of agreement about dose-time factors for SCCL can be found in a

Recent Trends in Radiation Oncology and Related Fields, Amendola and Amendola, Editors

review of existing prospective trials for SCCL:   total doses ranged from 30 Gy in two weeks to 75 Gy in eleven weeks.[3]

A retrospective study of patients who received radiation therapy alone for SCCL limited to the thorax, was made to determine if there was a dose-response relationship for local control.  The results suggested a dose-response curve similar to other carcinomas of the lung.  The median dose proved to be approximately 55 Gy in five and one-half weeks; below this dose, 46% (16/35) patients failed within the field of irradiation; above the median dose, 24% (4/17) recurred.[3]  The optimal dose-time factors for control of SCCL by radiation therapy alone could not be investigated further because of the increasing acceptance that a number of cytotoxic chemotherapeutic agents were capable of producing responses with SCCL.

The rapid development of chemotherapy for SCCL in the 1970's was unparalleled except perhaps by developments in therapy for testicular carcinomas. From a review of a large number of therapeutic trials, Bunn et al.[4] concluded that the use of multi-agent chemotherapy was clearly superior to single drugs, and three drugs seemed to provide maximum effectiveness. Patients with limited disease were more likely to have complete responses, and those who were ambulatory had higher response rates and longer survivals than those who had a poorer performance status.  Investigators from all disciplines came to accept the necessity to use combination chemotherapy in all patients with SCCL, and it was and still is questioned whether there is any role for radiation therapy, except for sanctuary sites that do not receive sufficient concentrations of the drugs.[5]

Data from prospective, centrally randomized, phase III trials comparing systemic chemotherapy alone versus chemotherapy plus thoracic irradiation are few, and they have produced conflicting results.  There may be many reasons for the discrepancies.  End-points have been used that only partially assess the value of the therapy.  Median survival is the most common end-point in trials of treatment of SCCL: yet median survival is a palliative end-point, and it is influenced more by patient characteristics, such as performance status and extent of disease, than by differences in therapy.  Long-term survival, at least survival beyond the median, or perhaps, three-year survival, may be a much more important measure of effectiveness of therapy. There are many examples of treatments which resulted in a better short-term survival, but yielded poorer long-term survivals.  Studies have often neglected to look at patterns of failure, especially following chemotherapy alone, so assessment of the effectiveness of local treatment was made only indirectly. Even when patterns of failure have been analyzed, all failures within the chest have often been reported; true recurrences within the field of irradiation have not been separated from peripheral extensions outside the volume irradiated and pleural effusions. Quality control in radiation therapy has been lacking and inadequate fields of treatment or inadequate doses may have been administered.

## PATTERNS OF FAILURE AFTER RADIATION THERAPY AND/OR CHEMOTHERAPY WITH ONE OR TWO DRUGS

A retrospective evaluation of the patterns of failure after treatment of carcinomas of the lung limited to the chest was made in a Veterans Administration Lung Group (VALG) trial which compared radiation therapy alone versus radiation therapy plus hydroxyurea and lomustine. There were no differences in patterns of failure when small cell carcinoma was compared to the other cell types, although the interval to failure was slightly longer with SCCL.[6] A more detailed evaluation of patterns of failure was undertaken prospectively in a subsequent VALG trial,[7,8] in which patients with "limited disease" received only radiation therapy. Only 10% of the patients who failed had local recurrence alone, although 40% had both local and distant failure; 31% died with clinical evidence of distant metastases without local failure. Three hundred autopsies from VALG studies included 57 patients with SCCL: thirty percent of these patients died from complications of the intrathoracic tumor with no evidence of extrathoracic dissemination.

## PATTERNS OF FAILURE AFTER COMBINATION CHEMOTHERAPY WITH THREE OR MORE DRUGS

In general, patients treated with intensive chemotherapy alone tend to fail in sites of original disease with or without failure in sites not previously involved. Despite the volume of data from chemotherapy trials for SCCL, specific chest failure rates are often missing. Cohen et al.[9] reviewed data from six trials which relied upon combination chemotherapy alone; 46% of 71 patients failed in the chest. In addition, they reported 9 of 14 patients (64%) who were complete responders to chemotherapy in trials of the National Cancer Institute-Veterans Administration Medical Oncology Branch, recurred in the chest; 4 had also had extrathoracic metastasis.

At the Medical College of Wisconsin, a prospective trial was undertaken to determine if combination chemotherapy was sufficiently effective to control the intrathoracic tumor.[10] Patients received cyclophosphamide, 900 mg/M2, doxorubicin, 60 mg /M2 and vincristine, 2 mg/M2, intravenously every three weeks for six cycles. Patients received prophylactic cranial irradiation, but thoracic irradiation was withheld until there was failure of continued response during the six cycles or there was any evidence of residual thoracic tumor, by chest roentgenograms or computed tomograms at the end of six cycles; evidence of progression or recurrence at any time warranted irradiation of the chest. Patients who were complete responders, by clinical and radiologic procedures were followed with no further treatment until progression. Thirty-one consecutive patients were entered into the study. Eleven of 12 with limited disease, and six of 19 with extensive disease responded completely. Of the 17 complete responders, 14 (82%) failed at the primary site from 22 to 87 weeks after the start of treatment. Eight of 11 with limited disease, and all six of those with extensive disease, had failure to control the primary tumor.

In a review of the literature up to 1979, Salazar and Creech[11] found the reported frequency of failure at the primary site in patients with limited disease treated with chemotherapy to be 82%, but they observed that many articles did not evaluate the intrathoracic failure rate. Patients with extensive disease have at least as high a risk of chest relapse as those with limited disease. In trials of chemotherapy for extensive disease, Cohen et al.[12,13] reported failure rates in the chest alone of 42% to 63%, and rates of failure in the chest plus distant sites of 63% to 81%. These high intra-thoracic failure rates occurred in spite of complete response rates of 55% to 69% to combinations of cyclophosphamide, 1000 mg/m2, lomustine 100 mg/m2 and methotrexate, 15 mg/m2, with or without additional drugs.

Lininger et al.[14] reported a prospective study at the Mayo Clinic of alternating non-crossresistant combinations of chemotherapy for patients with extensive SCCL. Despite high response rates (80% to 90%), 46% of patients progressed first at the site of the primary tumor.

Harper et al.[15] observed a direct correlation between the initial size of the intrathoracic tumor, as assessed by total cross-sectional area seen on computed tomograms, and both response and survival following treatment with cyclophosphamide, methotrexate, and lomustine. When the measured area of the tumor exceeded 30 cm$^2$, there were no complete responses: eight of 21 tumors less than 30 cm$^2$ responded completely. These results of direct measurements corroborate the clinical impression that bulky tumors are more likely to recur after chemotherapy.

PATTERN OF FAILURE AFTER COMBINATION CHEMOTHERAPY AND CHEST IRRADIATION.

There are two fundamentally different types of failure within the chest when results of chemotherapy and radiation therapy to the chest are evaluated. Failure within the volume adequately encompassed by the field of irradiation is failure of combined treatment; moreover, it is a primary failure of radiation therapy since the whole justification for thoracic irradiation is the elimination of tumor within the treated volume. Another variation on radiotherapeutic failure is recurrence at the edge of the field; this is a failure to appreciate the volume at risk and encompass it with adequate margins. The other fundamental type of intrathoracic failure is relapse in the peripheral lung, well beyond the field of irradiation, in areas not initially thought to contain tumor. In addition, failure in the pleura, especially with effusion is common. These latter types of intrathoracic failure are not due to inadequacy of irradiation, but are due to failure of control with the systemic chemotherapy.

Mira and Livingston[16] were among the first investigators to differentiate between types of intrathoracic failure. Of 17 patients with limited disease treated with systemic chemotherapy and thoracic irradiation, two (12%) recurred within the field of irradiation. However, another seven (41%) recurred in the chest, outside the field of irradiation, without evidence of regrowth at the primary site. Intrathoracic spread of cancer of the lung in general, and SCCL in particular, is not fully understood. Retrograde lymphatic metastasis to the periphery of the lung and to the pleura may be more prevalent than previously appreciated. Failure to fully evaluate the extent of disease in the chest may, in part, be overcome by the systematic use of computed tomography.

As a consequence of the high failure rate at the primary site when chemotherapy alone was used (MCW Study III), a prospective phase I/II study of consolidation thoracic irradiation was initiated (Study IV). After the initial staging procedures, including computed tomography, patients received prophylactic cranial irradiation, (25 Gy in two weeks), and combination chemotherapy with the same drugs and doses as in Study III. In the second through the sixth cycle, intravenous methotrexate was administered, 60 mg/M2 given in a bolus followed by 80 mg/M2 by infusion over a four hour period; calcium leucovorin was started 24 hours after the methotrexate, 75 mg by infusion over a one hour period, and 6 mg orally, every 6 hours for 48 hours.[17] Following the sixth cycle, complete re-evaluation of patients with clinical complete responses was carried out: all tests that were abnormal at the time of initial evaluation were repeated. Three weeks after completion of chemotherapy, "consolidation" irradiation was administered to the chest with a target volume designed to encompass the original extent of disease. The total dose received at the point of intersection of the multiple fields of irradiation was 37.5 Gy in 15 fractions in three weeks. This dose was chosen on the basis of previous studies of the dose-tumor control relationships for thoracic radiation therapy with and without systemic chemotherapy[18]: these studies had shown that total doses of 27.5 Gy to 37.5 Gy at 2.5 Gy per fraction could be expected to control only 20% of tumors without chemotherapy, whereas more than 80% were controlled when similar doses were administered in conjunction with cyclophosphamide, doxorubicin, and vincristine.

A total of 46 patients were evaluable for thoracic irradiation following chemotherapy: 20 initially had limited disease and 26 had extensive disease. At the completion of chemotherapy, complete responses were seen in 19 (95%) and 15 (58%) respectively. One patient with extensive disease refused thoracic irradiation. With these patients at risk from 18 to 49 months (median of 32 months), six of nineteen (31%) with limited disease, and one of fourteen (7%) with extensive diseases had recurred within the field of irradiation. Recurrences were seen from five and one-half to sixteen months after completion of treatment. Thus, by comparison with Study III, in which patients received only chemotherapy and 82% (14 of 17) of the complete responders failed at the primary site, with radiation therapy following complete response to chemotherapy, only 21% (7 of 33) failed at the site of the original tumor.

SURVIVAL AFTER CHEMOTHERAPY WITH AND WITHOUT THORACIC IRRADIATION.

In spite of high response rates with the best chemotherapeutic regimens, and in spite of the addition of thoracic irradiation, the prognosis for patients with SCCL is still very grave. Most patients may be considered cured if they are alive and continuously free of SCCL 30 months or more after treatment.[19] A small proportion may develop late recurrence, and another group may develop a new primary carcinoma of the lung, clearly different from SCCL.

There are several impediments to the evaluation of the effect of chest irradiation upon survival in patients with SCCL. Many studies have reported thoracic failure rates after irradiation of the local-regional tumor that are unacceptably high. This may be due to insufficient total dose, inadequate fields of treatment, delivery of irradiation in a manner which reduces the efficacy in regard to tumor control (such as split-course therapy), or timing or sequencing of the two modalities such that subclinical recurrence may already have started. Furthermore, it is important to choose the proper endpoint to evaluate the effect of irradiation of the chest for SCCL.

Williams et al.[20] reported a randomized comparison of chest irradiation versus none, in patients with disseminated SCCL who received cyclophosphamide, vincristine, lomustine, and procarbazine. Irradiation was started after two or three cycles of chemotherapy: 30 Gy were delivered in 10 fractions in two weeks. Eight of 13 patients failed within the thorax. The choice of patients with extensive disease, the initiation of irradiation after only two or three cycles, and the lack of specification whether thoracic failures were within the field of treatment prevent any meaningful conclusions from this study.

In another study of patients with extensive disease (WP-L 72-22), The Working Party in Lung Cancer found no advantage of radiation therapy to the chest compared with chemotherapy alone. However, the total dose administered was only 20 Gy,[5] a dose that would not be expected to control even exquisitely radiosensitive tumors.

The effectiveness of radiation therapy should, in principle, be tested more appropriately in patients with tumor limited to the chest. However, a large randomized trial which studied the use of thoracic irradiation combined with cyclophosphamide, vincristine, lomustine, and methotrexate, showed there to be no advantage over chemotherapy alone.[5,21] The irradiation used was a split-course regimen, 20 Gy in one week-two week interruption-20 Gy in one week, which has now been shown to be suboptimal in squamous carcinomas, adenocarcinomas, and large cell carcinomas of the lung.[22] The other inherent disadvantage of split-course radiation therapy for SCCL is the second half of the therapy may be treating tumors which are already regrowing. Even much more intensive split-course regimens have been associated with high local recurrence rates. As previously noted, control within the field of irradiation has been seen in approximately 80% of patients treated with combinations of chemotherapy and thoracic irradiation at the Medical College of Wisconsin; others have observed similar local control rates.[24-27]

The survival of patients with SCCL is dependent upon many factors including: pretreatment characteristics, the effectivenss of the systemic chemotherapy and the effectiveness of local irradiation. Radiation therapy would be expected to have its greatest impact on survival with the most highly effective systemic treatment. Bunn and Ihde[28] reviewed a large number of tudies with widely variable chemotherapy and radiotherapy: among 492 patients with limited disease treated with both modalities, 17% were alive and free of cancer at two years, compared with 7% of 246 patients who received only chemotherapy.

Choi et al.[29] evaluated survival beyond the median in 276 patients with SCCL; they found that all long-term survivors had been treated with chest irradiation alone or chest irradiation plus chemotherapy. None of thirty patients treated with chemotherapy alone for limited disease, with irradiation reserved for local failure, survived beyond 24 months. Among 111 patients with limited disease reported by Looper et al.[30] the absolute survival four years after treatment was 10% for patients with no thoracic irradiation compared with 20% with irradiation of the primary tumor in addition to chemotherapy.

In a prospective, randomized trial of the Southwest Oncology Group, patients who received 45 Gy in 15 fractions survived longer than those who received 30 Gy in 10 fractions. Survival was significantly influenced by the accuracy of radiotherapy delivery: patients with major protocol deviations survived shorter periods than those with minor or no protocol deviation. In fact, the technical adequacy of the irradiation was the most important prognostic factor.[31]

Computed tomography (CT) has made a considerable impact upon the initial assessment of the extent of disease, and it may contribute substantially to the delivery of radiation therapy. In a review of fifty-one patients who underwent CT as part of the pretreatment diagnostic studies, 49% were found to have more extensive primary tumors than appreciated by standard imaging studies, and 63% were determined to have more advanced nodal disease in the chest. CT of the upper abdomen showed unsuspected metastases in the adrenal glands, retroperitoneal lymph nodes, and other infradiaphragmatic sites in 29% of patients. CT is very useful in delineating the tumor from secondary changes due to bronchial obstruction; it has proved to be the most important study upon which to base "consolidation" thoracic irradiation after complete response to chemotherapy.

SUMMARY

Small cell carcinoma of the lung (SCCL) is radiocurable in a small proportion of patients. In spite of its great responsiveness to radiation therapy, total doses similar to those required for other histopathologic types of carcinoma of the lung are required for permanent control. Due to its great propensity for dissemination beyond the thorax, systemic chemotherapy has become the mainstay of treatment. SCCL is very responsive to many cytotoxic drugs, but ultimate control with chemotherapy alone has been very infrequent. Most patients who fail chemotherapy recur in areas which originally contained tumors of considerable mass: at least three-quarters recur at the site of the primary tumor and regional lymph nodes. Radiation therapy which adequately encompasses the intrathoracic tumor and which is carried to sufficient total doses, can reduce the failure rate within the field of treatment to approximately twenty percent. Short-term (median) survival is not influenced by irradiation of the chest, at least with currently available chemotherapy. However, long-term survival (two to five years) is significantly increased by the use of thoracic irradiation in addition to chemotherapy. Technical factors -- total dose, continuous rather than split-course regimens, custom blocking with adequate margins -- and full appreciation of the original extent of the intrathoracic tumor, aided greatly by computed tomography, are important determinants of the outcome of radiation therapy. Improved delivery of radiation can be expected to improve control rates and survival. The importance of chest irradiation is likely to increase as systemic chemotherapy improves.

REFERENCES

1. Fox, W., and Scadding, J.G. Medical Research Council trial of surgery and radiotherapy for primary treatment of small-celled or oat-celled carcinoma of bronchus: ten year follow-up. Lancet 2:62-65, 1973.
2. Scadding, J.G. Comparative trial of surgery and radiotherapy for primary treatment of small-cell carcinoma of the bronchus. Lancet 2:979-9, 1966.
3. Cox, J.D., Byhardt, R.W., Wilson, J.F., Komaki,R., Eisert, D.R., and Greenberg, M. Dose-time relationships and the local control of small cell carcinoma of the lung. Radiology 128:205-208, 1978.
4. Bunn, P.A., Jr., Cohen, M.H., Ihde, D.C., Shackney, S.E., Matthews, M.J., Fossieck, B.E., Jr., and Minna, J.D. Lung Cancer (Progress in Therapeutic Research, Vol. 11), Muggia, F., and Rozencweig, M., eds, Raven Press, New York, pp. 549-558, 1979.
5. Bleehen, N.M., Bunn, P.A., Jr., Cox, J.D., Dombernowsky, P., Fox, R.M., Host, H., Joss, R., White, J.E., and Wittes, R.E. Role of radiation therapy in small cell anaplastic carcinoma of the lung. Cancer Treatment Reports, 67:11-19, 1983.
6. Cox, J.D., Eisert, D.R., Komaki, R., Mietlowski, W., Petrovich, Z. Lung Cancer (Progress in Therapeutic Research, Vol. 11), Muggia, F., and Rozencweig, M., eds, Raven Press, New York, pp. 279-288, 1979.
7. Stanley, K., Cox, J.D., Petrovich, Z., and Paig, C. Patterns of failure in patients with inoperable carcinoma of the lung. Cancer 47:2725-2729, 1981.
8. Cox, J.D. and Yesner, R.A. Causes of treatment failure and death in carcinoma of the lung. The Yale Journal of Biology and Medicine, 54:195-200, 1981.
9. Cohen, M.H., Fossieck, B.E., Jr., Ihde, D.C., Bunn, P.A., Jr., Matthews, M.J., Shackney, S.E., Minna, J.D. Lung Cancer (Progress in Therapeutic Research, Vol. 11), Muggia, F. and Rozencweig, M., eds, Raven Press, New York pp. 559-566, 1979.

10. Byhardt, R.W., Libnoch, J.A., Cox, J.D., Holoye, P.Y., Kun, L.E., Komaki R., and Clowry, L. Local control of intrathoracic disease with chemotherapy and role of prophylactic cranial irradiation in small cell carcinoma of the lung. Cancer, 47:2239-2246, 1981.

11. Salazar, O.M. and Creech, R.H. "The state of the art" toward defining the role of radiation therapy and the management of small cell bronchogenic carcinoma. Int J Radiation Oncology Biol Phys 6:1103-1117, 1980.

12. Cohen, M.H., Creaven, P.J., Fossieck, B.E., Jr., Broder, L.E., Selawry, O.S., Johnston, A.V., Williams, C.L., Minna, J.D. Intensive chemotherapy with small cell bronchogenic carcinoma. Cancer Treat Reports 61:349-354, 1977.

13. Cohen, M.H., Ihde, D.C., Bunn, P.A., Jr., Fossieck, B.E., Matthews, M.J., Shackney, S.E., Johnston-Early, A., Makuch, R., and Minna, J.D. Cyclic alternating combination chemotherapy for small cell bronchogenic carcinoma. Cancer Treat Reports 63:163-170, 1979.

14. Lininger, T.R., Fleming, T.R., Eagan, R.T. Evaluation of alternating chemotherapy and sites and extent of disease in extensive small cell lung cancer. Cancer, 48:2147-2153, 1981.

15. Harper, P.G., Souhami, R.L., Spiro, S.G., Geddes, D.M., Guimaraes, M., Fearon, F., Smyth, J.F. Tumor size, response, and prognosis in small cell carcinoma of the bronchus treated by combination chemotherapy. Cancer Treat Reports 66:463-470, 1982.

16. Mira, J.G., Livingston, R.B. Evaluation and radiotherapy implication of chest relapse patterns in small cell lung carcinoma treated with radiotherapy-chemotherapy. Cancer, 46:2557-2565, 1980.

17. Byhardt, R.W., Cox, J.D., Holoye, P.Y., Libnoch, J.A. The role of combined modality therapy of small cell carcinoma of the lung. Int J Radiation Oncol Biol Phys 8:1271-1276, 1982.

18. Cox, J.D., Byhardt, R.W., Komaki, R., Wilson, J.F., Libnoch, J.A., Hansen R. Interaction of thoracic irradiation and chemotherapy on local control and survival in small cell carcinoma of the lung. Cancer Treat Reports 63:1251-1255, 1979.

19. Matthews, M.J., Rozencweig, M., Staquet, M.J., Minna, J.D., and Muggia, F. Long-term survivors with small cell carcinoma of the lung. Europ J Cancer 16:527-531, 1980.

20. Williams, C., Alexander, M., Glatstein, E.J., and Daniels, J.R. Role of radiation therapy in combination with chemotherapy in extensive oat cell cancer of the lung: A randomized study. Cancer Treat Reports 61:1427-1431, 1977.

21. Dombernowsky, P., Hansen, H.H., Hansen, M. (Abst) Treatment of small cell anaplastic bronchogenic carcinoma. Results from 2 randomized trials, II World Conference on Lung Cancer, Amsterd Excerpta Medica, p. 149, 1980.

22. Perez, C.A., Stanley, K., Grundy, G., Wanson, W., Rubin, P., Kramer, S., Brady, L.W., Marks, J.E., Perez-Tamayo, R., Brown, G.S., Concannon, J.P. and Rotman, M. Impact of irradiation technique and tumor extent in tumor control and survival of patients with unresectable non oat cell carcinoma of the lung. Report by the Radiation Therapy Oncology Group, Cancer, 50:1091-1099, 1982.

23. McMahon, L., Herman, T., Manning, M., Dean, J. Patterns of relapse in patients with small cell carcinoma of the lung treated with Adriamycin-cyclo-phosphamide chemotherapy and radiation therapy. Cancer Treat Reports, 63:359-362, 1979.

24. Cooksey, J., Bitran, J., Desser, R., Kinnealey, A., Mintz, J., Colman, M., Cimochowski, G., Griem, M., Demeester, R., Golomb, H. Small cell carcinoma of the lung: the prognostic significance of stage on survival. Europ J Cancer, 15:859-865, 1979.

25. Fox, R.M., Woods, R.L., Brodie, G.N., Tattersall, M.H.N. A randomized study: small cell anaplastic lung cancer treated by combination chemotherapy and adjuvant radiotherapy. Int J Radiation Oncology Biol Phys 6:1083-1085, 1980.

26. Greco, F.A., Richardson, R.L., Snell, J.D., Stroup, S.L., Oldham, R.K. Small cell lung cancer - complete remission and improved survival. Am J Medicine 66:625-630, 1979.

27. van Houtte, P., Tancini, G., Dejager, R., Lustman-Marechal, J. Small cell carcinoma of the lung: a combined modality treatment. Europ J Cancer 15:1159-1165, 1979.

28. Bunn, P.A. and Ihde, D.C. Small cell bronchogenic carcinoma: a review of therapeutic results. in Livingston, R.B., ed., Lung Cancer, Boston, Martinius, Nijhoff, pp. 169-208, 1981.

29. Choi, N.C., Kaufman, S.D., Carey, R.W., Sohier, W.D., Younger, J. Evaluation of the long-term survival of patients with small cell carcinoma of the lung beyond their median survival time in relation to therapeutic modalities and stages of tumor. Int J Radiation Oncology Biol Phys, (Abst), 8:70, 1982.

30. Looper, J.D., Joe, B.T., Shidnia, H., Hornback, N.B. The role of chest irradiation in limited small cell carcinoma of the lung treated with combination chemotherapy. Int J Radiation Oncology Biol Phys, (Abst) 8:69, 1982.

31. White, J.E., Chen, T., McCracken, J., Kennedy, P., Seydel, H.G., Hartman, G., Mira, J., Khan, M., Durrance, F.Y., Skinner, O. The influence of radiation therapy quality control on survival, response, and sites of relapse in oat cell carcinoma of the lung. Preliminary report of the Southwest Oncolo Group Study, Am Assn Cancer Research, 21:339, 1980.

NUCLEAR MAGNETIC RESONANCE:  PHYSICAL PRINCIPLES AND INSTRUMENTATION

ALEX M. AISEN, M.D.

INTRODUCTION

Nuclear magnetic resonance imaging is an outgrowth of nuclear magnetic resonance spectroscopy, a discipline developed during the 1940's and 1950's and widely applied in the fields of chemistry and biochemistry.  During the 1970's, Paul Lauterbur suggested and began developing the field gradient approach currently used for NMR imaging.  During the mid-1970's, developmental work was performed on practical imaging instruments at several university research centers.  By the late 1970's, these pioneering efforts began to reach fruition, and practical, whole body size, medical imaging devices became feasible.  At the end of the 1970's and in the early 1980's, industry began to invest in the technique, and commercial development began.  Today, virtually all major radiologic imaging companies, among others, have introduced, or will shortly introduce, NMR imaging instruments capable of producing pictures of essentially any part of the human body.

PHYSICAL PRINCIPLES

Atomic nuclei with an odd number of protons or neutrons possess the property of nuclear spin.  Such nuclei include the dominant isotopes of hydrogen ($^1$H), sodium ($^{23}$Na), and phosphorus ($^{31}$P), among others. Nuclei with spin will have two physical properties: angular momentum and (because they consist of spinning electrically charged particles) magnetic moments.  As a consequence of these two properties, they will exhibit interesting, and as we shall see, useful, behavior when exposed to a magnetic field.  Hydrogen nuclei are usually selected for NMR imaging because they are abundant and give a strong NMR signal.

The nuclei can be thought of as spinning about an axis, and this axis can be described as having an orientation, e.g. up or down, depending on the orientation of the north and south poles of their magnetic fields.

In the absence of an externally applied magnetic field, the orientation of the axes of a collection of atomic nuclei will be random.  However, if an external magnetic field is applied, for example by a large superconducting

Recent Trends in Radiation Oncology and Related Fields, Amendola and Amendola, Editors

electromagnet, there is a tendency for the nuclear spins to align themselves with the magnetic field. In a manner analagous to the behavior of toy bar magnets and compass needles, there is a slight tendency for the north poles of the spinning nuclei to align themselves with the south pole of the externally applied field; i.e., there is a preferred direction for the alignment of the nuclear axes. This preferred direction represents a low energy state of the nuclear spin system. The reason the tendency is "slight" is that ordinary thermal molecular motion at room or body temperature is great enough to flip many of the nuclei from one spin state to another.

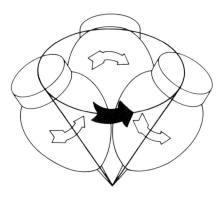

Fig. 1. Spinning toy top in vertically oriented gravitational field precessing in a circle (dark arrow).

As a consequence of their angular momentum, the nuclei experience another effect in the presence of an externally applied magnetic field: the phenomenon of precession. Consider the behavior of a spinning toy top in the Earth's gravitational field. Immediately after the top is set in motion, its axis is vertically aligned. But the axis begins to move, and it moves in a small circle about the vertical; this motion of the axis is called precession (Figure 1). The time it takes the axis to describe a complete circle depends on the precessional frequency. It must be noted that this precessional frequency is distinct from, and in the case of the toy top, significantly smaller than, the spin frequency of the top. As with toy tops in a gravitational field, spinning nuclei in a magnetic field will also precess. This is illustrated in Figure 2. The precessional frequency is given a name: the Larmor frequency. This unique frequency is essentially the same for all nuclei

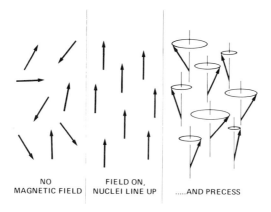

NO
MAGNETIC FIELD

FIELD ON,
NUCLEI LINE UP

.....AND PRECESS

Fig. 2. Spinning atomic nuclei (represented by the arrows) lining up and prescessing in a vertically oriented magnetic field.

of a given type in a given magnetic field; however, it does vary with, and is in fact proportional to the strength of the externally applied magnetic field. This can be represented mathematically by the following simple equation:

$$\omega = \gamma H$$

Where $\omega$ is the precessional frequency, $\gamma$ is a constant called the gyromagnetic ratio which varies from element to element, and H is the strength of the externally applied magnetic field. Most practical NMR imagers use a magnet with a field strength of between 1 and 5 kilogauss (a gauss is a unit of magnet field strength; for example, the earth has a magnetic field of about 0.5 gauss). For magnetic fields in this range, hydrogen nuclei will precess with a frequency of between 4 and 20 megahertz; by coincidence, this is in the same range as the FM radio band.

Next, we come to the phenomenon of resonance. As noted above, the spinning nuclei will tend to align themselves in a low energy state, that is, with the north poles of the nuclei tending to line up with the south pole of the externally applied magnetic field. If, however, an external source of energy is applied at exactly the right frequency, the nuclei can absorb energy. This absorption of energy is manifested by a flipping of the nuclear spins from a low energy state to a high energy state; in effect, energy is used to flip the north poles of the nuclear magnet from their "natural" alignment with the south pole of the external field, to the reverse direction: the north poles of some of the nuclear spins are now aligned with the north pole of the external magnetic field. How must this energy be applied in order for this absorption to be possible? It must be applied at the resonant frequency of the nuclear magnets, the Larmor frequency.

As a consequence of the rules of quantum mechanics, individual hydrogen nuclei can have one of only two possible spin states: up or down. However, when dealing with a large collection or ensemble of hydrogen nuclei (as we always are in any biological system), we are only concerned with the summed or average nuclear magnetism; this is what we can actually measure. This bulk magnetization can be thought of as behaving in a "classical" (referring to classical, or pre-quantum mechanical physics) manner; that is, of being able to take on any orientation. This is the assumption we employ in the subsequent discussion.

If we think of nuclear magnets in the low energy state as having a precessional angle of $0^\circ$ (that is to say, the spin axis is aligned with the axis of the external magnetic field), and then apply a suitable energy pulse, the precessional angle will gradually increase as the nuclear spins begin to reorient themselves as they absorb energy. The precessional angle of a collection of nuclear magnets will gradually increase from $0^\circ$ to $90^\circ$ and then to $180^\circ$ as the nuclear magnets absorb energy and reorient themselves so that they point in a direction $180^\circ$ apart from their initial low-energy state.

In order for this energy absorption to occur, the source of energy must be at the correct frequency. As noted above, this frequency varies with the

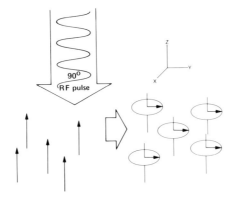

Fig. 3.    Effect of a $90^\circ$ RF pulse on the nuclear spin ensembles.    The external magnetic field is in the vertical, or z, direction.

strength of the externally applied magnetic field. For hydrogen nuclei in a magnet of practical construction, the frequency is in the radiofrequency range. Hence, the source of external energy will typically be a radio-frequency electromagnetic pulse, applied, in practice, by a radiofrequency antenna coil surrounding the patient.

The longer the excitatory RF pulse is left on, or the greater its intensity, the more energy will be absorbed by the collection of atomic nuclei. This is manifested by increasing changes in the average precessional angle. Certain RF pulses will produce a $90^{\circ}$ increase in the precessional angle (as some of the nuclei reorient their spins), RF pulses twice as long will produce a $180^{\circ}$ change in the average precessional angle. The effects of a $90^{\circ}$ pulse are illustrated in Figure 3; in the figure, the external magnetic field points in the z direction.

Immediately after the excitatory RF pulse is turned off, the high energy nuclei will "relax" back to their low energy state. As they do so, a radio frequency signal (called a free induction decay or FID), which is at the Larmor frequency, can be detected by a suitably placed radiofrequency antenna. This is illustrated in Figure 4. Typically, the same coil used to "broadcast" the excitatory radio frequency pulse is used to receive the emitted FID. It is by analying the emitted free induction decay that an NMR image is produced.

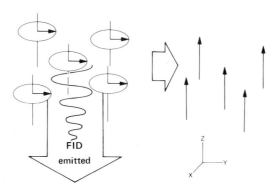

Fig. 4. The "excited" nuclear spin ensembles emit a radiofrequency signal termed an FID as they "relax" back to the ground state.

Again, the longer the excitatory radiofrequency pulse is left on, or the greater its intensity, the more energy the hydrogen nuclei will absorb. There is one other factor that will influence the amount of energy absorbed: the concentration of hydrogen nuclei. Not surprisingly, the greater the density of hydrogen nuclei, the more energy the system can absorb during a given pulse, and the greater the strength of the radiofrequency signal that will be re-emitted when the excitatory pulse is turned off. Thus, NMR techniques can be used to image hydrogen density. Tissues which have a low hydrogen concentration (such as aerated lung) will produce a weak signal; tissues with a larger hydrogen density will yield a stronger signal.

When the excitatory pulse is turned off, the absorbed energy is not released at a constant, predetermined rate. Rather, the rate of return to the low energy, or ground, state is determined by the chemical and physical environment of the hydrogen nuclei. This return to the ground state is termed "relaxation", and the speed with which it occurs is the relaxation rate. As it happens, the relaxation rate varies greatly from tissue to tissue, and between normal and diseased states. In fact, the tissue-specific variation in relaxation rate is generally much greater than the variation in simple hydrogen density. Thus, it is often much more productive to measure relaxation time than simple hydrogen density.

Actually, there are two kinds of relaxation time, termed $T_1$ and $T_2$, and they can be measured independently. It is not necessary to understand the physical differences between the two relaxation times, as long as one understands that there are two rate constants, and that they may vary in different ways. A brief explanation of the physical basis follows.

$T_1$ is, perhaps, the more obvious of the two; it is simply the overall rate at which the nuclei return from an excited state to the ground state. Figure 5 (left) shows a group of local nuclear magnetization vectors after a $90^{\circ}$ pulse; Figure 5 (right) shows the vector a short time later, after they have returned to the ground state. The rate constant for this process is $T_1$. $T_2$, which is always less than or equal to $T_1$, is the dephasing time. After a collection of hydrogen nuclei experience a $90^{\circ}$ pulse, they will all be pointing in the same direction in three dimensional space; this is illustrated in Figure 6 (on the left). As the nuclei relax, two things occur: they begin to move back towards the z direction; this is the $T_1$ relaxation described earlier. But also, they begin to get out of phase with one another in the x-y plane. This dephasing is illustrated in Figure 6 (on the right). For biological systems the $T_2$ dephasing ($T_2$ relaxation) generally occurs

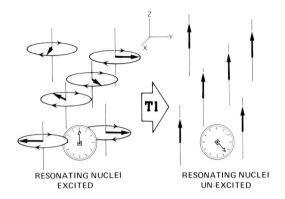

Fig. 5. $T_1$ relaxation time: the rate at which the excited nuclear ensembles return to the ground state. In this case, the left-hand diagram shows the nuclear spin ensembles previously excited by a 90° FR pulse, in an out-of-phase state; i.e., after $T_2$ relaxation has already occurred.

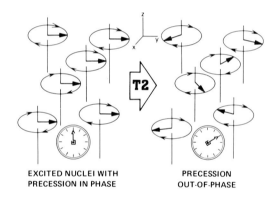

Fig. 6. The nuclear spin ensembles, shown on the left immediately after a 90° excitatory pulse, lose phase coherence; the rate at which they do so is given by $T_2$.

much faster than the reorientation towards the z direction ($T_1$ relaxation). Because $T_1$ relaxation occurs along the direction of the main magnetic field, it is often called longitudinal relaxation; $T_2$ relaxation is termed transverse relaxation.

$T_1$ and $T_2$ relaxation occur simultaneously. As noted above, $T_2$ relaxation is always equal to or faster than $T_1$ relaxation and in biological systems it is usually a substantially faster process. Hence the spins go out of phase ($T_2$ relaxation) before they have moved significantly away from the

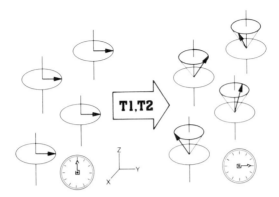

Fig. 7. The figure on the left illustrates the nuclear spin ensembles immediately after a 90° excitatory pulse; the diagram on the right shows them after partial $T_1$ and complete $T_2$ relaxation have occurred.

x-y plane ($T_1$ relaxation). Figure 7 illustrates the state of the nuclear spins following a 90° excitation pulse after "complete" $T_2$ relaxation and partial $T_1$ relaxation have occurred.

In summary, there are 3 different properties of matter which one can measure with NMR:

     1) The hydrogen density
     2) The two relaxation times, $T_1$ and $T_2$
     3) The nature of the movement or flow in the case of liquids such as blood. (This has not been discussed).

(There are others as well, but these are the ones important in imaging applications.) These quantities can be measured by applying radiofrequency pulses, or sequences of pulses, to an object or patient, and then observing the radiofrequency signal reemitted afterwards. In practice, many pulse sequences are used, depending on which parameter, or combinations of parameters, are of interest. The sequences differ in the strengths of the RF pulses and in the lengths of the intervals between them. For example, the saturation-recovery sequence is generally used to yield a signal heavily dependent on the simple hydrogen density; the inversion recovery sequence generates a signal largely determined by $T_1$, and the spin-echo sequence largely depends on $T_2$.

The foregoing discussion describes in brief how NMR might be used to analyze a homogeneous substance, for example, a test tube containing a pure sample of a chemical unknown. It does not describe how NMR can be used to provide "local" information on a heterogeneous substance, such as a human patient. The principles of NMR imaging will now be described.

If an object is placed in a uniform external magnetic field, all the nuclei of a given NMR isotope (for imaging, the common hydrogen nuclei or protons) will have the same Larmor frequency. A radio frequency pulse applied at this Larmor frequency would excite all hydrogen nuclei in the object equally. Local excitation, however, can be obtained by placing the object in a spatially varying external magnetic field. This is achieved through the use of gradient coils. These gradient coils will add a spatially varying magnetic field to the external magnetic field produced by a large superconducting or resistive electromagnet. With a suitable gradient coil, the external magnetic field would be slightly stronger, for example, near the patient's head, and then gradually decrease to a slightly lower value near the patient's feet. Because the Larmor frequency is proportional to the external field strength at a given point, the Larmor frequency would also vary with location. This is illustrated in Figure 8. Hydrogen nuclei located in the upper portion of the patient would have a different (in this case, slightly higher) resonant frequency from those at the patient's feet. Hence, if the applied radiofrequency pulse has only a single frequency component, only a portion of the hydrogen nuclei in the patient will be able to absorb RF energy and become excited. These resonant nuclei would be those in a transverse plane such that

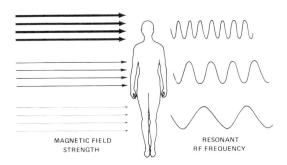

MAGNETIC FIELD
STRENGTH

RESONANT
RF FREQUENCY

Fig. 8. The effects of a spatially varying magnetic field on the resonant Larmor frequency are illustrated. (Note: The amount of variation shown in this figure is very much greater than would be used in an actual imager.)

282

the external magnetic field strength produced a Larmor frequency exactly matching that of the applied excitatory RF pulse. This process is known as selective excitation.

A similar effect can be employed during receipt of the free induction decays. If a gradient field is applied during the relaxation phase, nuclei exposed to different external magnetic field strengths will have slightly different resonant frequencies, and the emitted FID's will vary in frequency. Nuclei closer to the patient's head, for example, might emit RF signals with a higher frequency than those at the patient's feet. By performing a frequency analysis, or Fourier analysis, of the emitted free induction signal, spatial localization in one dimension can be achieved.

The techniques for obtaining three-dimensional spatial localization are varied and complex. Some are based on back projection techniques similar to those employed in computed tomography. Others are based on the use of "phase encoding" gradient signals applied in the x, y, and/or z directions. A detailed analysis is beyond the scope of this presentation. Suffice it to say that using suitably applied gradients and mathematical techniques such as back projection or multi-dimensional Fourier transformation, production of clinically useful images is eminently feasible. An abbreviated description of one scheme follows.

In this typical NMR device, the imaging process would begin with the application of a selective excitation sequence to excite the nuclei in one plane of the patient. This sequence might consist of a narrow frequency range RF pulse applied in the presence of a linear magnetic field gradient oriented in the

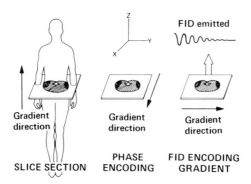

Fig. 9. A scheme for imaging is illustrated, refer to the text for details.

cranial-caudad direction. After selection of this transverse imaging plane (Figure 9, left), the initial magnetic gradient would be turned off, and a second magnetic gradient applied in one of the two remaining directions, for example, the antero-posterior direction. No RF pulse would be applied at this time (Figure 9, center). As a result of this second gradient, a phenomenon called "phase encoding" occurs. This permits subsequent mathematical analysis to determine where, in the AP direction, a given "bit" of signal arises. It still remains to obtain information on location in the medial-lateral direction. This is done by application of a third magnetic field gradient during the actual readout of the RF signal reemitted by the hydrogen nuclei in the patient (Figure 9, right). During this phase of the imaging process, nuclei experiencing a higher field emit a higher frequency signal than nuclei experiencing a lower field. In order to obtain a complete image, it is necessary to repeat the above process many times, each time with a different magnitude phase encoding pulse. After computer processing, an image of the selected transverse slice is obtained.

The preceeding summary is rather complex, but it is not necessary to understand the details. The process can be summarized by stating that there are two aspects to the NMR imaging process: making NMR measurements through the use of radiofrequency pulse sequences, and obtaining spatial localizaton through the use of magnetic field gradients. There are different pulse sequences and different imaging methods.

In general, it takes 4 to 8 minutes to produce an image; efficiency can be improved by "overlapping" pulse sequences so that several slices are imaged concurrently. Thus, as many as 10 or more slices might be imaged during a 4-minute period. It is not possible to break up the time and make one (high quality) image in one-tenth of 4 minutes.

INSTRUMENTATION

There are several components to a clinical NMR imaging device:
1) The large magnet for generating the external magnetic field.
2) A radiofrequency antenna, which surrounds the patient.
3) A set of magnetic gradient coils.
4) A computer system for reconstructing and displaying the images.
5) Power supplies for the magnetic and radiofrequency systems.
6) A patient bed and suitable restraining devices.

The most expensive portion of the NMR system is the magnet. Currently, three types of magnets are used in "commercial" NMR imagers: superconducting electromagnets, air core resistive electromagnets, and permanent magnets.

Superconducting magnets are significantly more expensive than resistive magnets. A typical superconducting magnet might cost approximately $500,000. They do not require electricity to operate, but they must be continually filled with liquid helium and liquid nitrogen to maintain superconductivity. This requires a staff adequately trained in the handling of these cryogens, and well versed in their hazards. Superconducting magnets offer the advantages of greater field strength and greater field homogeneity, both of which result in better clinical images.

Resistive magnets are also used; they are limited to a maximum field strength of about 1.5 kilogauss. They do not require liquid nitrogen or liquid hydrogen, but they require a large amount of electricity while operating, and a large cooling system. In general, the cost of electricity roughly equals the cost of cryogens for the superconducting system. The purchase price of the magnet alone is generally under $100,000. Because of the lower field strength and lower field homogeneity typical of air core resistive magnets, the pictures produced are usually of a somewhat lower quality.

Experimental work is now being done on permanent magnets for NMR imagers, and in fact, one clinical imager based on a large, 3 kilogauss, permanent magnet is already available. The role of permanent magnet technology remains to be determined. One of its roles may be in "low end" NMR imaging systems. Work on hybrid magnet designs and designs using iron or steel "field return paths" (which reduce extraneous fields around the imager) is also underway.

Siting of an NMR system is rather more complex than with other imaging devices because of the large magnetic fields involved. Extreme caution must be taken to prevent magnetic objects from coming close to the magnet, where they can be turned into flying missiles with potentially serious effects. Often, installations are equipped with metal detectors at the doors. There is no known biologic hazard from the magnetic field, except to patients with implanted cardiac pacemakers (which often have magnetic controls), or ferromagnetic implants such as certain types of surgical clips. Siting problems for future NMR systems may be mitigated if work on new magnet designs is successful.

In general, for a 5 kilogauss magnet, pacemakers must be kept approximately 26 feet from the center of the magnet. Large metal stretchers should be kept about 20 feet from the magnet, small hand tools about 10 feet from the magnet, and certain electronic devices such as image intensifiers, about 45 feet from the magnet to ensure their normal operation.

The gradient power supplies and RF systems pose fewer problems than the magnets themselves; these subsystems are essentially the same in all types of NMR imagers, regardless of the magnet type. The computer console is quite similar to the type of system used in computed tomography scanners. The components of a typical NMR scanner are shown in Figure 10.

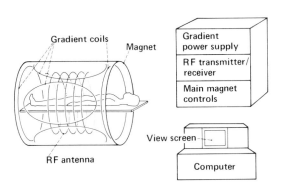

Fig. 10. The components of a "typical" NMR imager.

SAFETY CONSIDERATIONS

NMR imaging is believed to be safe and without hazard (save that from moving magnetic objects accidentally permitted too close to the magnet). Three potential areas of hazard have been raised, all have been studied and thus far, no actual danger has been demonstrated. The three potential areas for hazard are: 1) effects of the large external magnetic field, 2) effects of the RF system and 3) effects of the time varying magnetic fields produced by the gradient coils. As far as is known, large, nonchanging, static magnetic fields, even considerably in excess of those used in NMR imagers, produce no harmful effects in man. Radiofrequency fields, if strong enough, can produce local heating. Care is taken in the design of NMR imagers to keep the power levels in a clinical imaging device below harmful levels.

The area of greatest concern is the time-varying gradient fields used to produce spatial localization. Here, the possibility of inducing (by the same principle as an electrical generator) electrical currents in conductive tissues does exist. If great enough, such current might be able to induce cardiac arrhythmias, and possibly seizures in the central nervous system. Much work has been performed studying such effects, and the gradients used in

NMR imagers do not produce any of the aforementioned deleterious responses. It is believed that the first such effects which might be discernible are phantom flashes of light or phosphenes, induced in the retina by gradients with a high enough rate of change. The levels used in clinical imagers are well below even this threshold.

In summary, the fields employed in clinical imaging machines have been studied extensively and are without known biological hazard. Thus, NMR shares with ultrasound the virtue of safety, lacking the slight potential for harm that exists with imaging modalities employing ionizing radiation.

BIBLIOGRAPHY

1. Partain, C.L., James, A.E., Rollo, F.D., Price, F.R., eds. Nuclear Magnetic Resonance Imaging. W.B. Sanders, Philadelphia, 1983.
2. Kaufman, L., Crooks, L.E., Margulis, A.R., Nuclear Magnetic Resonance Imaging in Medicine. Igaku-Shoin, New York, 1981.
3. Farrar, T.C., Becker, E.D. Pulse and Fourier Transform NMR: Introduction to Theory and Methods. Academic Press, New York, 1971.
4. Pykett, I.L. NMR Imaging in Medicine. Scientific American, 246(5):78-88, May, 1982.
5. Gore, J.C., Emery, E.W., Orr, J.S., Doyle, F.H. Medical Nuclear Magnetic Resonance Imaging. I. Physical Principles, Invest Radiol 16:269-274, 1981.
6. Pykett, I.L., Newhouse, J.H., Buonanno, F.S., et al. Principles of Nuclear Magnetic Resonance Imaging. Radiology 143:157-168, 1982.
7. Steiner, R.E. The Hammersmith Clinical Experience with Nuclear Magnetic Resonance. Clin Radiol 34:13-23, 1983.
8. Bradbury, M.D., Radda, G.K., Allen P.S. Nuclear Magnetic Resonance Techniques in Medicine. Annals of Internal Medicine 98:514-529, 1983.

NUCLEAR MAGNETIC RESONANCE:  CLINICAL APPLICATIONS

MARCO A. AMENDOLA, M.D. AND ALEX M. AISEN, M.D.

INTRODUCTION

The development of nuclear magnetic resonance in medical diagnosis is already being touted as the most revolutionary advance in imaging techniques of the 20th century.[1] In the following pages we will try to review some of the facts that make this a highly provocative prediction.

The images produced by an NMR device are cross-sectional; in fact, at first glance, transverse NMR images bear some resemblance to computed tomographic images. However, while computed tomographic images demonstrate x-ray attenuation, NMR images demonstrate several different parameters. Almost all NMR imaging is done with devices tuned to the resonance of hydrogen; this is by far the most abundant NMR nucleus within the body. Hence, these NMR images demonstrate the properties of hydrogen and since most body hydrogen is in the form of water, NMR images demonstrate various forms of water. As noted in the earlier chapter, several parameters are imaged:

1. The hydrogen density
2. The two relaxation times, $T_1$ and $T_2$
3. The nature of the movement or flow for liquids such as blood.

Which of these parameters is demonstrated in a given NMR image depends on the settings on the imaging device; different radiofrequency pulse sequences produce images which emphasize these parameters differently. Images made using the "saturation recovery" pulse sequence are basically maps of the hydrogen density. The appearance of tissue on the image depends relatively little on the $T_1$ and $T_2$ values. Images made using the inversion recovery method depend much more heavily on $T_1$; images made using the spin echo pulse sequence depend most heavily on $T_2$.

Saturation recovery imaging is probably more easily and quickly performed, but it has been found that these images provide less diagnostic information than inversion recovery and spin echo images. Most imagers today use either the inversion recovery or the spin echo methods. Images made using any of the three previously mentioned methods are not pure hydrogen density, $T_1$ or $T_2$ images; they are merely dominated by the respective parameters. Using several

Recent Trends in Radiation Oncology and Related Fields, Amendola and Amendola, Editors

images, it is possible to obtain enough information to calculate actual values for the hydrogen density, $T_1$ or $T_2$; in certain limited cases this has been found to be useful.

NMR OF THE CENTRAL NERVOUS SYSTEM

The nature of NMR imaging is such that imaging can be performed in any desired plane.[2] Currently available NMR imagers are capable of imaging in the direct transverse, coronal, and sagittal planes; some more advanced devices can perform direct imaging in oblique planes as well. Finally, certain advanced NMR scanners are capable of imaging entire volumes at once. The sagittal plane is ideally suited to display certain anatomic structures like the brain stem, the cerebral ventricles in the mid-line and the area of the craniospinal junction (Figure 1). The ability to obtain detailed coronal and sagittal images is quite advantageous for localization of tumors in the suprasellar region and in the roof of the orbit. This can be achieved with NMR without the penalty of the increased radiation dose needed for sagittal and coronal reconstruction in the case of x-ray CT.[3,4] The potential use of NMR for radiation therapy localization and treatment planning in those areas is easily realized.

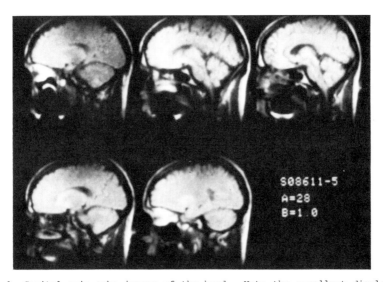

Fig. 1. Sagital spin echo images of the head. Note the excellent display of anatomic structures of the posterior fossa including the 4th ventricle, cerebellum and brain stem and upper portion of the spinal cord (illustration courtesy of Dr. Alexander Margulis, Department of Radiology, University of San Francisco California, and Diasonics Corporation).

The initial major clinical triumph of NMR imaging was the demonstration of the demyelinization characteristic of multiple sclerosis (MS). Such lesions are often missed on CT examination, and they are detected on NMR studies with far greater frequency. This is because NMR is able to differentiate white matter from gray matter with remarkable contrast. The loss of lipid material (myelin) and the subsequent increase in water content in the demielinating plaque which is characteristic of MS, is easily seen and apparently yields a strong signal in the NMR images obtained with "spin-echo" techniques.

In the work of Young et al.[5] ten patients with MS were scanned with x-ray CT with and without intravenous contrast enhancement and by NMR using an inversion-recovery sequence. A total of 19 lesions, varying in size between 5x7 mm and 8x13 mm were demonstrated by CT all situated in the periventricular region. NMR scans demonstrated 112 additional lesions. These varied in size from 3x4 mm to 7x12 mm and were particularly well seen in the periventricular region and brain stem. The authors concluded that NMR demonstrated abnormalities in MS on a scale not previously seen except at autopsy.[5]

NMR is also proving useful in the diagnosis of various other inflammatory lesions, in many cases detecting lesions missed or seen with less clarity on CT. One preliminary study suggests that NMR demonstrates more accurately the degree of brain involvement in systemic lupus erythematosus (SLE) than x-ray CT. Vermess et al.[6] studied 8 patients with clinical evidence of cerebral involvement by SLE. In 2 patients with negative CT examination, NMR showed sizable brain lesions. In 6 patients the CT scans were abnormal. In 3 of these patients the NMR scans were equally abnormal (demonstrating the same number of lesions). In the other 3 patients, NMR showed additional lesions not seen by CT. There were no lesions seen on CT which were not recognizable or which were less well seen on NMR.

NMR is able to diagnose tumors of various organ systems based on both the distortion of normal anatomic structures caused by the mass and on the intrinsic NMR properties ($R0$, $T_1$, $T_2$) of the neoplastic tissue.[7] For example, the high sensitivity of NMR for lipids (short $T_1$) makes tumors with fatty components easily discernible by NMR. In 4 patients with glioma and 12 cases of metastatic tumor to the brain studied by Bydder et al.,[8] the T1 values were generally increased. NMR was generally better at defining mass effect because of the well visualized grey and white matter anatomy. In this study, however, there was often difficulty in differentiating tumor from surrounding edema. Unlike CT, NMR images of the posterior fossa are not degraded by bone artifacts, and lesions of the posterior fossa particularly within the cerebellum and brain stem have been readily distinguished. Hemorrhage within brain tumors is well demonstrated but calcifications do not produce an NMR signal and are generally not as well shown as with CT.[7,9] It has been suggested that radiation damage of the brain is more readily demonstrated with NMR than with CT.[9] It is already clear that for optimal evaluation of brain tumors and other CNS pathology, a combination of different NMR imaging sequences (spin echo, inversion recovery, etc.) and of all three NMR parameters (R0, Tl, T2) will be needed.[10-12]

Due to the lack of signal from rapidly flowing blood, NMR has produced detailed images of the vasculature supplying and draining arteriovenous malformations (AVM).[7] Even "cryptic" AVM's not revealed by bilateral internal carotid angiography have been detected with NMR.[13]

X-ray CT is a proven accurate modality for the detection and follow-up of intracranial hemorrhage. However, isodense subdural hematomas may pose significant diagnostic problems.[14] NMR imaging can help significantly in this area: the medial margin of the hematoma is not likely to be isodense with both gray and white matter unless there is considerable concomitant cerebral edema. The lateral margin of the hematoma will not be obscured by bone artifact.[8]

The spinal cord is directly imaged by NMR without the need to inject intrathecal contrast material as in conventional radiology. Gray and white matter differentiation within the cord is possible by NMR. Sagittal and coronal images of the spine already appear to be superior in quality when compared with similar CT reconstructions.[15] Clearly detailed NMR sagittal images of intramedullary tumors have already appeared in the literature.[12,16]

## NMR OF THE CHEST

NMR is good at imaging the mediastinum. The normal mediastinal fat gives an intense NMR signal on spin echo imaging. In 9 patients with bronchogenic carcinoma studied by Gamsu et al.,[17] separation of mediastinal tumor from blood vessels, airways and mediastinal fat was readily accomplished. Vascular compromise was more easily demonstrated than on CT scans.

In the pulmonary hila absence of NMR signal from flowing blood reduces the hila to simple vascular and bronchial outlines, with a small amount of surrounding fat. On NMR hilar masses and lymphadenopathy can be easily discerned from blood vessels without the need for using large bolus of intravenous contrast material as an x-ray CT.[15,17]

In the case of the pulmonary parenchyma, respiratory motion is a far greater problem in NMR imaging, which involves a much greater imaging time than CT; hence, CT examination will probably prove superior to NMR studies in the detection of small pulmonary nodules, at least until improvements in technique such as respiratory gating or decreased acquisition times are feasible.

CARDIOVASCULAR NMR IMAGING

The application of NMR imaging to the cardiovascular system can be divided into three categories: the use of gated or ungated NMR imaging to study the anatomic structure of the heart and the larger blood vessels; the use of the tissue characterization capabilities of NMR to detect abnormalities such as infarction, ischemia, and atherosclerotic abnormalities; and the use of the flow sensitivity of NMR to measure normal and abnormal blood flow in the heart and great vessels.

Early clinical NMR images through the heart showed clear differentiation between myocardium and blood; measurement of chamber dimension and wall thickness was possible;[18] one study demonstrated the ability to visualize the papillary muscles, moderator bands, and the wall of the left ventricle.[19] With the addition of ECG-gating circuitry, additional detail is visible, including the valve leaflets.[15,20] Several groups have noted the feasibility of measuring changes in myocardial wall thickness and chamber dimension through the cardiac cycle.[21-23]

Initial work in animals has provided encouraging evidence that it should be possible to detect myocardial infarction in vivo on the basis of the NMR relaxation times. Several reports have demonstrated this to be the case in canine hearts following ligation of one or more of the major coronary arteries.[9,24] An additional report suggests that the ability to differentiate normal from abnormal myocardium will be greatly enhanced through the use of paramagnetic contrast agents.[25] To date, little work has been done with human patients. One potential problem using NMR to study myocardial infarction is the fact that metal objects cannot be brought near the imager; this may pose a problem for acutely ill patients with monitoring or life support systems. The study of chronic myocardial infarction will likely prove the easier task.

It is well known that NMR images display flow dependence, and numerous groups have suggested using this to study the motion of blood.[15,19] The flow characteristics shown on an NMR imager are heavily dependent on the nature of the pulse sequence and imaging method employed. To date, however, little or no quantitative in vivo work with humans has appeared in the literature. Much vascular anatomy can be seen on NMR images, and reports demonstrating abnormalities, including aneurysms and atherosclerotic disease have been described.[19]

It is worth noting that patients with pacemakers will probably not be able to undergo NMR imaging because of possible interference with their device.[26]

NMR OF THE LIVER, GALLBLADDER AND PANCREAS

In the abdomen, too, NMR is proving remarkably useful (Figure 2.). It is sensitive in the detection of metabolic abnormalities, as well as structural lesions. Although disease has traditionally been regarded in patho-anatomic terms, NMR techniques may allow investigation in chemical and physiologic

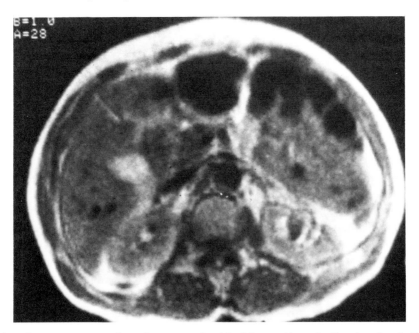

Fig. 2. Transverse spin echo mage of mid abdomen through the level of the kidneys and lower portion of the liver. Note lack of signal from flowing blood in aorta and inferior vena cava (illustration courtesy of Alexander Margulis, M.D., University of California at San Francisco, and Diasonics Corp.).

terms. Since such alterations precede changes in anatomy, NMR may become an especially useful and unique diagnostic method.[27] For example, certain forms of cirrhosis can be differentiated because of chemical differences in the liver parenchyma resulting from the diseased states. In Laennec's cirrhosis $T_1$ is prolonged, however, in biliary cirrhosis and Wilson's disease (in which abnormal deposits of copper, a paramagnetic material, are present) $T_1$ is diminished.[28]

In certain metabolic diseases like hemochromatosis and hemosiderosis there is evidence of reduced Tl relaxation times, probably reflecting increased liver iron contents.[28,29] Saturation recovery images show little anatomic detail within the liver, but inversion recovery (IR) images show great soft tissue contrast, enabling the hepatic veins, inferior vena cava portal veins, bile ducts and gallbladder to be seen as dark structures against the much lighter liver parenchyma.[28] Dilated bile ducts are distinguishable from portal veins by analyzing flow rates.[9] Both metastatic liver tumors and hepatomas are well shown as masses with prolonged Tl relaxation times.[9,28,29] Liver infarcts and localized focal liver atrophy have been shown with NMR in cases not demonstrable with x-ray CT.[9]

According to Hricak et al.[30] calcified gallstones have a very low intensity NMR spin echo signal, showing as filling defects of negative contrast in bile that has a more intense signal. These authors also found that concentrated bile in the gallbladder emits a high intensity spin echo signal (SE) while hepatic bile in the gallbladder produces a low intensity SE signal. NMR may prove to be a simple and safe test of gallbladder function.[20]

The normal pancreas has a Tl comparable to the liver and diseases like pancreatitis and neoplasms produce an increase in Tl values.[31,32] As with CT, it may be difficult to separate the abnormal pancreas from adjacent loops of bowel. Oral contrast agents may be necessary for this purpose; dilute ferric chloride has already been used as an oral contrast.[2] Active research is being conducted in the development of potential oral and intravenous paramagnetic contrast agents for NMR imaging.[33,34] Further investigations are needed to find the true accuracy of NMR of the pancreas.

NMR OF THE GU TRACT

Excellent anatomic detail of normal intrarenal structures has already been demonstrated by NMR without the administration of any intravenous contrast material.[2,9,31,35,36] The renal cortex and medulla are strikingly differentiated. In the work of Hricak et al.[35] the renal cortex was of higher intensity than the medulla, but was less intense than the hilar or perirenal adipose tissue. The intensity and prominence of the renal medulla was dependent upon the state of hydration. During forced diuresis the distinction between cortex and medulla became more apparent.[35]

Because of the presence of sinus fat the renal hilum presents as a high intensity area. Due to the effect of flowing blood, renal veins and arteries are seen as low intensity tubular structures in the hilar region. The collecting system and ureters are also of low intensity due to the long Tl and T2 values of urine (similar to water).

NMR has been able to distinguish simple renal cysts from other renal masses. On SE images the simple cyst appears as a round or slightly oval, homogeneous, low intensity mass with characteristically long Tl and T2 values. Hemorrhagic cysts have been depicted as high density lesions.[36] Five patients with renal carcinoma studied by Hricak et al.[36] were accurately staged by NMR. In comparison with x-ray CT, NMR provided additional information regarding tumor invasion into the intrarenal veins and inferior vena cava. The tumor itself showed a spectrum of intensities on SE images ranging from hypointense to hyperintense.

The possibility of diagnosing rejection of a transplanted kidney by NMR is intriguing.[2] The main drawback of NMR in studying renal pathology is its inability to recognise calcifications. It is possible that the major impact of NMR in nephro-urology may be in the investigation of medical renal disease.

Preliminary work suggests that NMR compares well with CT on its ability to delineate the normal as well as the abnormal adrenal gland without ionizing radiation or intravenous contrast.[37] Furthermore, in some patients NMR may differentiate cortex from adrenal medulla, since the adrenal cortex has a much higher lipid content and is expected to show a higher intensity signal than adrenal medulla.[38]

Images of the abdomen and pelvis of remarkable anatomic detail are routinely available by NMR. The promise for its use in the delineation of portals for radiation therapy treatment planning cannot be over-emphasized.

In the pelvis the lack of significant motion artifact allows for excellent demonstration of anatomical detail in health and disease.[9] Direct sagittal and coronal views add a new dimension to the study of the relationship between bladder, prostate and rectum.[2,38] The prostate gland and seminal vesicles are well displayed. The prospect of identifying with NMR small foci of carcinoma in the prostate and differentiating malignancy from benign prostatic hyperplasia is an exciting possibility which awaits further investigation.

NMR OF THE MUSCULO-SKELETAL SYSTEM

Scant information is available regarding NMR imaging of bone and bone tumors.[39-41] In a recent study of patients with giant cell tumors of bone[40] these lesions showed a lower NMR signal intensity suggesting that these tumors either possess lower proton concentration or a reduction in the $T_2/T_1$ ratio. In that report NMR imaging could detect lesions using information present in the images relating to both structural changes (bone marrow replacement and cortical bone destruction) and changes in NMR relaxation times. NMR was highly successful in defining the extension of a giant cell tumor in the marrow cavity.[40]

At the time of this writing little has been reported regarding NMR imaging of metastatic tumor to bone. However, impressive examples have been published of direct sagittal NMR scans of a metastases from a renal cell carcinoma to a thoracic vertebral body depicting the destroyed bone and tumor mass extending posteriorly into the spinal canal and compressing the spinal cord (which was directly visualized without any type of contrast material).[39] Given the ability of NMR to demonstrate tumor involvement of the bone marrow, this certainly represents a potentially useful area of research in order to complement the highly sensitive but poorly specific radionuclide bone scan in the search for bone metastases.

According to Moon, et al. the dramatic soft tissue contrast inherent to NMR imaging techniques makes it highly advantageous for musculo-skeletal diagnosis.[39] For example muscle, tendon and ligament, nerves and blood vessels, all of which have roughly similar gray scale values on nonenhanced X-ray CT, demonstrate entirely different NMR imaging characteristics.

It is likely that NMR will add a new dimension to the investigation of intervertebral disk disease. NMR appears able to differentiate the annulus fibrosis from the nucleus pulposus. Lumbar disk protrusion has been demonstrated in patients with CT evidence of the disease.[39]

In general, NMR is less sensitive than CT examination in the detection of calcification. NMR is not attenuated by bone and there is no problem with beam hardening artifacts. Hence, NMR is more sensitive in the evaluation of bone marrow, or soft tissues within bone (for example, the posterior fossa of the brain), as compared to x-ray CT.

Another potential clinical application of NMR is in the study and flow quantification of organic fluids like blood, urine, or CSF. The implications for noninvasive study of vascular diseases, for example, are significant.

NMR OF THE BREAST

Since the orignial suggestion by Damadian that NMR could be able to differentiate benign and malignant disease due to a longer Tl of cancerous tissue[42] considerable in vitro work has been done including the study of mammary tumors.[43-45] The study by Beall et al.[43] found that normal, preneoplastic and neoplastic primary cell cultures of mouse mammary epithelial cells were distinguishable on the basis of either relaxation time, Tl or T2. Goldsmith et al.[44] reported 95% discrimination of malignant and non-malignant breast tissue based on the combination of Tl and T2. Bovee et al.[45] studying dissected samples of mammary tissue, demonstrated Tl images of breast cancer lesions which were clearly differentiable from the nonmalignant surrounding breast. Preliminary in vivo clinical obervations,[46] indicate that cysts of the breast can be identified on NMR images and can be easily distinguished from other types of lesions by their high Tl values. Normal breasts and breasts with extensive fatty replacement were found to have the lowest Tl values, whereas Tl values of malignant tissue were elevated. However, in the work of Ross et al. Tl values for malignant and fibrocystic disease were found to overlap.[46]

Pilot clinical studies are under way, however, at present there is no meaningful experience regarding NMR imaging of small non-palpable breast cancer in vivo. It appears that x-ray mammography, a relatively inexpensive and highly accurate technique, will not be replaced by NMR in the near future.

CONCLUSION

In summary, NMR is proving to be very useful in examination of all parts of the body. However, because of its newness, it is not yet clear what its ultimate role will be in an era in which x-ray computed tomography has already achieved great advances. Prospective studies comparing NMR to other imaging modalities and especially CT are already under way at several institutions throughout the world. It is, however, clear that there are many cases in which NMR will surpass x-ray CT.

REFERENCES
1.   Baltaxe, H.A., Geokas, M.C., Nuclear magnetic resonance. Editorial, Ann Int Med 98:540-541, 1983.
2.   Holland, G.N., Hawkes, R.E., Moore, W.S. NMR tomography of the brain: coronal and sagittal sections. J Comput Assist Tomogr 4:429-433, 1980.
3.   Worthington, B.S. Clinical prospects for nuclear magnetic resonance. Clin Radiol 34:3-12, 1983.

4. Hawkes, R.C., Holland G.N., Moore, W.S., Worthington, B.S. Nuclear magnetic resonance (NMR) tomography of the brain: a preliminary clinical assessment with demnstration of pathology. J Comput Assist Tomogr 4:577- 586, 1980.

5. Young, I.R., Hall, A.S., Pallis, C.A., Legg, N.J., Bydder, G.M., Steiner, R.E. Nuclear magnetic resonance imaging of the brain in multiple sclerosis. Lancet, 2:1063-1066, 1981.

6. Vermess, M., Bernstein, RM., Bydder, G.M., Steiner, R.E., Young, I.R., Hughes, G.R.V. Nuclear magnetic resonance (NMR) imaging of the brain in systemic lupus erythematosus. J Comput Assist Tomogr 7:461-467, 1983.

7. Mills, C.M., Brant-Zawadzki, M.D, Crooks, L.E., Kaufman, L., NEwton, T.H., Norman, D. Nuclear magnetic resonance imaging of the central nervous system. in Diagnostic Radiology, Margulis, A.R., Gooding, C.A., eds, University of California Printing Department, San Francisco. pp 341-346, 1983.

8. Bydder, G.M., Steiner, R.E., Young, I.R., et al. Clinical NMR imaging of the brain: 140 cases. AJR 139:215-236, 1982.

9. Steiner, R.E. The Hammersmith clinical experience with nuclear magnetic resonance. Clin Radiol 34:13-23, 1983.

10. Buonanno, F.S., Pykett, I.L., Brady, T.J., et al. Clinical relevance of two different NMR approaches to imaging of a low grade astrocytoma. J Comput Assist Tomogr 6:529-535, 1982.

11. Crooks, L.E., Mills, C.M., Davis, P.L., et al. Visualization of cerebral and vascular abnormalities by NMR imaging. The effects of imaging parameters on contrast. Radiology 144:843-852, 1982.

12. Huk, W., Heindel, W., Deimling, M. Stetter, E. NMR tomography of the central nervous system: comparison of two imaging sequences. J Comput Assist Tomogr, 7:468-475,1983.

13. Brasch, R.C. Nuclear magnetic resonance imaging in children: initial experience. In Diagnostic Radiology, Margulis A.R., Gooding, C.A., eds. University of California printing office, San Francisco, p 1-10, 1983.

14. Amendola, M.A., Ostrum, B.J. Diagnosis of isodense subdural hematomas by computed tomography. AJR 129:693-697, 1977.

15. Alfidi, R.J., Haaga, J.R., Yousef, S.J., et al. Preliminary experimental results in humans and animals with a superconducting whole-body, nuclear magnetic resonance scanner. Radiology 143:175-181, 1982.

16. Margulis, A.R., Crooks, L.E., Kaufman, L. Clinical applications of nuclear magnetic resonance. in Diagnostic Radiology, Margulis, A.R., Gooding, C.A., eds, University of California Printing Office, San Francisco, p 125-128, 1983.

17. Gamsu, G., Webb, W.R., Sheldon, P., et al. Nuclear magnetic resonance of the thorax. Radiology 147:473-480.1983.

18. Hawkes, R.C., Holland, G.N., Moore, W.S., Roebuck, E.J., Worthington, B.S. Nuclear magnetic resonance (NMR) tomography of the normal heart. J Comput Assist Tomogr 5:605-612, 1982.

19. Herfkens, R.J., Higgins, C.B., Hricak, H., et al. Nuclear magnetic resonance imaging of the cardiovascular system: Normal and pathologic findings. Radiology 147:749-759, 1983.

20. Yeung, H.N., Kramer, D.M., Hunter, W.N., Hinshaw, W.S. Application of NMR imaging in cardiology. Abstracts and Scientific Program: Society of Magnetic Resonance in Medicine, First Annual Meeting, 154 Boston, MA, August 16-18, 1982.

21. Go, R.T., McIntyre, W.J., Meany, T.F., et al. Cardiac nuclear magnetic resonance imaging for visualization of heart chambers, myocardial and valvular structures, and ventricular wall motion. Abstracts and Scientific Program: Society of Magnetic Resonance in Medicine, First Annual Meeting, 63-64, Boston, MA, August 16-18, 1982.

22. Goldman, M.P., Pykett, I.L., Brady, T.J., Pohost, G.M. Gated proton NMR imaging in dogs with experimental myocardial infarction. Abstracts and Scientific Program: Society of Magnetic Resonance in Medicine, First Annual Meeting, 63-64, Boston, MA, August 16-18, 1982.

23. Heidelberger, E., Peterson, S.B., Lauterbur, P.L.: 3D Synchronized proton NMR images of the beating heart. Abstracts and Scientific Program: Society of Magnetic Resonance in Medicine, First Annual Meeting, 72-73, Boston, MA, August 16-18, 1982.

24. Williams, E.S., Kaplan, J.I., Thatcher, F., Zimmerman, G., Knoebel, S.B. Prolongation of proton spin lattice relaxation times in regionally ischemic tissue from dog hearts. J Nucl Med 21:449-453, 1980.

25. Brady, T.J., Goldman, M.R., Pykett, K., et al. Proton nuclear magnetic resonance imaging of regionally ischemic canine hearts: Effect of paramagnetic proton signal enhancement. Radiology 144:343-347, 1982.

26. Pavlicek, WE., Geisinger, M., Castle, L.O.N., et al. The effects of nuclear magnetic resonance on patients with cardiac pacemakers. Radiology 147:149-153, 1983.

27. James, A.E., Partain, C.L., Holland, G.N., et al. Nuclear magnetic resonance imaging: the current state. AJR 138:201-210, 1982.

28. Doyle, F.H., Pennock, J.M., Banks, L.M., et al. NMR imaging of the liver: initial experience. AJR 138:193-200. 1982.

29. Smith, F.W., Mallard, J.R., Reid, A., Hutchison, J.M.S. NMR tomographic imaging in liver disease. Lancet 1:963-966, 1981.

30. Hricak, H., Filly, R.A., Margulis, A.R., et al. Work in progress: NMR imaging of the gallbladder. Radiology 147:481-484, 1983.

31. Young, I.R., Bailes, D.R., Burl, M., et al. Initial clinical evaluation of a whole body NMR tomograph. J Comput Assist Tomogr 6:1-18, 1982.

32. Smith, F.W., Reid, A., Hutchison, J.M.S., Mallard, J.R. NMR imaging of the pancreas. Radiology 142:677-680, 1982.

33. Runge, V.M., Stewart, R.G., Clanton, J.A., et al. Work in progress: potential oral and intravenous paramagnetic NMR contrast agents. Radiology 147:789-791, 1983.

34. Brasch, R.C., London, D.A., Wesbey, G.E., et al. Work in progress: NMR study of a paramagnetic nitroxide contrast agent for enhancement of renal structures in experimental animals. Radiology 147:773-779, 1983.

35. Hricak, H., Crooks, L., Sheldon, P., Kaufman, L. NMR imaging of the kidney. Radiology 146:425-432, 1983.

36. Hricak, H., Williams, R.D., Moon, K.L. NMR imaging of the kidney: renal masses. Radiology 147:765-772, 1983.

37. Moon, K.L., Hricak, H., Crooks, L.E., et al. NMR imaging of the adrenal gland: a preliminary report. Radiology 147:155-160, 1983.

38. Hricak, H., Moon, K.L. NMR imaging of the genitourinary system. in Diagnostic Radiology, Margulis, A.R., Gooding, C.A., eds, University of California Printing Office, San Francisco, p 97-103, 1983.

39. Moon, K.L., Genant, H.K., Helms, C.A., Chafetz, N.I., Crooks, L.E., Kaufman, L. Musculo-skeletal applications of nuclear magnetic resonance. Radiology 147:161-171, 1983.

40. Brady, J.J., Gebhart, M.C., Pykett, I.L., et al. NMR imaging of forearms in healthy volunteers and patients with giant-cell tumor of bone. Radiology 144:549-552, 1982.

41. Hinshaw, W.S., Andrew, E.R., Bottomley, A., et al. An in vivo study of the forearm and hand by thin section NMR imaging. Br J Radiol 52:36-43, 1979.

42. Damadian, R. Tumor detection by nuclear magnetic resonance. Science 171:1151-1153, 1971.

43. Beall, P.T., Asch, B.B., Chang, D.C., Medina, D., Hazlewood, C.F. Distinction of normal, preneoplastic, and neoplastic mouse mammary primary cell cultures by water nuclear magnetic resonance relaxation times. J Natl Cancer Inst 64:335-338, 1980.

44. Goldsmith, M., Koutcher, J.A., Damadian, R. NMR in cancer XIII: application of the NMR malignancy index to human mammary tumors. Br J Cancer 38:547-554, 1978.

45. Bovee, W.M., Creyghton, J.H., Getrewer, K.W., et al. NMR relaxation and images of human breast tumors in vitro. Philos Trans R Soc Lond (Biol) 289:535-536, 1980.

46. Ross, R.J., Thompson, J.S., Kim, K., Bailey, R.A. Nuclear magnetic resonance imaging and evaluation of human breast tissue: preliminary clinical trials. Radiology 143:195-205, 1982.

ACTIVITIES OF THE RADIATION THERAPY ONCOLOGY GROUP


H. GUNTER SEYDEL, M.D.




The Radiation Therapy Oncology Group (RTOG) was founded in 1971 and has since grown to involve over 40 teaching hospitals which are participating in more than 50 active randomized protocols and pilot studies including Phase I/II studies. There has been a growth in patient entered on studies to over 1500 in 1982 with a previous accession of approximately 20,000 patients to registries.

The goals of the RTOG have been defined since its inception as the advancement of knowledge of the role of radiation therapy in the management of cancer, the improvement of control of local tumor both in the primary and regional areas, the reduction of morbidity from treatment including a decrease in complications and interdisciplinary management through cooperation with other oncologic disciplines.

When the RTOG was organized in 1971, in the form of a national clinical cooperative group to conduct radiation therapy research and multidisciplinary investigations, Dr. Simon Kramer, Professor and Chairman of the Department of Radiation Therapy and Nuclear Medicine at Thomas Jeferson University, became its first chairman. Dr. Luther Brady, Profesor and Chairman of Radiation Therapy and Nuclear Medicine at Hanneman Medical College is the current Chairman of the RTOG.

Since its inception, the RTOG has strived to enter patients on protocols which address the goals, of improvement of curative and palliative management of cancer and reduction of side effects. Because of the type of modality offered through radiation therapy, the control of primary and regional node involvement is one of the main objectives of the studies into which patients are entered. Collaboration with other oncologic disciplines has taken place especially in areas where radiation therapy plays a significant role in the primary management of patients with cancer.

Long term statistical information has been collected through registries with reference to complications and patient survival and other aspects of

This paper represents the opinion of the author and does not state official policies or data of the Radiation Therapy Oncology Group.

Published 1983 by Elsevier Science Publishing Co., Inc.
Recent Trends in Radiation Oncology and Related Fields, Amendola and Amendola, Editors

statistical information. Through the various committees in RTOG, cooperation between surgical specialties, medical oncologists, pediatric oncologists among others has been fostered as part of the multidisciplinary effort of the capitalized group.

The administrative structure of RTOG allows the priorization of protocols with an aim of integrating radiobiological developments into clinical radiation therapy protocols and to thereby secondarily provide additional training experience for those instutitions in whom residents participate in protocol treatment.

Since 1971, the membership in RTOG has more than doubled, presently numbering over 50 university hospitals who are participating in multidisciplinary research and in significant randomized studies. The majority of the randomized Phase III studies of potentially curable disease were palliative applications of radiation therapy. The case accession has significantly increased since the group's beginning and has grown to over 1500 in 1982, having started with approximately 500 cases in 1971. It is estimated that well over 50% of the patients entered on studies are potentially curable because of the type of cancers involved in studies as well as the extent of disease which is being investigated. A registry performed functions of registration of patients seen in radiation therapy departments participating in RTOG and by its closure, had accessioned well over 25000 patients. Interdisciplinary management of patients has found expression in the intergroup protocols such as those addressing the question of treatment of localized mesothelioma and in this manner, RTOG has been able to influence other clinical cooperative groups such as the Eastern Cooperative Oncology Group, the SouthWest Oncology Group, the Gynecology Oncology Group and Childrens Cancer Study Group. Quality control for some of the intergroup protocols are being carried out through RTOG for other groups, indicating the expertise which has been developed in the headquarters office.

Through programs of the National Cancer Institute, RTOG has extended its activities to community hospitals who are affiliated with member institutions of RTOG and since May 1977, the Group has maintained a cancer control program for clinical cooperative groups. This has led to a major influence of community physicians on cancer care through RTOG activities. It has led to a reinforcement of multidisciplinary patient management in the participating institutions as well as in the RTOG member hospitals, and thus is not only a research but also an educational tool. Early cancer control program support for data collection quality control as well as educational efforts at the community hospitals are supported.

The development of neutron therapy and other particle therapy in the United States has been significantly influenced by RTOG. The institutions who are performing these studies in the United States are expected to access approximately 1000 patient into studies per year including both Phase I/II and randomized clinical trials. RTOG has taken a leading role in data management and quality control for these institutions.

The Quality Control Committee has established mechanisms to assure compliance in all spectra of radiation therapy such as dose prescription, dose delivery and compliance with protocol prescriptions. Day to day quality control is part of this effort through randomization procedures, treatment planning review, data management as well as review of pathology, medical oncology and forms information.

Among the studies which have spearheaded RTOG efforts are those which are traditionally part of radiation therapy and include head and neck cancer, glioma, lung cancer and metastatic lesions especially bone and brain metastases. In affiliation with other groups such as the Gynecology Oncology Group, gynecologic cancer, breast cancer, endocrine, genitourinary, hematopoietic cancer and soft tissue sarcomas are being studied. The new developments in radiation biology such as radiation sensitizers and protectors, hyperthermia and the above mentioned High-LET therapy also are major efforts on the part of the capitalized group. The design on the protocols follows two lines of scientific inquiry. Phase III studies compare a current accepted management protocol to alternative radiation therapy techiques or a combination of radiation therapy with other means of treatment, i.e. chemotherapy. Through the developments of Radiation Biology and the Modality Committee, Phase I/II studies are developed to investigate new research areas according to the need to test the feasability with respect to complications and the potentials of newly introduced treatment methods prior to their introduction into randomized Phase III studies.

Examples for cooperative Phase III studies are the completed protocols on the treatment of gliomas where radiation therapy was compared to radiation therapy and chemotherapy, and head and neck cancer protocols which compare radiation therapy with pre- and post-operative radiation and surgery. The initial efforts to enter chemotherapy into a closed study of radiation therapy effectiveness addressed the question of the use of methotrexate in head and neck cancer. This was one of the milestones in the development of cooperative clinical studies. Much of the experience gained from studies as these mentioned above have led to a refinement of the techniques of both Phase I/II design and Phase III implementation in the group.

Priorities in protocol development in RTOG are directed to high LET radiation, sensitizers and protectors, biologic response modifiers, modifications of time-dose-volume relationship in tradiation therapy techniques, combined modality treatment, especially combining chemotherapy and radiation therapy, and special facility protocols such as those involving hyperthermia and radioactively tagged immunoglobulins.

The LET studies involve neutrons and pions, and contain approximately 30 Phase I, II and III protocols, covering both the high LET radiation itself as well as mixed beams of photons and LET. The sites which are being addressed involve the head and neck area, gynecology, genitourinary sites, lung, GI tract, and central nervous system among others.

Sensitizers studies employing misonidazole and protector studies involving WR-2721 comprise a significant number of Phase I, II, and II protocols including sites in the lung, head and neck, pelvic malignancies, brain and liver metastases, central nervous system, and the genitourinary tract among others.

The biologic response protocols have in the past used the drug levamisole in lung cancer and are now developing a randomized study employing thymosin in lung cancer as well as other sites.

Studies involving the comparison of treatment regimens with various time dose volume schemes, have addressed questions of metastatic disease, involving liver, brain and bone metastases, as well as the newly developed studies with two fractions per day in the treatment of lung cancer, head and neck cancer, and the central nervous system primary tumors. Combination chemotherapy, radiation therapy has been employed in the definitive treatment of localized non-metastatic non-oat cell carcinoma of the lung, as well as in various presentations of head and neck cancers.

Immunoglobulin studies involve liver tumors and more recently non-oat cell lung cancer.

Hyperthermia is being developed in selected number of institutions and has addressed the study of recurrent previously treated lesions while additional studies are in the developmental stages.

The results of the registries for soft tissue sarcoma, early breast cancer, head and neck tumors and others are being analyzed at this time and will continue to produce significant information for the community of therapeutic radiologists in the United States. Studies such as the analysis of the various fractionation schemes in treatment of brain and bone metastases have made an impact on the practice of radiation therapy through optimizing effectiveness and speed of administration. The extent of the RTOG's influence on the oncologic community as a whole has been remarkable. The total annual patient load of all participating institutions is more than 36,750 and the clinical trials therefore influence a significant number of practicing physicians in the oncology field.

It is expected that the Radiation Therapy Oncology Group will continue to develop significant information for the practicing radiaton therapist with the aim to optimize achievement of local tumor control and results of palliative treatment. In this manner, it is expected that the entire oncologic community will benefit from the trials which will allow the medical oncologist to better control systemic disease and the oncologic surgeon to provide appropriate procedures for maximum benefit to the patient.

RADIATION THERAPY IMMOBILIZATION AND PORT REPRODUCTION TECHNIQUES
FOR HEAD AND NECK TUMORS


CYNTHIA A. COLWELL, R.T.(T.)


When evaluating immobilization and positioning techniques for the head and neck area, there are many factors to consider in order to choose the method(s) that best suits the patient, as well as the individual institution. Since no single method or technique seems to meet all the requirements of every situation, it seems appropriate to sometimes combine methods and be open to alternative ways of achieving the best results.

Factors affecting immobilization and port reproduction techniques can be broken down into four categories: 1) patient considerations, 2) operational considerations, 3) technical considerations, and 4) facilities available at each hospital or clinic. It may not always be feasible to give each equal consideration.

In the planning stages of any particular treatment, it is necessary to assess each patient individually to determine what device, if any, or technique is most appropriate. The physician, nurse and technologist may collectively do this, which seems to be the ideal situation. During this assessment, the following considerations must be evaluated:

1. Age of the patient.
2. Patient's physical condition and other limitations (i.e. tracheostomy, presence of other life support devices, disorientation).
3. Location and size of the tumor (anterior, posterior, lateral).
4. Cosmetic effects on the patient.
5. Psychological impact (social interaction with skin marks).
6. Possible skin reactions due to scattered radiation from the immobilization device.
7. Overall comfort of the patient.

Many institutions have one way of immobilizing all patients and there is little if any flexibility in changing that method to help meet the above considerations. No two people are alike, so why choose to standardize when there are other options available? It may be that operational and technical considerations or the facilities prevent them from doing otherwise.

The two main operational concerns are: 1. labor expense - the personnel and time necessary to fabricate and implement a treatment aid, including daily set-up time, and 2. commodity expense - the cost of materials.

In many well-meaning departments where personnel wish they could use a different immobilization technique, there are budgetary restraints. In this age of hospital cut-backs and cost containment programs, certain new ideas may have to be abandoned in favor of those less costly or that require less personnel.

Technical considerations, the third category, are as follows:
1. Duplication of patient's original position.
2. Accurate daily reproduction of treatment ports.
3. Ease of use on a daily basis.
4. Flexibility of the method.

Most people would agree that accurate daily reproduction of the treatment port is essential to every patient no matter what method/technique is employed to get the end result. Part of that process is duplicating the patient's original position on a day-to-day basis. However, it is easy to get wrapped up solely in the treatment aid and forget that the effectiveness of any treatment with respect to treatment aids and port reproduction is really a function of the technologist performing the job. In other words, no matter how fancy or simple the treatment aid is, it is the technologist who creates the end result: daily accurate reproduction of the treatment port. What one technologist considers an "easy to use" method, another finds cumbersome. A negative attitude toward the device/method may be a direct result of the technnologist's educational training as well as previous experience. This does not imply that the technologist is right or wrong but merely suggests that in-services, training and experience will promote further understanding of the total picture as to why one treatment aid was chosen over another in a given situation. Nevertheless, it is hoped that the conscientious technologist will adapt to whatever method is used.

Flexibility of the treatment aid may also be necessary, especially in clinics/institutions where operational concerns are of utmost importance (i.e. if only one device is chosen, this device must be flexible enough to accomodate the majority of patient positions and diseases).

Lastly, facilities can be a great enemy. After having chosen one or more methods that meet all of the necessary patient, operational and technical requirements, lack of space and equipment may prohibit carrying out any of these plans.

Some treatment aids used throughout the country are as follows:
1. Ann Arbor Headholder Device
2. Plaster casts, Vacuform system
3. Polyform-Thermoplastic
4. Alpha Cradle
5. Tape and neckrest
6. Biteblock device

TABLE 2                     PLASTER CASTS, VACUFORM SYSTEM

(Casts and molds are used predominantly in larger institutions

and less frequently in small clinics.)

| Advantages | Disadvantages |
|---|---|
| 1. May be advantageous with children and elderly patient. | 1. May not work well for disoriented patients or patients who cough frequently (the entire cast must be removed to allow the patient to sit up). |
| 2. Minimal cosmetic and emotional effects if marks/tattos are not used. Usually the port is accurately cut out, thus no marks are needed. | |
| 3. Minimal skin reaction unless treatment is given through shell. | 2. Increased personnel--at least one extra techonlogist needed to work in mold room. Aproximately 45-60 minutes is needed for initial cast set up. Takes 1.5 to 2 hours vacuform cast initial set-up time. |
| 4. Patient is usually comfortable unless claustrophobic or airway is semi-blocked (fear of entrapment and inability to breathe). | |
| 5. Generally no emotional or psychological effects, unless used in conjunction with marks or tattoos. | 3. Duplication of work or modification of cast ecah time tumor shrinks or patient position changes. New shells must be made to assure proper fit. |
| 6. Generally regarded as easy to use because of individual fitting. | |
| 7. Good daily duplication of patients' original position. | 4. Needs a lot of space for both fabrication of molds and extra space in treatment room for storage. |
| 8. Provides accurate reproduction of the port if used in conjunction with marks, tattoos, landmarks or if an accurate "window" is cut out of shell to match treatment port. | 5. Accessory equipment necessary includes vacuform machine, cast cutter and various other tools. |
| 9. Location of tumor does not really affect set-ups since casts are quite adaptable. | 6. Extensive work-up time due to forming, setting and drying of mold. Should allow 16-24 hours for planning, molding and other work-up time. |
| 10. Fast daily treatment set-up of approximately 3-5 minutes. | |

COST

1. Vacuform machine:  $7,800
2. Approximate cost for plaster cast: $23-55/cast (materials and personnel)
3. Approximate cost for Vacuform:  $50-55 (materials and personnel)

The following tables relate the above mentioned considerations to each system as advantages and disadvantages.

---

TABLE 1                          ANN ARBOR HEADHOLDER

(The Ann Arbor Headholder was developed in 1959 at the University of Michigan Hospital and is still used today for many patients.)

---

Advantages

1. Meets majority of requirements for location of tumor.

2. Has no serious cosmetic effects unless used in conjunction with marks/tattoos. Special advantage is that marks do not need to be used since it is based on measurements.

3. Minimal psychological/emotional effects, except for claustrophobia in some patients.

4. No skin reactions.

5. Minimal personnel time: takes average of 5 minutes for set-up time both in simulator and treatment room.

6. Accurate reproduction of treatment ports, provided the patient is positioned properly in device each day (lasers and geographic landmarks may be used for alignment).

7. Is quite flexible in that it will accomodate the majority of head and neck cases where patient is lying supine.

8. Minimal space is needed since one headholder/room may be used for all patients.

9. No additional equipment is required.

10. Relatively easy to use but technologists from other institutions sometimes have difficulty adjusting to the system.

Disadvantages

1. Does not accomodate patients under the age of 5 because of ear clamps.

2. Headholder does not work well for disoriented patients or those who are in poor condition (may injure ears).

3. Many patients express discomfort when tightening ear clamps.

4. Does not always fit patients' ears well because ears are not symmetrical.

COST

1. Initial expense of building headholder is approximately $1,200-$1,500.
2. Ongoing materials cost is minimal as plastic pieces need replacing only once every 1-2 months (approximately $1.50/piece).

TABLE 3                         POLYFORM-THERMOPLASTIC

(This is a thermoplastic which becomes soft and pliable when heated to 70  C)

Advantages

Disadvantages

1.  Can be used on any age patient--
    particularly useful for children and
    elderly patients.

2.  Has no cosmetic effects if accurate
    "window" is cut out to exact perimeter
    of the treatment field, thus eliminat-
    ing marks or tattoos which many
    patients find undesirable.

3.  No known skin reactions if treatment
    is not done through plastic shell.

4.  Relatively comfortable to patient.

5.  Daily set-up time is low (3-5 min.).

6.  Easy to use.

7.  Duplicates patient's original posi-
    tion on a daily basis and effectively
    immobilizes for the duration of the
    treatment.

8.  Found to accurately reproduce treat-
    ment port.

9.  Does not require large mold room or
    extra equipment but does require more
    space in treatment room for storage.

1.  Patients experience minor
    discomfort when mask is applied
    (heat).

2.  May not work well on disoriented
    patients or those with breathing
    difficulties as they may not be
    able to hold still while mold is
    being formed.

3.  Requires 20-30 minutes to
    fabricate.

4.  If no mold room is available, it
    ties up the simulator room.

COST

Approximately $11-$13 per patient, including materials and personnel.

Table 4                       ALPHA CRADLE

(A patient immobilization system that expands to take on the form
of the patient utilizing a pre-cut form and chemicals.)

| Advantages | Disadvantages |
|---|---|
| 1. Meets any age requirement. | 1. Cannot be used for patients who have emphysema or asthma. |
| 2. Suits most patients regardless of condition. | 2. Chemicals can cause reaction if contact with skin is made. |
| 3. Tumor, if anterior or lateral, can be easily treated. | 3. Bulky and not always easily handled by technologists. |
| 4. Comfortable to patient. | 4. Must have storage space for pre-cut unused forms as well as adequate storage space for forms currently under use. |
| 5. Has no serious cosmetic effects unless used with marks/tattoos. | 5. May not accomodate all neck treatment areas well, i.e. post obliques. |
| 6. Allows repeated duplication of original first day position. | 6. Procedure takes 15 minutes to set-up (ties up simulator room), modification takes additional 15 minutes. |
| 7. No additional equipment needed. | |

COST

Approximately $50 to $60 per patient including materials and personnel.

TABLE 5                      TAPE AND NECKREST

| Advantages | Disadvantages |
|---|---|
| 1. Accomodates any age. | 1. Does not allow accurate repeated duplication of original patient |
| 2. Used especially for patients in poor condition who cannot tolerate any other treatment aid. | position without use of geographic landmarks. |
| 3. No psychological impact unless marks are used. | 2. Does not allow for accurate reproduction of treatment port |
| 4. No cosmetic effects unless marks or tattoos are used (marks are generally used). | without use of marks, tattoos or geographic landmarks. |
| 5. Location of tumor makes no difference. | |
| 6. No skin reactions noted from tape itself. | |
| 7. Generally comfortable to patient. | |
| 8. Relatively fast procedure: 3 minutes. | |
| 9. Easy to use. | |
| 10. Requires no extra space or equipment. | |

COST

Materials: $80 for one set of 5 different sizes of neckrests.

---

TABLE 6                                BITEBLOCK DEVICE AND NECKREST

---

Advantages                                          Disadvantages

1.  Has no cosmetic effects unless used      1.  Pediatric or elderly patients
    with marks or tattoos.                       may not tolerate system easily.

2.  No psychological impact.                 2.  Patients in poor condition
                                                 cannot easily tolerate biteblock
3.  Generally comfortable to most patients.      (coughing , etc.).  Also, system
                                                 cannot be used for patients with
4.  Minimal personnel time in both initial       pulmonary distress due to airway
    set-up during planning (5 min) and           blockage.
    set-up for treatment (3 min).
                                             3.  Increased skin reaction in oral
5.  Relatively easy to use.                      cavity has been noted at Univer-
                                                 sity of Michigan Hospital, but
6.  Accurate daily duplication of original       not elsewhere; possible causes
    patient position.                            are under investigation.

7.  Accurate reproduction of treatment       4.  Cannot accurately reproduce
    port with use of marks, tattoos              treatment ports without use
    and/or geographic landmarks.                 of marks, tattoos or landmarks.

8.  Requires minimal space: 1 device per
    room, different mouthpiece used for
    each patient.

---

COST

1.  Materials:  Approximately $80 for one set of different-sized neckrests.
2.  Equipment:  Approximately $1000 for initial fabrication of biteblock
                device.

---

Skin marks, though often cosmetically unacceptable to the patient, are very
commonly used.  Gentian violet ink contained in fine-tip pens or applied from
a bottle with a fine applicator is the most popular type of ink used.  It is
very important that lines delineating treatment fields be thin and accurate.
It is suggested that port films be taken regularly, at least once a week, to
make sure marks do not shift.  Before marking the patient a quick evaluation
of the patient's skin condition should be made.  This will help determine how
useful and effective skin marks will be.  The cosmetic and emotional effects
of the marks are very important concerns.  The skin marks serve as a constant
reminder to the patient of his disease, as well as announcing it to friends,
relatives and co-workers.  In some cases, the use of marks could seriously
hinder a patient's ability to carry on a normal life while undergoing

treatments, or could even cause the patient to refuse treatment. Therefore, skin marks should be used cautiously in the head and neck area, especially for patients where the emotional impact could far outweigh the clinical benefits.

Tattoos may be a better alternative to surface skin marks for some patients, especially those who have trouble maintaining marks from day to day (oily skin condition, heavy perspiration). Tattoos in the head/neck area should be done as inconspicuously as possible. The center and at least one (preferably two) corners could be tattooed for good alignment. Remembering that skin may change in the neck due to weight loss or tumor shrinkage, check films should be taken regularly, preferably once a week or at any time a change is suspected or noted.

Measurements may be used to enhance a treatment aid to at least minimally determine the height of the beam from the table to a specified border or the central axis and at best localize the entire port every day.

Use of geographic/anatomical landmarks requires adequate surface anatomical knowledge on the part of the technologist. Some common sites to base anatomical landmarks upon in the head and neck area are: eye, ear, nose, mouth, and neck or base of the skull.

The anatomical landmarks about the eye include superior, inferior and lateral orbital margins, inner and outer canthus. It is preferable to take bony landmarks of the eye since they are radiographically visible.

Anatomical landmarks about the ear include the superior, inferior and anterior tragal notch, tragus, tragal notch, superior junction of the ear and face and the inferior junction of the ear and face. It is preferable to use the tragal notches for anatomical landmarks since they are not subject to change.

The nose has some useful landmarks which include the lateral and inferior ala nasi. The nasion and glabella are also used if prominent in the patient.

The anatomical landmarks about the mouth are not considered to be very accurate due to movement of the mouth. They include the commissure of the mouth, muco-cutaneous junction and the columella. Whenever possible, landmarks of other anatomical sites should be recorded.

The skull has landmarks such as the tip of mastoid and chin and external occipital protuberance, which are helpful only if they are prominent and can be palpated easily.

In the neck area, the superior and inferior borders of the clavicle, thyroid notch, tip of mastoid and spinous process are commonly used as anatomical landmarks.

In general, whether marks, tattoos, measurements or anatomical landmarks are used, it is very important to have accurate documentation in the treatment records.

Immobilization of the head/neck area and duplication of the treatment port has been and continues to be one of the primary concerns in the field of Radiation Therapy. With so many options available, it is important to take the time and effort to find the system that best fits the majority of needs.

SELECTED READINGS

1. Dickens, C.W. A Radiotherapy Mold Room Manual. London & Surrey, 1971.
2. Gerber, R., Marks, J., Purdy, J. The Use of Thermal Plastics for Immobilization of Patients during Radiotherapy. .Int J Radiation Oncol Biol Phys 8:1461-1462, 1982.
3. Hauskins, L., Thompson, R. Patient Positioning Devices for External-Beam Radiation Therapy of the Head and Neck. Radiology 106:706, March 1973.
4. Latourette, H.B., Simons, C.S., Lampe, I. A Localization Scheme for Radiation Therapy Planning with the Theratron. Radiology 73:762-770, November, 1959.
5. Mulvaney, T. Utilizing Anatomical Landmarks for Patient Positioning and Field Location. (Personal communication), 1983.

# Index

A

Abdominal failures, 114

ABVD regimen, 48

Adenocarcinoma, 188

    large bowel, 111

Adrenal lymphoma, 68-71

Alkylating agent, 47

Anatomical landmarks, 314

Angular momentum, 274

Ann Arbor staging classification, 43-44

Artificial sweeteners, 187

Autologous marrow, 49

Axillary node,

    dissection, 234

    sampling, 234


B

Beam energy, 237

Benign prostatic hyperplasia (BPH),169

Bichloroethylnitrosourea (BCNU), 95

Biologic hazard, 284

Biopsy, 53

Bite block device, 313

Bladder cancer, 187, 197-206

    superficial, 198

Bladder neoplasms,

    advanced, 202

Bolus, 237

    administration, 95-96

Bone,

    lymphoma, 76

    marrow transplantation, 49

Breast carcinoma, 221,231, 249, 296

Brain stem gliomas, 83-85

Burkitt's lymphoma, 39, 63


C

Cancer, See individual entries.

    breast, 221, 231, 249, 296

    cervical, 209

    colorectal, 131

    management, 301

    prostate, 159

Cardiovascular system, 291

Carotoid artery infusion, 97

    continuous, 97-98

    intermittent, 96-97

Cavitron Ultrasound Aspirator (CUSA),103

Cell kill, 215

Central nervous system (CNS),

    lymphoma, 43

    neoplasms, 95

    tumors, 83

Central tandem, 217

Cerebellar Astrocytoma, 101, 106

Cervix,

    barrel shaped, 213

Chemotherapy, 44, 267, 303

    adjuvant, 88

    Fluorouracil (5-FU), 140

    intra-arterial, 142

    intra-vesical, 192, 203

Choriocarcinoma, 102

318

Chromosomal rearrangements, 40

Cirrhosis, 293

Classifications of NHL,
   international, 40-42
   Rappaport, 40-42
   working formulation, 40

Clonogenic assays, 202, 205

Cold wedge, 254

Colon, 113
   local recurrence, 113

Combination therapy, 45

Combined approach, 214

Colorectal carcinoma, 111
   metastatic, 131

Computed tomography (CT), 53, 156, 169,
      249, 268
   assisted biopsy, 76, 106
   scanning, 101
      pitfalls, 258
      upper abdomen, 268
      whole body, 250

Computerized assisted tomographic
      scanning (CAT), 226

COP, 45, 47

Craniopharyngioma, 89, 93, 104-105

Cyclophosphamide, 45

Cystectomy, 200
   salvage, 192, 201

Cytocentrifuged cerebrospinal fluid
      (CSF), 86


D

Differentiation,
   degree, 153

Diffuse lymphoblastic cell, 49

Disease-free survival, 88

Distant,
   failures, 121
   metastatic disease, 233

Downstaging, 202

Doxorubicin, 47, 204

Dyes, 187

Dysgerminomas, 84


E

Edema,
   arm, 243

Electron beam, 239
   boost, 119

Embryonal cell tumors, 102

Endocervical canal, 213

Endometrial extension, 213

Epstein-Barr virus, 39

Ernst applicator, 214

Excisional biopsy, 249

Exocervix, 213

Exophytic tumors, 218

External beam irradiation, 217
   techniques, 140
   therapy, 174
   whole abdominal, 144

External contour, 259

Extrahepatic tumor, 129

Extranodal,
   disease, 43
   lymphoma, 43-44


F

Floating-aorta sign, 55

5-fluorouracil, 127

FIGO, 211

Fourier transformation, 282

Fractionation schemes, 304

FUDR, 129


G

Gastric lymphoma, 66

Gastric outlet obstruction, 144

Gastrointestinal lymphoma, 43, 66-68

Gastrojejunostomy, 144

Gentian violet ink, 313

Glioma, 289, 303

  brain stem, 83-85, 101, 104

  deep, 106

  hypothalmic, 105

  opticochiasmatic, 105

  thalamic, 101

GU tract lymphoma, 71


H

Headholder, 310

Head and neck cancer, 303

Hepatic artery,

  chemotherapy, 128

  infusion of FUDR, 135

  lymphoma, 64-65

  metastases, 127

Hepatitis,

  chemical, 136

High grade lymphomas, 41-42

High-LET therapy, 303

Histiocytic lymphoma, 63

Hodgkin's disease, 21-36, 43, 58

  chemotherapy, 30

  combined modality approach, 33

  hilar disease, 22

  irradiation,

    hepatic, 21

    lung, 25

    prophylactic, 33

    whole lung, 21

  laparotomy staged, 21-36

  mediastinal disease, 22

  nodular sclerosing, 27

  radiation,

    hepatitis, 33

    pneumonitis, 27

  radiotherapy, 21

  recurrence, 32

  -free survival, 24

  survival, 24

  total nodal irradiation (TNI), 28

  "Y" fields,

    inverted, 21, 28

    mantle, 21

Human T cell leukemia/lymphoma virus

  (HTLV), 40

Hydrogen density, 278, 287

Hypogastric lymph nodes, 176

Hyperthermia, 303

Hysterectomy,

  extrafascial, 217


I

$^{125}$I implantation, 165

$^{125}$I seed distribution, 181

Imaging techniques, 287

Immobilization techniques, 307-315

Immunologic evaluation,

  urothelial tumors, 205

Immunotherapy, 204

Implantable pump, 96

  system, 99

Interdisciplinary management, 301

Intergroup protocols, 302

Internal mammary lymph nodes (IMLN),

  73, 249, 254

International formulation, 42

Interstitial implantation, 180, 190, 236

  Iridium use, 192

Intra-arterial,

  BCNU, 96

  complications, 96-97

  chemotherapy, 95

  infusions, 127

Intracavitary applicators, 214

Intracavitary irradiation, 214, 217
Intacranial hemorrhage, 290
Intracranial pressure, 89
Intraoperative,
  electron(s), 140
    boosts, 123
  irradiation, 119, 140
  management, 102, 104
  ultrasonography, 103
Intrathoracic lymphoma, 72-74
Intraventricular injections, 98-99
Intravesical BCG, 204
Inversion recovery, 287
  sequence, 280
Iodine$^{125}$ implants, 140
Irradiation,
  adjuvant, 122-123
  postoperative, 192
  preoperative, 191
Isodense subdural hematomas, 290
Isodose distribution, 254


L

Larmor frequency, 281
Levamisole, 304
Liver perfusion, 135
Local,
  control, 267
  failure, 213, 217
  recurrence, 211, 241
Longitudinal relaxation, $T_1$, 279
Low grade tumors, 41-42
Lung,
  cancer, 303
  inhomogeneity, 249
Lymph node,
  involvement, 150
  metastases, 188, 223
Lymphadenectomy, 167, 174

Lymphadenectomy,
  total, 215
Lymphangiography (LAG), 160, 174
  bipedal, 58
Lymphatic,
  invasion, 209
  pathways, 209
Lymphoma, 53
  adrenal, 68-71
  bone, 76
  CNS, 43
  computed tomography in, 53-76
  extranodal, 43-44
  gastrointestinal, 43, 66-68
  GU tract, 71
  hepatic, 64-65
  high grade, 41-42, 47-49
  intermediate grade, 41-42
  intrathoracic, 72-74
  large cell, 49, 63
  low grade, 45-47
  non-Hodgkin's, 39-50
  renal, 68-71
  thoracic, 73


M

Magnetic field, 273
Malignant Astrocytomas, 95-98
Manchester Philosophy, 209
Mastectomy,
  modified radical, 249, 250
  radical, 221
  total, 221
Mediastinal,
  adenopathy, 53
  lymphadenopathy, 72
  nodes, 54
Medulloblastoma, 83, 85-89, 101, 104
Megavoltage, 217

Meningeal carcinomatosis, 98-99

Mesenteric adenopathy, 53

Metastatic,

   disease, 204, 233

   lesions, 303

Methotrexate, 47

Midbrain gliomas, 83

Misonidazole, 304

Mitomycin C, 129

Monoclonal antibody, 49, 205

MOPP, 48

Multiple sclerosis (MS), 289

Myelography, 86

Mycosis fungoides, 42

Myocardial infarction (MI), 291


N

NCI trial, 143

Nephrectomy, 71

Neutron therapy, 303

Nitrates, 187

Non-Hodgkin's lymphoma (NHL), 39, 58

   clinical characteristics, 42-43

   diagnostic evaluation, 43-44

Nuclear Magnetic Resonance (NMR), 273-286

   clinical applications, 287-296

   imaging,

      bone, 295

      gated, 291

      ungated, 291

     isotope, 281

     signal, 273

     spectroscopy, 273

Nuclear magnets, 276


O

Obturator, 176

Optic nerve gliomas, 84

P

Palliative biliary bypass, 139

Pancreatic cancer, 139-146

   biliary obstruction, 139

   curative resection, 139

   failures, local-regional, 145

   median survival, 140, 142

   palliation,

     long-term, 140

   peritoneal seeding (PS), 139

   recurrence, local-regional, 139

   survival, 143

   systematic failures, 146

Pancreatic lymphoma, 68

Para-aortic lymph nodes, 174

Paravertabral nodes, 73

Particle therapy, 303

Patterns of failure, 263-266

Pelvic,adenopathy, 54

   adenopathy, 54

   failure, 156

   lymph nodes, 176

   lymphadenectomy, 176

   lymphatic metatasteses, 164

   recurrence, 118

Percutaneous needle biopsy, 53, 176

Performance status, 262

Pericardial lymphoma, 74

Peritoneal seeding, 114

Permanent magnets, 284

Phase I/II/III studies, 303

Pilot studies, 301

Pinealoma, 105-106

Plaster casts, 309

Polyamines, 107

Port reproduction techniques, 307-315

Posterior,

   mediastinal nodes, 73

   thalamic lesions, 106

Postoperative,

  chemotherapy, 117

  irradiation, 192

  radiation (XRT), 115-118

Precessional frequency, 275

Prednisone, 45

Preoperative,irradiation, 191

  irradiation, 191

  radiation (XRT), 115

Primary Immunodeficiency, 39

Procarbazine, 47

Prognostic,

  factor, 189, 212

  features in NHL, 44

Progressive extrahepatic disease, 134

Prospective randomized trial, 249

Prostate, 180

  mucinous adenocarcinoma, 170

Prostatic,

  carcinoma, 149, 169

  sarcoma, 172

Protector studies, 304

Pulmonary nodules, 74


Q

Quality control, 263, 303

Quantum mechanics, 276


R

Radioactive $^{125}$I seeds, 174

Radiation, 214

  damage of the brain, 290

  dose, 288

  megavoltage, 156

  postoperative, 221

  sensitizers, 124, 303

  therapy, 44-45, 200, 267, 301, 303

    breast, 221-245

    definitive, 229

therapy cont.

  ports, 53

  protocols, 302

  research, 301

  stage IB carcinoma of cervix, 209-219

  techniques, 87, 235

  treatment planning, 169

Radiation Therapy Oncology Group (RTOG), 301-305

Radiofrequency,

  fields, 285

  pulse, 278

Radionuclide scanning, 129

  bone, 76, 160

Radiotherapy, 267

  preoperative, 200-201

  treatment planning, 249

Randomized,

  protocols, 301

  studies, 302

Rappaport classification, 40-42

Rectal cancer, 113

Recurrence, late, 266

Recurrent grade I and II astrocytomas, 96

Regional chemotherapy, 95

Regsitries, 301

Relaxation time, 287  See $T_1$ and $T_2$.

Renal,

  carcinoma, 294

  lymphoma, 68-71

  transplant recipients, 39

Residual disease, 123

Resonance, 275

  hydrogen, 287

Retrocrural lymph nodes, 58

Retroperitoneal adenopathy, 55

S

Salvage,

   cystectomy, 192, 201

   surgery, 241-242

Saturation-recovery, 287

   sequence, 280

Segmental resection, 189

Seizures, 107

Seminal vesicle(s), 172-173

   angle sign, 172

Sezary syndrome, 42

Shrinking field technique, 155

Shunt, 102

Simulator lines, 250

Skin marks, 313

   gentian violet ink, 313

   tattoos, 314

Small bowel obstruction, 122

Small cell carcinoma of the lung (SCCL), 261-269

   patients,

      prognosis, 266-267

Southwest Oncology Group, The, 49

Spin-echo sequence, 280, 287

Spinal cord, 290

Splenic lymphoma, 65

Split-course therapy, 266-267

Squamous cell carcinoma, 188

Staging, 53, 189

   classification, 112

   laparotomy, 63

   systems, 149-150, 160-161, 197

Stromal invasion, 212

Subcarinal nodes, 72

Sublethal damage, 215

Substages, 216

Superficial bladder tumors, 202

Supraclavicular adenopathy, 74

Surgical resection, 140

Surveillance abdominal films, 64

Survival, 202


T

T cell lymphoblastic lymphomas, 40

$T_1$, 287

$T_2$, 287

Tattoos, 314

Thalamic gliomas, 83

Therapeutic ratio, 121-122

Therapy,

   new approaches, 49

Thio-tepa, 203

Thoracic,

   irradiation, 261

   lymphoma, 73

Three-dimensional display, 258

Thymosin, 304

Tissue inhomogeneity, 258

Total body irradiation (TBI), 44-45

Total cystectomy, 189

Tracheobronchial compression, 74

Transitional cell carcinoma, 188

Transurethral resection, 198

   bladder (TURB), 189

Transverse relaxation $T_2$, 279

Treatment,

   port, 308

   portals, 60

   program, 223

   response, 75

Tryptophan, 187

Tumor,

   localization, 152

   size, 231-232


U

Ultrasound, 64, 249

Underdosage, 256

Urinary diversion, 200

V

Vaginal colpostats, 217
Vascular invasion, 212
Vincristine, 45
VM26, 203

W

Wedge compensation, 236, 258
Wedged tangential fields, 257
    complications, 257
Whole body irradiation(WBI), 45
Workup, 223

X

X-ray CT, 288, 295